Progress in Drug Research

Volume 68

Series editor

K. D. Rainsford, Sheffield Hallam University,
Biomedical Research Centre, Sheffield, UK

For further volumes:
http://www.springer.com/series/4857

Omar M. E. Abdel-Salam
Editor

Capsaicin as a Therapeutic Molecule

Springer

Editor
Omar M. E. Abdel-Salam
Department of Toxicology and Narcotics
National Research Center
Cairo
Egypt

ISBN 978-3-0348-0827-9 ISBN 978-3-0348-0828-6 (eBook)
DOI 10.1007/978-3-0348-0828-6
Springer Basel Heidelberg New York Dordrecht London

Library of Congress Control Number: 2014934672

Printed on acid-free paper

Springer Basel AG is part of Springer Science+Business Media (www.springer.com)

Preface

Capsaicin, a homovanillic acid derivative (8-methyl-N-vanillyl-6-nonenamide), is the pungent ingredient in red peppers of the plant genus *Capsicum*, including chillies and jalapenos. Capsaicin has long been used as a probe for sensory neuronal mechanisms. This is because capsaicin selectively stimulates, and at large doses, defunctionalizes a subset of primary afferent neurons with unmyelinated C fiber or thinly myelinated Aδ fibers. Most capsaicin-sensitive fibers are polymodal nociceptors (which respond to a range of sensory stimuli including noxious heat, pressure, and chemical irritation) as well as heat nociceptors, mechano-heat insensitive chemonociceptors, and warm receptors. The molecular site of action of capsaicin and other structurally related substances have been identified and cloned. This receptor, the transient receptor potential vanilloid 1 (TRPV1), formerly vanilloid receptor subtype 1 (VR1), forms a nonselective cation channel in the plasma membrane that is highly expressed in peripheral and central terminals of these primary sensory neurons. Capsaicin application at submicromolar concentrations activates the subset of polymodal nociceptor fibers that express its receptor; this leads to release of neuropeptides, such as substance P and calcitonin gene-related peptide, from nerve terminals and burning pain. Higher concentrations or the repeated application of low concentrations of capsaicin leads to desensitization, i.e., decline in response to capsaicin and also to other stimuli of polymodal nociceptors. This desensitizing action has made capsaicin attractive for use as a peripherally acting analgesic for chronic painful syndromes.

Capsaicin has moved toward clinical applications and is used currently in topical creams and gels to relieve intractable neuropathic pain, uremic pruritus, and rheumatoid arthritis. Capsaicin also proved of value in nonallergic (vasomotor) rhinitis, migraine, cluster headache, herpes zoster, and bladder overactivity and interstitial cystitis. Resiniferatoxin is an ultrapotent capsaicin analog isolated from the dried latex of the cactus-like plant *Euphorbia resinifera*. In patients with overactive bladder, intravesical resiniferatoxin improves bladder function without having significant irritancy and/or toxicity. Intrathecal resiniferatoxin is currently undergoing clinical trials in patients with intractable cancer pain. Capsaicin and capsaicin-like molecules have thus remarkable potential as pharmaceutical agents for treating various human aliments.

The intended purpose of this volume is to compile the available knowledge and the most recent achievements pertaining to the application of capsaicin and capsaicin-like molecules in the management of various human aliments. It also seems timely to cover basic issues on the capsaicin receptor, the mechanisms of its action, and its role in physiological and pathological processes and provide the latest perspectives on these issues. The book aimed to combine both basic science on the pathophysiological role of sensory nerves and TRPV1 in the disease process itself, in addition to covering current knowledge and highlighting the most recent progress in the use of capsaicin as a therapeutic agent. Each chapter is written by noted experts in their field of endeavor. In this way, it is hoped that the book will be useful for both clinicians and researchers and that it will stimulate their future research.

I would like to thank all the authors of this volume who worked diligently to produce such outstanding chapters that not only covered current knowledge but also discussed important potential pharmaceutical implications for further research in this field. This book has been only possible because of their efforts. I am most indebted to the Series Editor, Prof. Dr. Kim Rainsford, and the Senior Editor Dr. Hans Detlef Klüber for their idea that has led to this book, for kindly inviting me to produce this volume and for the invaluable support. I would also like to gratefully acknowledge the Springer's edition Staff and in particular the Project Coordinator Dr. Andrea Schlitzberger for her continued help and advice throughout the preparation and production of this book.

Omar M. E. Abdel-Salam

Contents

Chapter 1
Capsaicin and Sensory Neurones: A Historical Perspective

János Szolcsányi

Abstract Capsaicin, the pungent ingredient of red pepper has become not only a "hot" topic in neuroscience but its new target-related unique actions have opened the door for the drug industry to introduce a new chapter of analgesics. After several lines of translational efforts with over 1,000 patents and clinical trials, the 8 % capsaicin dermal patch reached the market and its long-lasting local analgesic effect in some severe neuropathic pain states is now well established. This introductory chapter outlines on one hand the historical background based on the author's 50 years of experience in this field and on the other hand emphasizes new scopes, fascinating perspectives in pharmaco-physiology, and molecular pharmacology of nociceptive sensory neurons. Evidence for the effect of capsaicin on C-polymodal nociceptors (CMH), C-mechanoinsensitive (CHMi), and silent C-nociceptors are listed and the features of the capsaicin-induced blocking effects of nociceptors are demonstrated. Common and different characteristics of nociceptor-blocking actions after systemic, perineural, local, intrathecal, and in vitro treatments are summarized. Evidence for the misleading conclusions drawn from neonatal capsaicin pretreatment is presented. Perspectives opened from cloning the capsaicin receptor "Transient Receptor Potential Vanilloid 1" (TRPV1) are outlined and potential molecular mechanisms behind the long-lasting functional, ultrastructural, and nerve terminal-damaging effects of capsaicin and other TRPV1 agonists are summarized. Neurogenic inflammation and the long-list of "capsaicin-sensitive" tissue responses are mediated by an unorthodox dual sensory-efferent function of peptidergic TRPV1-expressing nerve terminals which differ from the classical efferent and sensory nerve endings that have a unidirectional role in neuroregulation. Thermoregulatory effects of capsaicin are discussed in detail. It is suggested that since hyperthermia and burn risk due to enhanced noxious heat

J. Szolcsányi (✉)
Department of Pharmacology and Pharmacotherapy, University of Pécs
Medical School, Szigeti u. 12, Pécs H-7624, Hungary
e-mail: janos.szolcsanyi@aok.pte.hu

O. M. E. Abdel-Salam (ed.), *Capsaicin as a Therapeutic Molecule*, Progress in Drug Research 68, DOI: 10.1007/978-3-0348-0828-6_1, © Springer Basel 2014

threshold are the major obstacles of some TRPV1 antagonists, they could be overcome. The special "multisteric" gating function of the TRPV1 cation channel provides the structural ground for blocking chemical activation of TRPV1 without affecting its responsiveness to physical stimuli. A new chapter of potential analgesics targeting nociceptors is now already supported for pain relief in persistent pathological pain states.

1.1 Introduction

Capsaicin is the main pungent hot principle of the fruit capsicum species (*Capsicum annuum, Capsicum frutescent, Capsicum longum* etc.) of the genus *Solanaceae*. This plant originated from the Americas and has become a popular culinary spice of food throughout the world. Thus capsicum is known under various names such as chilli pepper, red pepper, paprika, cayane pepper, tabasco, jalapeno, or under its ancient name aji.

Archeological evidence from Mesoamerica documented that inhabitants of the Tehuacan valley consumed red pepper back to about 7000 BC. From burials from this age, pepper fruits and seeds were found in early settlements of Mexico. Ancient native people domesticated chilli around 5200–3400 BC, (Mac Neish 1964; Mózsik et al. 2009) and potteries from the Nazca Culture in Peru were decorated with figures of chilli fruits (Lembeck 1987). For further interesting readings see (Mózsik et al. 2009; Szállási and Blumberg 1999).

The written history of red pepper started with Christopher Columbus, who described in his log in 1493 that inhabitants of the New World commonly eat foods with chilli (Szolcsányi 1993). He named it red pepper because of its spicy taste resembling the black and white peppers of the *Piper* genus used in Europe as favorite and rather expensive spices. Red pepper was also popular in the Old World.

Beyond its culinary usage capsicum has been used also since centuries as folk medicine. Since the nineteenth century, extracts prepared from pungent pods were listed in Pharmacopoeia of the United States as *Oleoresin capsicin* since 1860 (Du Mez 1917), and an alcoholic extract, *Tinctura capsici* was used in Europe as topical counterirritant analgesic remedies (Nothnagel 1870; Geissler and Moeller 1887). Since these preparations with the burning sensation induced also cutaneous vasodilatation and reddening of the skin they were also called rubefacients. In tropical countries, chilli intake was used as folk medicine to cope with the hot climate by enhancing heat loss regulation with capsicum-induced skin vasodilatation and "gustatory sweating" (Lee 1954).

Isolation of the pungent principle and studies on the pharmacological effects of capsicum started in the early decades of the nineteenth century. Impure extract made by Christian Friedrich Bucholz was first named as *capsicin* and the oily impure ingredient isolated by Rudolf Buchheim was named *capsicol* since it was thought to be a nitrogen-free nonalkaloid compound. Thresh crystallized for the first time the active principle in 1876 and renamed it *capsaicin* (Geissler and

Moeller 1887; Thresh 1876; Suzuki and Iwai 1984). The chemical structure of capsaicin was determined by Nelson in (1919).

The chemical structure of capsaicin is 8-methyl-N-vanillyl-*trans*-6-nonenamide (Fig. 1.1). It is the main pungent ingredient of red pepper, but in capsicum species six further sharp tasting capsaicin-related compounds have also been isolated with similar pungency. These so called *capsaicinoids* differ in structure from the main hot ingredient of capsaicin only in the double bond, arborization, or length of the long aliphatic chain. In commercial capsicums, the following capsaicinoids were isolated: capsaicin 33–59 %, dihydrocapsaicin 30–51 %, nordihydrocapsaicin 7–15 %, and the remainder, less than 5 % are homodihydrocapsaicin homocapsaicin, nonanoyl-vanillylamide, and decanoyl-vanillylamide (Mózsik et al. 2009). The cis-isomer of capsaicin (Fig. 1.1) is a synthetic compound which is not produced by the plant.

The first paper on studying the pharmacological effects of capsaicin was published by Endre Hőgyes in 1878. His main findings include (1) In humans capsicol as counterirritant does not induce vesiculation in the skin in contrast to cantharidine commonly used at that time; (2) Oral intake of capsicol in gelatine capsules enhances gastrointestinal motility without gustatory effect; (3) In dogs capsaicin induces fall in body temperature. Owing to the lack of effects in various preparations innervated by efferent nerves his main conclusion was that "capsicol acts mainly on sensory nerves" (Hőgyes 1878). Although these observations were published in a well-recognized pharmacology journal they remained unnoticed for more than 60 years and did not form a starting point for the pharmacology of sensory nerve endings.

In striking contrast, at that time similar approaches on the selective actions of natural alkaloids such as curare, ergot alkaloids, nicotine, and atropine paved the way to the mechanism of efferent neurohumoral transmissions which led to the identification of their neurotransmitters of acetylcholine and noradrenaline. Thus the pharmacology of the efferent nervous system started with investigation the effects of these rather toxic herbal compounds. The pharmacology of nociceptors started decades after the discovery that nociceptors are the sites of capsaicin desensitization as described in Ref. (Szolcsányi 2005) (Fig. 1.2).

1.2 Capsaicin Desensitization

The phenomenon of "capsaicin desensitization" was discovered by Nicholas Jancsó in the 1940s of the last century (Szállási and Blumberg 1999; Szolcsányi 2005, 1984). It was a serendipitious observation in the course of experiments in which he studied the pivotal mediator role of histamine in mediation of inflammation and storage of macromolecules in endothelial and macrophage cells. During these years, antihistaminic drugs were inaccessible and therefore he used in rodents high histamine doses for desensitization of these receptors. He used by chance capsaicin instead of histamine for desensitization because he thought

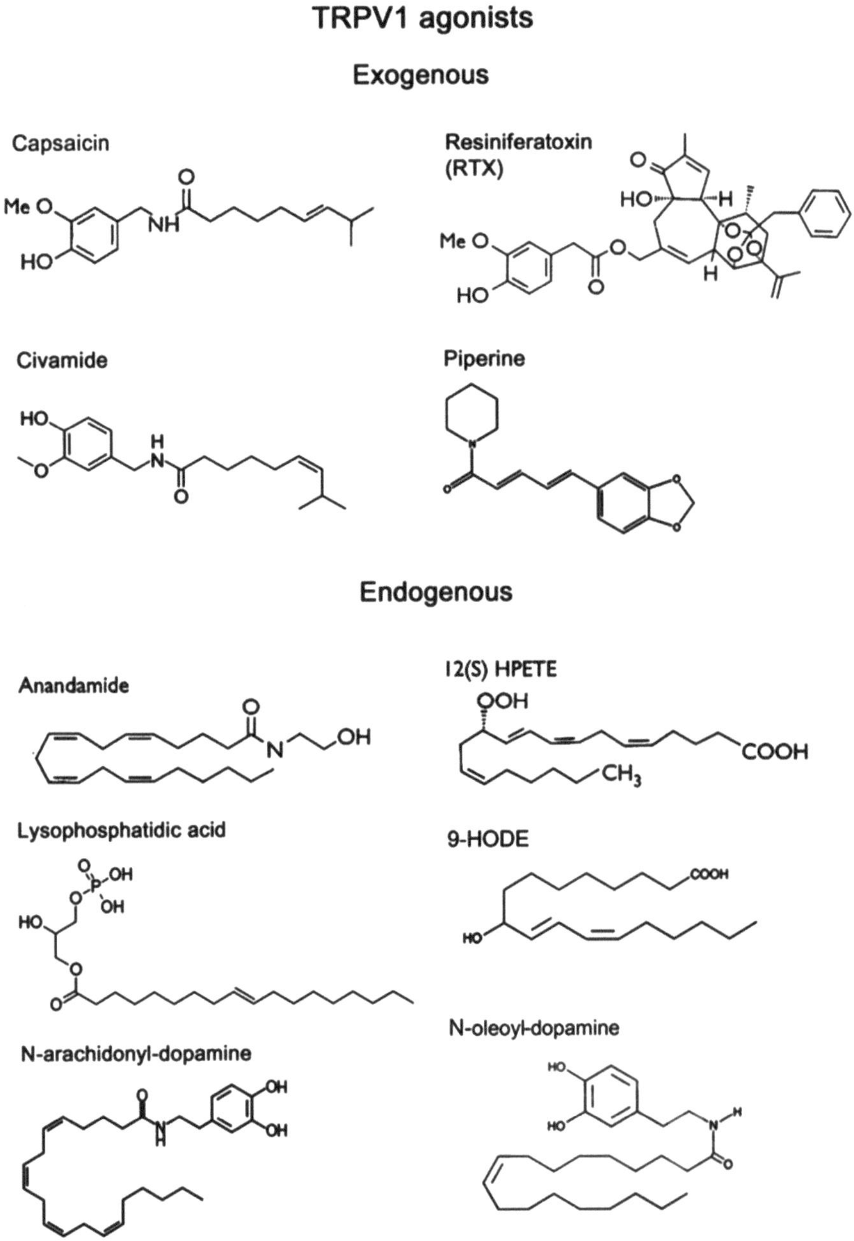

Fig. 1.1 Chemical structure of some exogenous and endogenous agonists of the transient receptor potential vanilloid type-1 (TRPV1) capsaicin receptor

that capsaicin acts as a potent histamine releasing agent. It turned out, however, that the "capsaicin desensitization" is a new phenomenon and it differs from the actions of histamine in its broad-spectrum antinociceptive effect. The perspectives

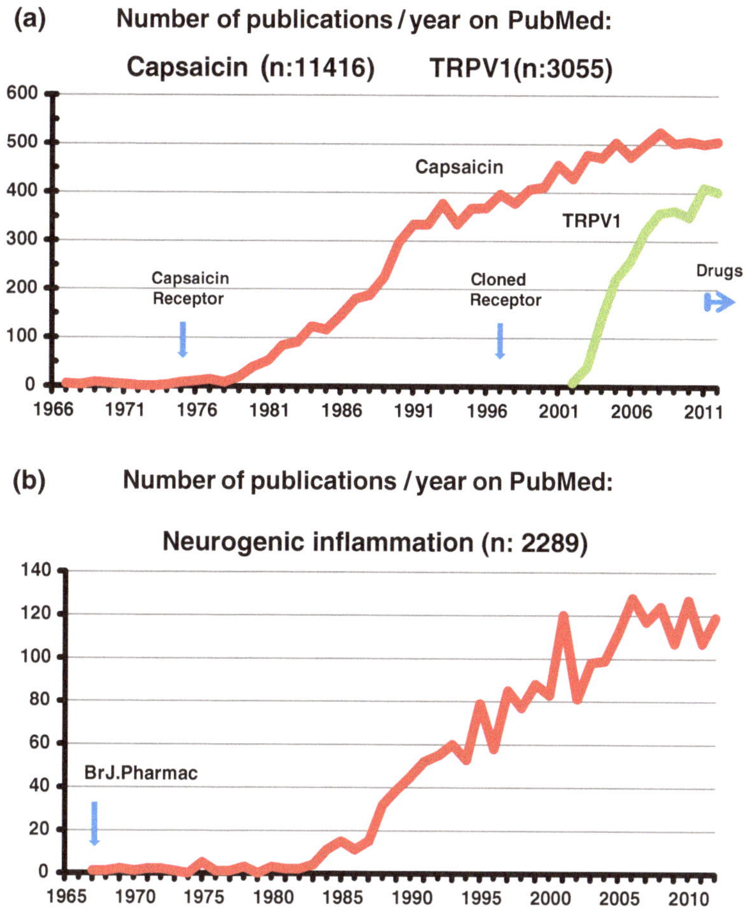

Fig. 1.2 Number of publications at keywords of *capsaicin* and *TRPV1* (**a**) or *neurogenic inflammation* (**b**) indicated in database of PubMed (2013 March); capsaicin receptor: first publication of a hypothetical receptor in 1975 (Szolcsányi and Jancsó-Gábor 1975a); cloned receptor: cloning the capsaicin receptor in 1997 (Caterina et al. 1997). Drugs: first FDA approval for a capsaicin containing drug (Qutenza). Br. J. Pharmac.: first direct evidence for the existence of neurogenic inflammation (Jancsó et al. 1967). For more details see text

of these early data, however, were not recognized by the editor of Experientia and the manuscript written by N. Jancsó with his wife Aurelia Jancsó-Gábor in 1949 on the discovery of capsaicin desensitization was rejected. Afterward the Jancsó couple focused on their main field of interest on storage of macromolecules in inflammatory cells and in the kidney which were published in the Nature and other journals. However, they never sent another manuscript on capsaicin to international journals. In 1955 Nicholas Jancsó wrote an excellent monograph in German on storage of macromolecules in the reticulonoendothelial system and in the kidney (Jancsó 1955). He took this opportunity to summarize all of his results and concept about "capsaicin desensitization." Since his views on actions of capsaicin have been often misinterpreted in recent reviews, I quote in English two sentences from the book: (1) "The resistance of eyes desensitized by capsaicin also against acidic, alkalic and even hypertonic salt solutions"... indicates "that the sensory nerve endings become unresponsive to chemical stimuli although their physical excitability remains"; (2) "Those receptors (denselben Receptoren) are apparently desensitization which remain responsive to physically evoked corneal or sneezing reflexes." In contrast to the desensitization of the nicotinic receptors "synaptotropen Verbindungen" he never considered the existence of a capsaicin receptor on sensory nerve endings (Jancsó 1955).

About 10 years later Jancsó 1964 briefly outlined his views for the last time in English in an abstract of an invited lecture: "Capsaicin induces in rats and guinea pigs a peculiar sensory disturbance lasting for weeks or even years. The animals become insensitive to pain by chemical substances while the perception of pain caused by physical means remains unimpaired. Capsaicin probably interferes with the synthesis of the mediator substance (of neurogenic inflammation JS) in the pain receptor or in the whole neurone. The mediator substance may be a bradykinin-like polypeptide, or the enzyme producing it" (Jancsó 1964).

The mechanism of this "peculiar" phenomenon remained enigmatic and without quantitative published data even his statements were questioned and challenged (Makara et al. 1967). After 4 years of experimental physiological background I joined the Jancsó's couple to work on capsaicin in 1962. We worked together until his demise in 1966. This period was very fruitful but the results were not summarized, completed and particularly were not prepared for publication. The first paper on capsaicin desensitization was sent to the Br. J. Pharmacol. Jancsó et al. (1967) 1 year later (Fig. 1.2) providing also the first direct evidence for the existence of neurogenic inflammation. Since my view about the role of bradykinin differed from Jancsó's interpretation, this part of experiments and his quoted conclusion on this aspect were omitted although the data with enhanced bradykinin-like activity obtained from the skin after antidromic nerve stimulation were convincing. I myself made the titration under his supervision on the isolated rat uterus preparation for several months. My impression was that this bradykinin-like activity is increasing in time at room temperature and therefore I attributed it to an enhanced bradykininogen extravasation and not to a release from the nerve endings. Few years later by using also the rat-isolated duodenal preparation, we obtained the first hint of evidence that substance P might be the mediator which is released from the stimulated sensory nerve endings: "The contraction of the rat duodenum could be attributed to the presence of another mediator: e.g. substance P" (Jancsó-Gábor and Szolcsányi 1972).

These results remained unnoticed for 10 years (Fig. 1.2). Neither the selective blockade of chemonociception in capsaicin-pretreated rats nor its blocking effect on neurogenic inflammation initiated further research although the sensory receptor-selective action of capsaicin was documented also by action potential recordings from the saphenous nerve of the capsaicin-desensitized rats (Jancsó et al. 1967). It is worthy to mention that until the mid-1960s there was no unequivocal evidence for the existence of nociceptors (Melzack and Wall 1965) although

Sherrington predicted their existence already in 1906 (Sherrington 1906). Thus, it remained elusive whether the long-lasting capsaicin desensitization is a neurotoxic effect which renders sensory nerve terminals in general unresponsive to chemical agents, or the effect is related to a loss of function of a subgroup of sensory receptors, notably nociceptors, which mediate chemonociception but not those which mediate mechano-nociception.

1.3 Selective Effect of Capsaicin on Cutaneous C-Polymodal Nociceptors

C-polymodal nociceptors in the skin, the major subgroup of unmyelinated afferent fibers were discovered by Bessou and Perl in 1969 (Bessou and Perl 1969). The coined name polymodal refers to responsiveness of these sensory end organs to three different modalities: noxious heat, moderate-high mechanical, and chemical (acids) stimuli. First evidence of a selective action of capsaicin on C-polymodal nociceptors was obtained by the capsaicin-evoked selective collision of the C_2 compound action potentials of the cat saphenous nerve which could be activated also by noxious heat (Szolcsányi 1977). In addition both electrophysiological and psychophysical evidence for the thermodependence of its sensory effects on animals and humans, respectively provided evidence that capsaicin selectively acts on C-polymodal nociceptors (Szolcsányi 1977). Psychophysical assessments on human tongue and skin also supported this conclusion. Immersion of the tongue into 1 % solution of capsaicin resulted in selective loss of chemonociception evoked by capsaicin, mustard oil or zingerone without altering the recognition threshold concentrations of menthol and taste stimuli evoked by NaCl, quinine, ascorbic acid, and glucose. These results provided the first evidence that capsaicin is not a general chemosensory blocking agent but its effect is restricted to physiologically well-defined groups of sensory receptors identified as the C-polymodal nociceptors. Temperature discrimination limens were inhibited in the warm and hot (44–45 °C) range, but sensation to tactile and cold stimuli remained intact. On the blister base on volar skin, the pain producing effect of capsaicin, bradykinin, or acetylcholine, but not that of potassium chloride solution, was inhibited after topical application of a high, desensitizing concentration of 1 % capsaicin solution (Szolcsányi 1977; Szolcsányi and Pintér 2013). The results provided the first set of evidence for a selective action of capsaicin on nociceptors and for the thermo- and chemoanalgesic effect of capsaicin pretreatment on human skin and tongue (Fig. 1.3).

Excitation and desensitization of cutaneous primary afferent units in the rabbit ear by close arterial injection of capsaicin fully supported its highly selective action on this group of nociceptors (Fig. 1.4). Capsaicin did not evoke over a 100-fold dose range action potentials of C-mechanoreceptors, A-delta (Aδ) mechanical nociceptors, and all types of Aδ and Aβ mechanoreceptors or C-afferent cooling receptors (Szolcsányi 1987, 1980). These sensory receptors were neither desensitized to their natural stimuli after high doses of capsaicin.

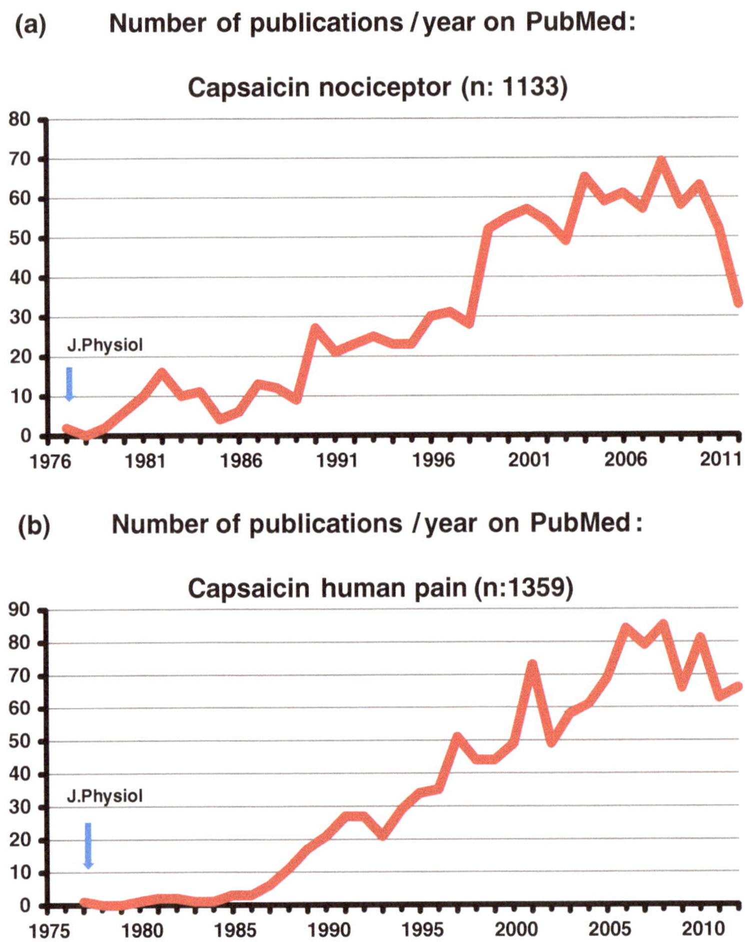

Fig. 1.3 Number of publications at keywords *capsaicin nociceptor* (**a**) and *capsaicin human pain* (**b**) *Arrows* first publication on the lists (Szolcsányi 1977)

It was interesting, however, that action potentials of C-polymodal nociceptors to all three modalities of mechanical, chemical (bradykinin, xylene, capsaicin), or noxious heat stimuli were suppressed or blocked. Desensitization of a single C-polymodal unit to one kind of stimulation often was not paralleled by similar changes in responsiveness to other modalities of stimulation and most units still responded to one type of stimulation. Thus, it seems that the transducer processes and not the conducting axons were impaired (Szolcsányi 1993, 1987). Notably, in contrast to earlier findings close arterial injection of bradykinin in low but not in high doses evoked action potentials exclusively on C-polymodal nociceptors but not on other types of afferent fibers (Szolcsányi 1987). Topical application of capsaicin in 50 % DMSO on the skin of rat (Kenins 1982), or on the burn-induced blister base in the cat (Foster and Ramage 1981), and on intact skin of humans

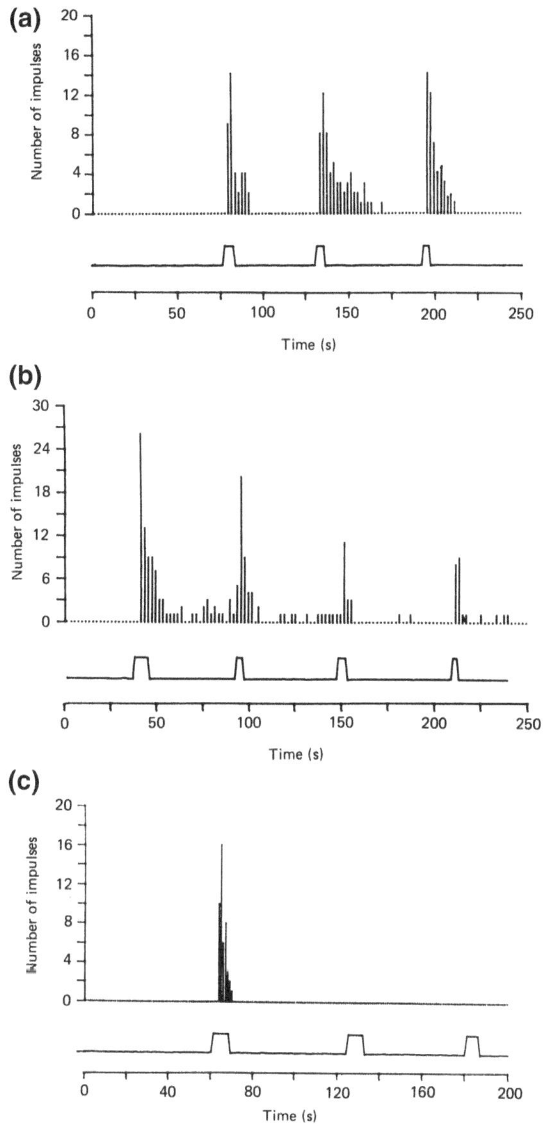

Fig. 1.4 Response of a C-polymodal nociceptor of the rabbit ear to repeated intra-arterial injections of capsaicin. Number of discharges in each 2 s period (**a** and **b**) and in 1 s (**c**). The marks below the graphs indicate the duration of capsaicin injection. Doses: 20 μg (**a**), 200 μg (**b**) and 600 μg (**c**). Note the reproducibility with the small dose and the desensitization after higher doses. (Reproduced from Szolcsányi 1987a with the kind permission of the editors of J. Physiology London)

(Konietzny and Hensel 1983) or monkeys (Bauman et al. 1991) as well single unit studies after intradermal injection in the rat (Martin et al. 1987) or monkey (Bauman et al. 1991) supported that capsaicin evoked action potentials only on C-polymodal nociceptors, on Aδ mechanoheat (polymodal) nociceptors, and also on mechano-insensitive (MiH) or silent C-nociceptors (Szolcsányi 1993, 1996). Interoceptors with axons conducting in C- and Aδ range and excited by bradykinin and in some cases also by mechanical stimuli were shown to be excited and desensitized by capsaicin. These results have recently been summarized elsewhere (Szolcsányi and Pintér 2013).

Beyond the mechano-heat sensitive C-polymodal nociceptors (CMH) in the skin of healthy human subjects, a smaller portion of C-nociceptors were mechanoinsensitive; most of them still responded to noxious heat (CH) but 6/67 units were insensitive to physical stimuli (CMiHi) (Weidner et al. 1999). Nevertheless, both C-polymodal nociceptor (CMH) (LaMotte et al. 1992; Schmelz et al. 2000a) and CH and CMiHi nociceptors were activated by intracutaneous injection of capsaicin (Schmelz et al. 2000a). Furthermore, topical application of mustard oil or capsaicin sensitized the CMi nociceptors and several of them afterward responded to mechanical stimuli (Schmelz et al. 1994). In another study, tonic pressure on the human skin sensitized most of the C-mechano-insensitive units and responded with action potentials after 20 s (Schmidt et al. 2000). It is important to note that there is clear evidence that capsaicin-sensitive CMH and CMi nociceptors mediate itch (Johanek et al. 2008; Han et al. 2013) and are mainly responsible to mediate the axon reflex flare in human skin (Schmelz et al. 2000b). Topical desensitization of the skin with high concentration of capsaicin abolished the itch sensation (Tóth-Kása et al. 1986). It is interesting that axon reflex flare could be evoked also in pigs (Pierau and Szolcsányi 1989), but not in rodents and it is also mediated by CMi fibers (Lynn et al. 1996). After UV-B irradiation these silent nociceptors are sensitized (Rukwied et al. 2008) as C-polymodal nociceptors (Szolcsányi 1987).

Taking together all these findings on the excitatory and blocking effects of capsaicin by recording activity of single sensory fibers the following conclusions can be drawn:

(1) Physiological well-defined types of sensory units with unmyelinated (C) or thin myelinated (Aδ) fibers are excited by capsaicin. The largest subgroup of these capsaicin-responsive units are the C-polymodal nociceptors but in monkeys, pigs, and humans considerable group of afferents are mechanically insensitive albeit they could be sensitized sometimes under inflammatory conditions to become mechanical responsive (Szolcsányi and Pintér 2013).
(2) Mechanoreceptors with unmyelinated or myelinated axons cannot be activated and there is no evidence for their long-term blockade after capsaicin application. Cold receptors are neither sensitive to capsaicin.
(3) After high capsaicin doses responsiveness of C-polymodal nociceptors is inhibited to mechanical, thermal, and chemical stimuli. Complete damage of these nociceptors, however, also could be elicited by higher doses of capsaicin (Szolcsányi and Pintér 2013). Nevertheless, there is functional evidence that after capsaicin pretreatment loss of responsiveness of capsaicin-sensitive nerve terminals is not necessarily due to loss of nerve fibers. Electrophysiological data support different stages of desensitization of the nerve endings to natural stimuli (sensory desensitization) (Szolcsányi 1993; Szolcsányi and Pintér 2013).
(4) Large group of capsaicin-sensitive sensory receptors release neuropeptides and induce neurogenic inflammation and other efferent tissue responses in internal organs. Thus, they have dual sensory-efferent function (see later).

1.4 Experimental Models for Capsaicin-Induced Blockade of Nociceptors

1.4.1 Terminology

The traditional descriptive term of "capsaicin desensitization" simply refers to the refractoriness of animals, human beings, or in vitro tissue preparations to capsaicin-type agents which is accompanied in rodents by chemoanalgesia and impaired thermoregulation in a warm environment (Szolcsányi 1993; Szolcsányi and Pintér 2013). Owing to the present state of knowledge on operations and modulation of TRPV1 channels the term is now obsolete. It might have been different meanings and therefore should be avoided. Here the long-term functional unresponsiveness of capsaicin-sensitive, TRPV1-expressing neurons and their sensory nerve endings are summarized which can be achieved by high doses of capsaicin or its congeners. Precise mechanisms at the molecular level of unresponsiveness, shift of threshold or thermal enthalpy, potency, or efficacy of agonists, modulators of the gating function of the integrative TRPV1 cation channel to various stimuli are discussed in another chapter of this book and see also recent references (Szolcsányi and Pintér 2013; Szolcsányi and Sándor 2012; Xia et al. 2011; Touska et al. 2011; Planells-Cases et al. 2011). In the pharmacology "desensitization" means a decreasing responsiveness or refractoriness to the action of a chemical agent, as declining gating of the TRPV1 or nicotinic receptors to the respective agonists by recording at cellular level of currents, ion fluxes, or other responses. For decreasing responsiveness to repeated application of an agonist compound in isolated organs or isolated cells, the term tachyphylaxis is used although in some publications they are also called desensitization. The term "desensitization" is an accepted term also in sensory physiology and pharmacology referring to the change of responsiveness of the sense organ to various stimuli (Szolcsányi 1993; Szolcsányi and Pintér 2013). In order to make it clear in this chapter for this functional blockade or diminished responsiveness of the capsaicin-sensitive primary afferent neurons, the term "sensory desensitization" is used. The importance of this differentiation is underlined by the fact that capsaicin-induced sensory desensitization involves all functions of the nociceptive nerve terminals, while pharmacological desensitization of the TRPV1 channel inhibits only those effects which are mediated by this cation channel.

1.4.2 Sensory Desensitization Induced by Capsaicin

Repeated application of capsaicin congeners in near threshold concentrations or low doses in vivo or in vitro induces reproducible effects without desensitization (Szolcsányi 1993; Szolcsányi and Pintér 2013; Szolcsányi and Jancsó-Gábor 1976). At higher concentration ranges, however, a dose-dependent sensory desensitization develops within minutes even under in vivo condition. Figure 1.4 (Szolcsányi 1987) shows that close arterial injection of capsaicin into the rabbit ear in doses of 20 μg elicited similar burst of discharges on a single unit of C-polymodal nociceptor, while a 10 times higher dose induced desensitization and further increment in dose resulted in unresponsiveness to capsaicin, although it still fired to an enhanced level of temperature or mechanical stimuli but not to bradykinin. Close arterial injection of 0.2 μg capsaicin into the hindleg of the rat also evoked reproducible number of spikes on C- or Aδ single unit fibers of polymodal nociceptors (Szolcsányi et al. 1988). Instillation of capsaicin congeners into the eye of rats produced similar reproducible nocifensive wiping responses at low threshold dose range of the compounds and induced sensory desensitization at higher doses. The sensory desensitization evoked by the compound was related to the chemical structure and not to magnitude of the nocifensive reaction. Thus, not excessive stimulation but strong binding of the agonist and lasting opening the cation channel is responsible for the sensory desensitizing effect (Szolcsányi and Pintér 2013; Szolcsányi and Sándor 2012). It is interesting that under these conditions no sensitization was observed although after subcutaneous (s.c.) injection of capsaicin under the skin of rat's hind paw (Szolcsányi 1977) or after topical capsaicin application on the skin of monkey (Bauman et al. 1991) or in an in vitro skin preparation (Guenther et al. 1999) sensitization of C-polymodal nociceptors to innocuous heat stimuli was observed.

For studying the sensory desensitizing effect of capsaicin there is a large scale of methods used in animal experiment:

(1) Topical application to the skin or instillation into the eye or applying to other mucosal areas of airways, gastric mucosa, or urinary bladder induces local desensitization. These latter scopes will be discussed in other chapters of the book owing to their potential therapeutic relevance.
(2) Close arterial injection. It has the advantage of studying dose-related effects with fast onset and short lasting exposure. Results of these treatments have been discussed and an example is shown in Fig. 1.4. Subcutaneous injection for regional sensory desensitization or neurotoxic damage of the cutaneous sensory nerve terminals can be achieved.
(3) Subcutaneous or intraperitoneal injections of capsaicin in large doses particularly in rats and mice is a common method for inducing long-term systemic sensory desensitization. The lasting effects observed after pretreatment of adult or neonatal animals—as has been compared mainly on rats—are qualitatively different. Therefore, they are discussed separately.
(4) Perineural application around various nerve trunks in rats, mice, guinea pigs, and other species.
(5) Intrathecal application.
(6) In vitro application to preparations of isolated organs, sensory nerve-peripheral tissues, sensory nerve-spinal cord preparation, tissue slices, cultured dorsal or trigeminal neurons and TRPV1 transfected cell lines are commonly used.
(7) TRPV1 gene-deleted mice and TRPV1 siRNA knockdown mice and recently gene modified animals using Cre-recombinant knock in mice have provided new scopes of evidence for the role of TRPV1 in various functions. Notably, TRPV1 transfected cell lines has become indispensable means in high throughput screening in drug development.

1.4.3 Systemic Application in Adult Animals

In rats the antinociceptive effect of systemic capsaicin pretreatment lasts for several days, weeks or months (Szolcsányi 1993; Buck and Burks 1986; Holzer 1991; Szolcsányi 1987b, 1990). In all reported studies the blockade of chemonociception to large scale of agents was clearly shown, but antinociceptive effect against noxious heat or mechanical stimuli resulted in controversial results. It could be due partly to methodical differences. It was particularly striking that although after topical application on the human skin there was a marked enhancement in noxious heat threshold (Szolcsányi 1990) in animal experiments when testings with conventional models of hot plate, tail flick, radiant heat or plantar tests which detect reflex latencies to suprathreshold stimuli the results were contradictory. Furthermore, often the eye-wiping test to capsaicin (Szolcsányi and Jancsó-Gábor 1976) was taken as a level of "desensitization" to noxious chemical stimuli, while physical stimuli were applied on other parts of the body. The first study (Holzer 1991) to measure the threshold for different nociceptive stimuli on the same skin area of the hind paw led to the following results. After a total s.c. dose of 400 mg/kg given in five successive days, the blockade of chemonociception to xylene was complete for a week, and it remained inhibited for 25 days while the enhanced noxious heat threshold returned slightly earlier. After pretreatment with 150 mg/kg nociceptive thermal threshold increased by 2.5 °C for one day, but returned to the control level on the fourth day. Slight enhancement in the threshold of cutaneous mechanical stimuli lasted only for 1 week (Szolcsányi 1987). Mechanical hyperalgesia due to chronic inflammation, however, was markedly reduced in capsaicin pretreated rats (Barthó et al. 1990). In contrast to all these findings antinociceptive effect of capsaicin pretreatment on the capsaicin-evoked eye-wiping test lasts after a dose of 50 mg/kg over 2 months (Szolcsányi 1993; Szolcsányi and Pintér 2013). Long-lasting antinociceptive effect of systemic capsaicin pretreatment of adult guinea pigs (Buck et al. 1981) and mice (Gamse 1982) were also reported. It is worthy to mention, that birds are not sensitive to the irritant effect of capsaicin and after high dose of close arterial capsaicin injection desensitization to nociceptive chemical stimuli was neither evoked (Szolcsányi et al. 1986).

The long-lasting antinociceptive effect of capsaicin pretreatment is accompanied by severe mitochondrial swelling of the small B-type neurons of the trigeminal or dorsal root ganglia (Joó et al. 1969; Szolcsányi et al. 1975; Chiba et al. 1986). This ultrastructural damage was described also in some corneal nerve endings after topical application of capsaicin (Szolcsányi and Pintér 2013; Szolcsányi et al. 1975) and could explain the functional loss of the affected nociceptors without frank degeneration. Peripheral and central nerve terminals of capsaicin-sensitive primary afferent neurons are more vulnerable to systemic or intra-arterial capsaicin doses. Thus in contrast to the cell body axon terminals but not the dorsal root fibers degenerate after capsaicin pretreatment (Chung et al. 1990, 1985; Pethő and Szolcsányi 1996; Palermo et al. 1981). Furthermore, impaired mitochondrial function with diminished ATP production could explain the characteristic fatigue of responsiveness of the affected sensory receptors (Szolcsányi and Pintér 2013; Szolcsányi and Jancsó-Gábor 1976; Szolcsányi 1990; Szolcsányi et al. 1975). The decreasing level of nocifensiveness to repeated application of a nondesensitizing vanilloid e.g. zingerone should be taken into account to avoid overlooking a partial desensitized state.

1.4.4 Systemic Treatment of Neonatal Rats

It was reported in 1977 by the group of Gábor Jancsó that rats treated s.c. on the second day of life with 50 mg/kg capsaicin produces within an hour massive acute necrotic cell death of small B-type of primary afferent neurons. These animals tested in the adult age failed to respond to capsaicin and in these animals neurogenic inflammation could not be elicited (Jancsó et al. 1977, 1987). One year later Thomas Jessell, Claudo Cuello and Leslie Iversen made the remarkable discovery (Jessell et al. 1978) that capsaicin pretreatment of adult rats selectively depleted the sensory neuropeptide substance P from the sensory ganglia but not from other tissues. Usage of capsaicin in neuropeptide research as a sensory neurotoxin was one of the main reason why interest to capsaicin research increased in the eighties as indicated on Fig. 1.2. For this purpose a model suggesting complete and selective loss of sensory neurons seemed to be more tempting than usage of rats treated in the adult age. Several quantitative morphological studies confirmed the original observation of Gábor Jancsó (1987) in respect of substantial loss of B-type neurons and sensory unmyelinated C-fibers in adult rats after neonatal pretreatment. It turned out, however, that loss of neurons is not restricted to the capsaicin-sensitive, i.e., C-polymodal nociceptive neuronal population and several secondary changes in the peripheral tissues and in the pain pathway was revealed which resulted in contradictory conclusions (Holzer 1991; Cervero and McRitchie 1981). Most importantly single unit studies showed an indiscriminate loss of sensory C-fibers (Welk et al. 1984) and the spectrum of destructed primary afferent neurons depended on the dose (Nagy et al. 1983). Selective degeneration of C-afferents has been described in a lower dose range of 20–30 mg/kg dose and the commonly used 50 mg/kg induced 18 % loss of the myelinated fibers. Furthermore, 34 % loss of large light RT96 labelled A-type neurons was also described (Lawson and Harper 1984). Further secondary changes are reviewed elsewhere (Szolcsányi 2005; Holzer 1991; Szőke et al. 2002a).

Acute necrotic cell death was not observed after neonatal treatment of rats with other TRPV1 agonists as resiniferatoxin (Szállási and Blumberg 1999; Szolcsányi et al. 1990) or anandamide (Szőke et al. 2002b) and in both cases again the selective, pronounced mitochondrial swelling in B-type sensory neurons was striking as in rats treated with capsaicin in adult age. Furthermore, quantitative morphometry provided strong evidence that there is no significant loss of neurons in trigeminal ganglia for 5 days after neonatal capsaicin treatment (Szőke et al. 2002a). The loss of neurons in trigeminal ganglia ensued on the next two weeks, but this loss was completely prevented by daily administration of 100 μg/kg s.c. NGF. The first dose was given one day after the capsaicin injection, to avoid the interference with the acute capsaicin effect.

It has been concluded that after neonatal capsaicin treatment few cells with necrotic or apoptotic signs of degeneration observed shortly after the treatment could be attributed to the asphyxia induced by capsaicin which evokes in this dose range pronounced reflex apnoea, fall in blood pressure and heart rate (Szolcsányi et al. 1990) leading dose dependently to mortality even after adult treatments (Szikszay et al. 1982). After treatment with other TRPV1 agonists as resiniferatoxin (Szolcsányi et al. 1990) or anandamide which do not evoke the Bezold Jarish reflex mitochondrial swelling in small type of neurons of dorsal root or trigeminal ganglia but not cell death was observed. In all cases of TRPV1 agonists these ultrastructural changes lasted for several weeks or months (Szállási and Blumberg 1999; Szolcsányi 1993; Szolcsányi and Pintér 2013; Szőke et al. 2002a; Szolcsányi et al. 1990; Szőke et al. 2002b). Except for these mitochondrial changes there are qualitative differences between the endpoints of adult or neonatal capsaicin treatments. An important difference should be underlined. Biological markers and sensory neuropeptides missing in rats pretreated in the neonatal age summarized in different reviews in several cases are not expressed in capsaicin-sensitive neurons (Buck and Burks 1986; Holzer 1991). Thus, in contrast to the listed data there is no evidence for expressing cholecystokinin, (CCK), vasoactive intestinal polypeptide (VIP), arginine vasopressin, bombesin, or galanin in TRPV1-expressing capsaicin-sensitive neurons (Szolcsányi et al. 1994). Another important point is the effect of capsaicin treatment on wound healing. Trophic lesions in the skin and cornea in rats pretreated at the neonatal but not in adult age were described by Carlo Maggi group (Maggi et al. 1987; Abelli et al. 1993). Wound healing was not affected after perineural capsaicin treatment (Wallengren et al. 1999) although epidermal immunoreactive CGRP and substance P fibers were markedly lost for at least 42 days (Dux et al. 1999).

1.4.5 Perineural Application

After perineural application of 1 % capsaicin the first evidence for a long-lasting functional impairment of capsaicin-sensitive afferent responses proposed to be due to substance P depletion was reported by Jancsó et al. (1980). Subsequent single unit studies revealed that after a non-selective axonal blockade of this high concentration of capsaicin lasting for 1–3 days, selective loss of C-polymodal nociceptors and an increased noxious heat threshold of the remaining units are together being responsible for the analgesic effect of this type of capsaicin treatment (Petsche et al. 1983; Pini et al. 1990; Szolcsányi 1993; Szolcsányi and Pintér 2013). The advantage of localized degeneration of capsaicin-sensitive afferents and the long-lasting effect due to degeneration of the fibers made this technique popular and was tested on sciatic, saphenous, or vagal nerve trunks mainly on rats but occasionally also on the guinea-pig, ferret, rabbit, cat, and monkey (Szolcsányi 1993; Szolcsányi and Pintér 2013).

After 1 % capsaicin application significant antinociception against noxious heat or mechanonociceptive stimuli lasted over 10 days (Szolcsányi 1987). In the concentration range of 0.1–1.5 % long-lasting depletion of substance P was reported (Wall 1987). Furthermore, for a potential therapeutical usage of the highly potent resiniferatoxin (RTX), perineural application was proposed in a concentration of 0.001 % which produced noxious heat analgesia for 2 weeks (Kissin 2008). In a recent publication (Browning et al. 2013), however, after perivagal capsaicin application degeneration of vagal efferent motoneurons was also demonstrated suggesting a "critical re-evaluation" in this field. Mechanism of neurotoxicity evoked by high concentration of capsaicin or RTX applied on nerve trunks remained enigmatic and could not be explained on the basis of cytotoxicity described in vitro when high concentration of capsaicin was applied to overexpressed cell lines or to cultured neurons of sensory ganglia (Kissin 2008).

1.4.6 Local Desensitization by Subcutaneous Pretreatment

Topical application of capsaicin is already in the analgesic therapy for some neuropathic and osteoarthritic pain states (Szolcsányi and Pintér 2013). Therefore this scope is discussed in other chapters of this book including the long-term loss of epidermal sensory fibers after subcutaneous injection of capsaicin in humans (Szolcsányi 1993; Szolcsányi and Pintér 2013). Under experimental condition in the rat, sc. injection of capsaicin (5 μg/50 μl) induced enhancement of noxious heat and mechanical nociception for 2 weeks (Szolcsányi 1987). In respect of noxious heat and noxious cold threshold changes induced, intraplantar injection of capsaicin, resiniferatoxin and N-oleoyldopamine (OLDA) were tested for several days. It has been found that injection of TRPV1 agonists of capsaicin and RTX induced an enhanced noxious heat threshold and shifted down the noxious cold threshold providing a clear desensitizing effect in a dose dependent manner. The recovery from the cold antinociception was, however, faster than that of the hot one indicating probably that the sensory desensitizing/damaging effect of the nerve endings lasted not as long as the vanilloid-induced diminished function of the noxious heat responsive TRPV1 thermotransducer. OLDA failed to elevate noxious heat threshold indicating its low sensory desensitizing potency (Bölcskei et al. 2010). Plantar incision-induced heat hyperalgesia was reduced by infiltration the plantar region by 0.025 and 0.1 % capsaicin similarly as after perineural capsaicin pretreatment while mechanical hyperalgesia was only slightly influenced (Hamalainen et al. 2009).

1.4.7 Intrathecal Application

The prolonged potent antinociceptive action of intrathecal capsaicin combined with depletion of substance P in the dorsal horn reported by the group of Tony Yaksh provided in 1979 the first evidence for the blockade of central terminals of capsaicin-sensitive nociceptors (Yaks et al. 1979). Damaged glomerular C-type terminals of the dorsal horn localized with ultrastructural technique proved the selective site of action (Palermo et al. 1981). Piperine and nonanoyl vanillyamide together with capsaicin enhanced the tail flick latency in parallel with the depletion of substance P and somatostatin, while the less pungent capsaicin congeners were less effective or ineffective after central application (Micevych et al. 1983) similarly as at the peripheral terminals for inhibition the eye-wiping responses (Szolcsányi and Jancsó-Gábor 1975). Structure–activity relationship between the potency of immediate neuropeptide release and long-term antinociceptive effect was observed (Jhamandas et al. 1984). The highly potent analgesic effect of intrathecal RTX application has been revealed in our laboratories in 1993 (Szolcsányi et al. 1993). More recent detailed analysis and therapeutical perspectives of intrathecal RTX application is discussed in a separate chapter of this book.

1.4.8 Effect on In Vitro Preparation

Until the mid sixties of the last century few papers were published on the in vitro effects of capsaicin on isolated preparations from mammals or on microorganisms (Fig. 1.5) (Molnár 1965; Szolcsányi 1982). Smooth muscle responses already reported seemed to me interesting to reveal some new type of neurogenic mechanisms mediated by some capsaicin-sensitive interoceptors. The first in vitro evidence reported in 1978 fully supported this hypothesis. Capsaicin selectively stimulated and subsequently abolished for hours the function of nerve endings of extrinsic neurons which elicited a new type of neural efferent mechanism (Szolcsányi and Barthó 1978; Barthó and Szolcsányi 1978). This unorthodox dual "sensory-efferent" function of "capsaicin-sensitive" nerve endings (Fig. 1.5) turned out to revise the classical axon reflex theory (Fig. 1.6) and will be discussed under a separate subheading. Subsequently several in vitro studies were reported on the role of substance P and other neuropeptides and about their possible mediator role in the spinal dorsal horn of the nociceptive pathway. Wide range of reports are summarized in several reviews (Buck and Burks 1986; Holzer 1991; Maggi 1995). The enhanced interest on capsaicin in the eighties (Fig. 1.2) could be attributed mainly to the high interest in neuropeptide-related research.

The first evidence that capsaicin (1–10 μM) selectively depolarizes and evokes spikes on dorsal root ganglion cells supplied by C fibers was reported by Heyman and Rang in (1985). A study on cell culture of dorsal root ganglia (DRG) cells revealed earlier a major subgroup of neurons which were selectively activated by bradykinin and as tested in some cases also to capsaicin (Baccaglini and Hogan 1983). The selective depolarization of vagal sensory C-fibers and cell bodies due to enhanced conductance to sodium and calcium ions was subsequently described together with the calcium-induced in vitro neurotoxic effect documented with ultrastructural pictures (Marsh et al. 1987). Furthermore, several seminal papers published by the Sandoz group from London analysed in detail the ion fluxes

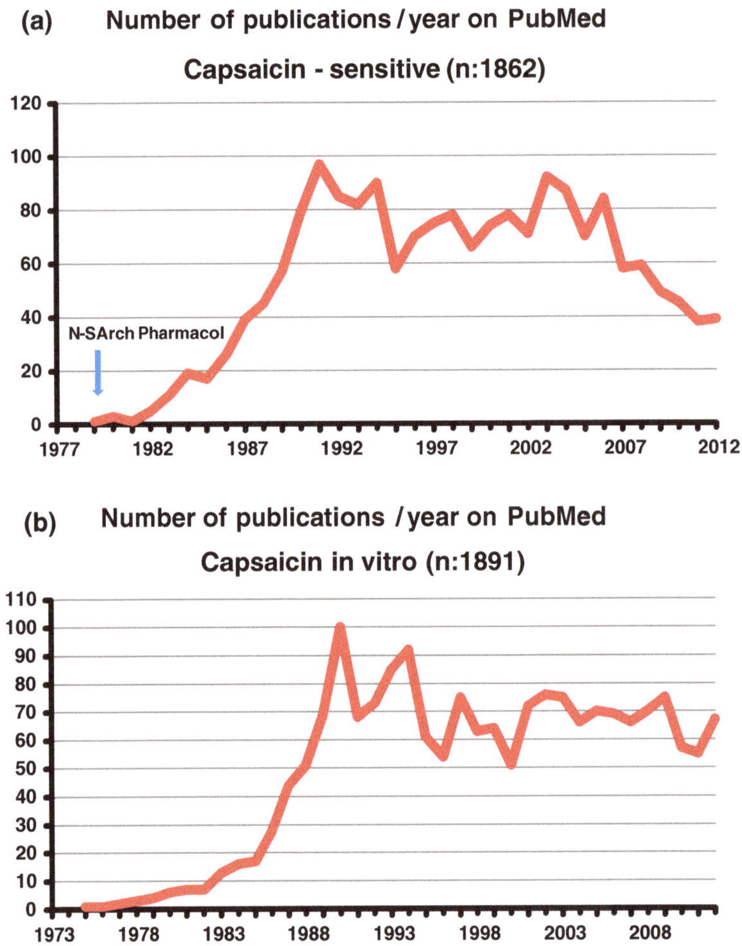

Fig. 1.5 Number of publications at keywords *capsaicin-sensitive* (**a**) and *capsaicin* in vitro (**b**). *Arrow* first publication on the list (Szolcsányi and Barthó 1979)

and their biochemical consequences (Wood et al. 1988; Winter et al. 1990) and electrophysiological effects of capsaicin (Bevan and Szolcsányi 1990; Bevan and Docherty 1993). In a rat saphenous nerve–skin preparation in vitro the selective excitatory effect of capsaicin on polymodal nociceptors was observed (Seno and Dray 1993) in accordance with the in vivo data discussed earlier. Threshold concentration of capsaicin was around 100 nM on C-MH and Aδ-MH (polymodal) fibers and up to 1–3 μM no other types of sensory receptors were excited.

Another seminal observation in studies on phorbol esters made by Peter Blumberg around the turn of the 1990s was the discovery that resiniferatoxin (RTX) a tricyclic diterpene isolated from the fresh latex of *Euphorbia resinifera* differs in actions from other phorbol esters and evoked responses on nociception and thermoregulation which resembled that induced by capsaicin. Capsaicin and RTX molecule share a common vanilloid moiety linked to apolar regions (Fig. 1.1). After the first in vivo studies were completed, a common spectrum of effects of these vanilloids revealed that RTX has several orders higher potency than capsaicin, but showed also some special features (Szolcsányi et al. 1990; De Vries and Blumberg 1989; Szállási and Blumberg 1989. Thus, RTX has become a promising tool and Árpád Szállási with Peter Blumberg introduced a H^3RTX binding technique and initiated a series of extensive investigations on the "vanilloid receptor" (Szállási and Blumberg 1990). Full account of these achievements (Szállási and Blumberg 1999) are discussed in two other chapters of this book. Nevertheless, it is worthy to mention that as early as in 1990 single patch recording from neurons of dorsal root ganglia showed evidence that capsaicin and RTX apparently gated the same ion channel (Bevan and Szolcsányi 1990). Furthermore, sympathetic neurons, neurofilament-containing (A-type) neurons and non-neural cells were not sensitive to RTX or capsaicin and the two compounds acted on the same cells (Winter et al. 1990) as an evidence also on a spinal cord-tail preparation (Dickenson et al. 1990).

Intrathecal application of capsaicin revealed the important scope of action of capsaicin on the central terminals of the capsaicin-sensitive afferents in the spinal cord (Dickenson et al. 1990). Two in vitro electrophysiological studies first supported these observations. The excitatory effect of capsaicin (10–20 μM) in a spinal cord slice preparation was followed by a loss of slow excitatory postsynaptic potentials (EPSP) (Urbán et al. 1985). In the isolated spinal cord of the neonatal rat dorsal root stimulation evokes a ventral root reflex on the conralateral side. The slow component of the ventral root reflex but not the fast one was abolished after local (1 μM for 30 min) or systemic (50 mg/kg s.c. 2 days before) capsaicin pretreatment (Akagi et al. 1985). More recently it has been described that capsaicin (1 μM) increased the glutaminergic miniature EPSP postsynaptic currents in lamina II dorsal horn second order nociceptive neurons while the amplitudes of the "inhibitory postsynaptic potentials" (IPSP-s) were inhibited (Pan and Pan 2004) or according to another study the GABAergic miniature IPSP-were not changed (Kim et al. 2009).

1.4.9 Action of Capsaicin on the Brain

The first functional and morphological evidence that capsaicin has a site of action in the brain was obtain more than 40 years ago within the series of analysing the thermoregulatory effects of capsaicinoids (Jancsó-Gábor et al. 1970a; Szolcsányi et al. 1971. This aspect will be discussed under a separate subheading since it forms the major obstacles for developing TRPV1 antagonist due to the common hyperthermic side effect of some otherwise promising drug candidates. Morphological evidence using radioimmunoassay, H^3RTX binding and in situ hybridization detections of TRPV1 mRNA resulted in positive effects in various brain regions although quantitative estimations revealed about a 30 times lower level of expression in brain areas than in the sensory ganglia (Caterina 2007). Using the TRPV1 reporter mice

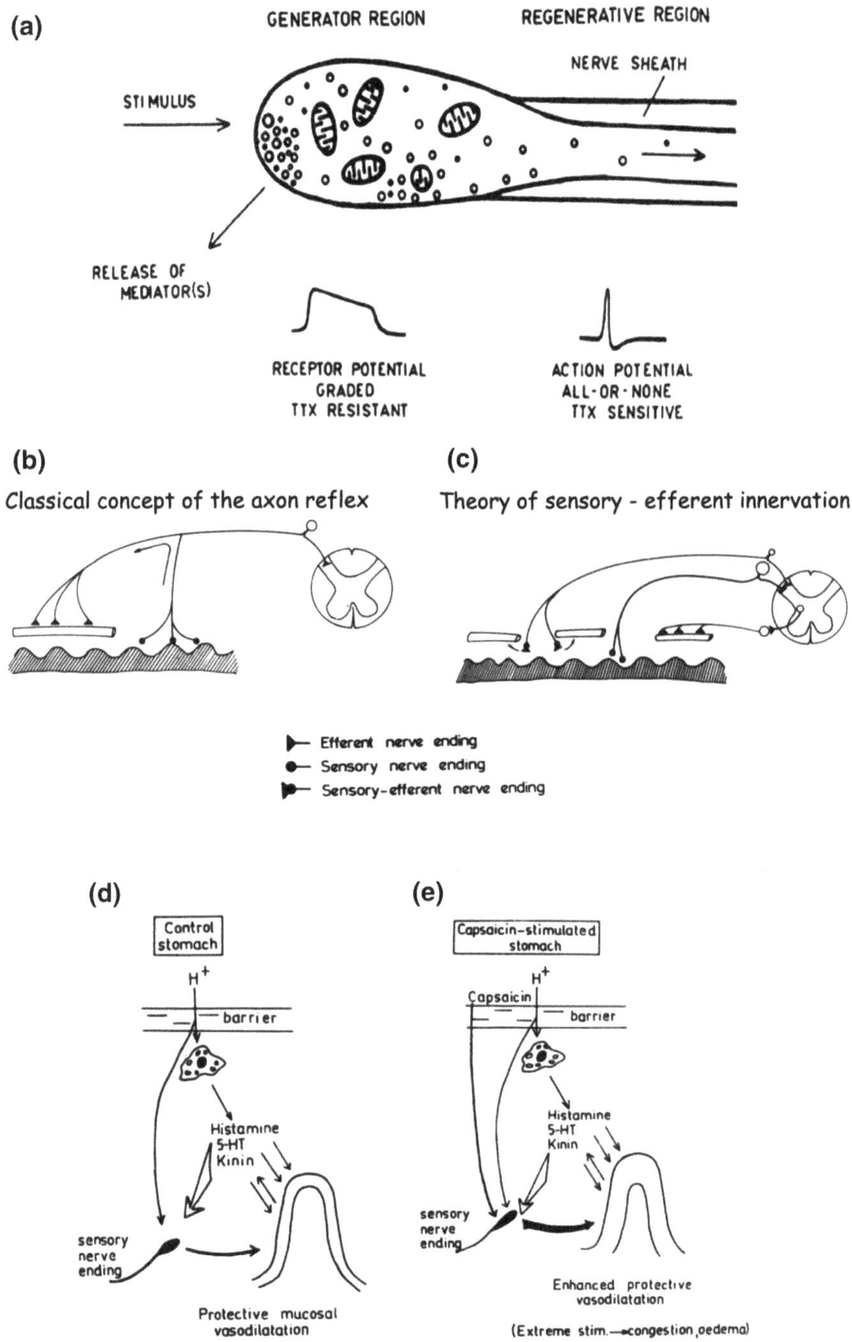
(a)
GENERATOR REGION
REGENERATIVE REGION
NERVE SHEATH
STIMULUS
RELEASE OF MEDIATOR(S)
RECEPTOR POTENTIAL
GRADED
TTX RESISTANT
ACTION POTENTIAL
ALL-OR-NONE
TTX SENSITIVE
(b)
Classical concept of the axon reflex
(c)
Theory of sensory - efferent innervation
Efferent nerve ending
Sensory nerve ending
Sensory-efferent nerve ending
(d)
Control stomach
H+
barrier
Histamine
5-HT
Kinin
sensory nerve ending
Protective mucosal vasodilatation
(e)
Capsaicin-stimulated stomach
H+
Capsaicin
barrier
Histamine
5-HT
Kinin
sensory nerve ending
Enhanced protective vasodilatation
(Extreme stim.→congestion, oedema)

◀ **Fig. 1.6 a** Theory of dual sensory-efferent function of capsaicin-sensitive nociceptors (Reproduced from Szolcsányi 1988 with the kind permission of Birkhäuser Publishing House). **b** Original concept of axon reflex theory. **c** Revised axon reflex theory (Reproduced from Szolcsányi 1984 with the kind permission of Akadémiai Kiadó, Budapest). **d** Role of capsaicin-sensitive nerve endings in gastroprotection. **e** Enhanced protection of gastric mucosa by intake of low concentration of capsaicin (Reproduced from Szolcsányi and Barthó 1981 with the kind permission of Akadémiai Kiadó, Budapest)

a highly sensitive technique TRPV1 was detected only in the posterolateral hypothalamus with strong presence in primary sensory ganglia (Cavanaugh et al. 2011). From the functional aspect particular attention was paid to sites of the descending inhibitory pain pathway and on the hippocampus. These unsettled issues on the actions of capsaicin in the brain are discussed in another chapter and in several recent reviews (Kauer and Gibson 2009; Steenland et al. 2006; Palazzo et al. 2008).

1.5 Efferent Function of Capsaicin-Sensitive Sensory Nerve Endings

It was discovered by Nicholas Jancsó that pain producing agents evoke inflammation by stimulation of nerve endings which could be desensitized by capsaicin pretreatment (Jancsó 1955, 1964). In a posthumous paper written by his wife Aurelia Jancsó-Gábor and myself as his coworker provided the first "direct evidence" for the existence of neurogenic inflammation (Jancsó et al. 1967). Cardinal signs of inflammation as plasma extravasation through the interendothelical gaps of the contracted endothelial cells of the post-capillary venules but not at the capillaries (Majno et al. 1961) and involvement tissue cells as histiocytes in storage of these proteins in response to orthodromic or antidromic electrical stimulation of sensory nerve endings were not shown earlier. Subsequently, in neurogenic inflammation of the airways the sites on postcapillary endothelial gaps were confirmed and adhered leukocytes (monocytes, neutrophils) and platelets were also detected (McDonald 1988). The axon reflex flare reddening was analysed in detail by Thomas Lewis (1927, 1937), antidromic vasodilatation described by Bayliss (1901) more than 100 years ago and even the loss of mustard oil-induced chemosis in the denervated eye could be attributed to responses of arterioles or in the last example the oedema could be due to the damaged capillaries (Szolcsányi 1996). Our studies in addition provided evidence for the mediating role of a subpopulation of nerve endings subserving chemogenic pain.

Could capsaicin-sensitive interoceptors also evoke similar dual sensory-efferent tissue responses? This was the intriguing next question to be answered. With my coworker Loránd Barthó we started these works on in vitro preparations of isolated organs. It turned out that on the classical preparation of the guinea-pig isolated ileum capsaicin and mesenteric nerve stimulation elicit a new type of nerve-mediated contraction (Szolcsányi and Barthó 1978; Barthó and Szolcsányi 1978). Subsequently we described capsaicin-sensitive neural responses in the rabbit ileum, guinea-pig taenia coli and airway smooth muscle preparations (Szolcsányi 1984, 1996;

Maggi 1995). On the other hand it was striking that neural responses to stimulation of vagal parasympathetic, mesenteric sympathetic, intramural cholinergic, purinerg or substance P mediated peptiderg neuroeffector transmissions were not affected. Thus the neuroselective action of capsaicin was proven for the first time under in vitro condition (Maggi 1995). Therefore the term "capsaicin-sensitive" neural system with characteristic "sensory-efferent" function was introduced in 1978 (Szolcsányi and Barthó 1978, 1979; Maggi 1995; Jancsó et al. 1968). Characteristic features of this type of capsaicin sensitivity are: (1) Fast response from nanomolar (10^{-8} M) concentrations of capsaicin; (2) Activation is followed after washing out the compound by lasting—after micromolar range irreversible—neuroselective blockade of the capsaicin-responsive neuroeffector responses to electrically or chemically induced stimulation without affecting neurotransmissions of classical autonomic nerves; (3) Responses evoked by capsaicin are absent after chronic denervation. Although up to 1 μM concentration of capsaicin smooth muscle responses to electrical stimulation of autonomic fibers remained unchanged, in the presence of high concentration (from 3×10^{-5} M) inhibition of responses to sympathetic nerve stimulation was observed. This non-selective effect, is however, fully reversible and recovers within minutes after washout the compound from the organ bath (Szolcsányi and Barthó 1978). On isolated neurons of the dorsal root ganglia a similarly reversible nonselective inhibition of outward currents was observed already in the presence of 1×10^{-5} M capsaicin (Szolcsányi 1990). These studies opened up high interest in the field of neuropeptide research particularly to shed light on the role of substance P, other tachykinins, CGRP or somatostatin as local regulatory peptides. The increase in the number of papers on capsaicin during the eighties under keywords of "capsaicin in vitro "or "capsaicin-sensitive" (Fig. 1.5) revealed several important scopes of this new type of neural mechanism (Maggi 1995).

In contrast to the classical axon reflex theory (Szolcsányi 1984; Caterina 2007; Cavanaugh et al. 2011; Kauer and Gibson 2009; Steenland et al. 2006; Palazzo et al. 2008; Majno et al. 1961; McDonald 1988; Lewis 1927) our results revealed that the mediator of the capsaicin-sensitive efferent responses is released from the sensory receptors and not through axonal collaterals from effector nerve terminals (Fig. 1.6).

More than 40 years ago we have shown that local anaesthetics instilled into the rat's eye did not inhibit the plasma extravasation evoked by capsaicin providing evidence for a mediator release from the nerve endings without involvement of axonal conduction (Jancsó et al. 1968). I have also shown on the guinea-pig isolated trachea that neurogenic contraction evoked by capsaicin ($3.3 - 330 \times 10^{-8}$ M), piperine ($3.5 - 350 \times 10^{-7}$ M) and two synthetic capsaicin congeners were neither inhibited by tetrodotoxin. Furthermore, under these conditions, potency of the compounds to evoke efferent response run parallel with their sensory receptor stimulating nociceptive effect (Szolcsányi 1983a). Thus, it has been suggested that capsaicin-sensitive sensory nerve endings have dual sensory-efferent functions (Szolcsányi 1984 ,1996, 1988) and in this way form a new type of nerve terminals different from the classical autonomic efferent and sensory afferent nerve endings which subserve unidirectional functions in neuroregulation (Fig. 1.6).

Further studies on effects of capsaicin in isolated organs supported (Maggi 1995; Németh et al. 2003; Maggi et al. 1988) or intended to modify slightly this concept (Lundberg 1996) suggesting that axon reflexes are needed at threshold concentration of capsaicin (10^{-8} M), but not at higher ranges. Jan Lundberg group reported inhibition by tetrodotoxin or omega-conotoxin in the guinea-pig perfused lung preparation (Lundberg 1996). We have revealed, however, (Németh et al. 2003) that release of sensory neuropeptides (substance P, CGRP, somatostatin) from the isolated rat's trachea evoked by 10 nM capsaicin was not inhibited by lidocaine (25 nM), tetrodotoxin (1 μM) omega-conotoxin GVIA (100–300 nM) and a low concentration (50 nM) of agatoxin TK while 250 nM agatoxin TK or cadmium (200 μM) inhibited or completely prevented the release of these neuropeptides. In the light of the preferential opening of the TRPV1 channel to Ca^{++} over Na^{+} (Caterina et al. 1997; Wood et al. 1988; Bevan and Szolcsányi 1990) the intracellular high Ca^{2+} concentration to TRPV1 activation could release neuropeptides probably even before the graded depolarization of generator potential open the voltage-gated Ca^{2+} and Na^{+} channels for spike initiation (Fig. 1.6). Beyond the conceptional novelty for neuroregulation this scope is important, since epidermal TRPV1-expressing arborizations of peptidergic fibers are also sites for neuropeptide release causing local effects on keratinocytes or on epithelial cells of the conjuctiva, airways and various organs. This would not be expected when the classical axon reflex theory—which still seems to be is reiterated (Chiu et al. 2012)—would be valid.

Further important point was, that antidromic stimulation of capsaicin-sensitive dorsal roots evoked also in internal organs neurogenic inflammation and enhancement of microcirculation. In rats segmental neurogenic inflammatory plasma extravasation was shown to antidromic stimulation of lumbosacral dorsal roots on genito-urinary organs and rectum (Pintér and Szolcsányi 1995) and enhancement of microcirculation not only in the skin but also in the striated muscle of the rat's hindleg was detected with laser-Doppler flowmetry (Pórszász and Szolcsányi 1994). It is important to note that in rodents where the receptive field of polymodal nociceptors is small, almost punctate no axon reflex flare could be seen, while in primates (see earlier) and pigs (Pierau and Szolcsányi 1989) the large receptive field indicating the wide arborization of the terminal axons was coupled with axon reflex flare evoked by capsaicin or other irritants.

In order to obtain some evidence for the functional significance of this efferent role of capsaicin-sensitive nerve terminals it seemed to be interesting to test the effects of capsaicin on the stomach where the mucose is in contact with high acidity of the gastric juice. Could capsaicin protect the mucosa by inducing enhanced mucosal microcirculation? Furthermore, capsaicin-pretreated rats are more prone for ulcer formation than the controls? Our results in fact fully confirmed that it is the case (Szolcsányi and Barthó 1981, 2001) and the scheme on Fig. 1.6d and e, from our first publication seems to be still valid. Afterwards extensive studies of Peter Holzer from Graz on the gastrointestinal mucosal protective effect of capsaicin in low concentration and on the role of CGRP released from TRPV1-expressing nerve endings were revealed several important new details in this field (Holzer and Sametz 1986). (For reviews

Holzer 1991, 2007; Szolcsányi and Barthó 2001). Clinical studies for gastroprotective effect of capsaicin are in progress in Pécs (Mózsik et al. 2009) and data obtained on humans are summarized by Gyula Mózsik in another chapter.

Final interesting point to refer here is the high efficacy of vasodilator efferent function of capsaicin-sensitive nerve endings. Both in humans to transcutaneous electrical stimulation and in rats to dorsal root stimulation the frequency optimum of enhancement in cutaneous microcirculation is much lower than that required to elicit pain or nociception (Szolcsányi 1996, 1988).

A serendipitous observation revealed an even more interesting neurohumoral regulatory role of the capsaicin-sensitive nerve endings. In the course of experiments to stimulation the cut peripheral end of dorsal roots in the rat a systemic antinociceptiv/antiinflammatory effect mediated by the capsaicin-sensitive nerve endings was discovered (Szolcsányi 1996; Szolcsányi et al. 2011). A subgroup of TRPV1-expressing sensory neurons store the neuropeptide somatostatin, which is also released when these polymodal receptors are activated and—as measured—access into the circulation producing a systemic "sensocrine effect." Inhibition of the function of immune cells, nociceptors, and neurogenic inflammation by nerve stimulation could be evoked via sst4 and sst1 somatostatin receptors. Synthetic stable peptide (TT-232) or nonpeptides analogues being selective agonists on these receptors are potential analgesic/antiinflammatory drug candidates without endocrine side effects which are mediated by the other three somatostatin receptors. High efficacy to inhibit by sst4 agonists neuropathic and complete Freund's adjuvant (CFA)-induced hyperalgesia underlines their potential usage as analgesics (Szolcsányi et al. 2011; Pintér et al. 2006).

1.6 Effects on Thermoregulation

The heat-loss effect of capsaicin was described already by Hőgyes (1878) and the loss of capsaicin-induced fall in body temperature in rats, mice and guinea-pigs was a good indicator for the state of "capsaicin desensitization" in early studies of Nicholas Jancsó (1955). Beyond the obvious effect of capsaicin on peripheral thermosensors the role of preoptic central warm sensitive thermodetectors was analysed with involvement of my help in these experiments (Jancsó-Gábor et al. 1970). Capsaicin activated several heat-loss thermoeffectors in rats as cutaneous vasodilatation, inhibition of oxygen consumption at cool but not at thermoneutral ambient temperature and in cats evoking sweating of the plantar skin and panting. Furthermore, in rats intrapreoptic microinjections of capsaicin interrupted shivering and induced fall in body temperature (Szolcsányi 1982; Szolcsányi and Jancsó-Gábor 1973, 1975b; Pierau et al. 1986).

Particularly striking was the effect of capsaicin on thermoregulatory escape behaviour from a warm environment. In the two setups we used the floor was covered with plastic sheet, to minimize the involvement of cutaneous receptors. In contrast to the controls after 1 mg/kg s.c. given capsaicin all rats escaped from the heat chamber (39–41 °C) and their body temperature decreased by 4 °C

(Szolcsányi and Jancsó-Gábor 1975b; Szolcsányi 2004). Rats pretreated 20 days before with high capsaicin doses (50 + 100 mg/kg s.c.) could not cope their body temperature to overheating (Szolcsányi 1982; Jancsó-Gábor et al. 1970) and remained in the heat chamber although their hyperthermia reached nearly lethal level of 42 °C (Szolcsányi and Jancsó-Gábor 1975b; Szolcsányi 2004. In striking contrast rats where the brain 5-HT level was depleted by p-chlorophenylanine (PCP) treatment although they also showed enhanced hyperthermia in the warm chamber their thermoregulatory behaviour was just the opposite to that of the capsaicin pretreated animals. All PCP-treated rats left faster the warm chamber than the controls indicating that their impaired physiological heat-loss regulation was compensated by behavioural means (Szolcsányi and Jancsó-Gábor 1975b). After desensitizing doses of capsaicin the rat's body temperature for 1–2 days was significantly higher at room temperature but after this period their body temperature does not differ from that of the controls (Szikszay et al. 1982; Szolcsányi 1982; Szolcsányi and Jancsó-Gábor 1973, 1970). Beyond capsaicin piperine, several vanillylamides and homovanilloylamides induced also long-term/irreversible impaired thermoregulation lasting for several months (Szolcsányi 1982; Jancsó-Gábor et al. 1970).

Thermoregulatory behaviour and physiological regulatory features of capsaicin pretreated rats do not support the concept that tonic activation of visceral TRPV1 by nonthermal factors is the adjustable reference signal in thermoregulations as proposed recently (Romanovsky et al. 2009). Temperature selection of rats between two compartments differing in 5 °C differences was not altered in capsaicin pretreated rats up to 25 °C ambient temperature. These rats were pretreated with 50 + 100 mg/kg s.c. capsaicin 3–120 days before testing and remained in the warmer chamber of 35 versus 30 °C, while the controls choose the 30 °C. There was no sign of recovery of the disturbed thermoregulatory behaviour for 4 months. Slight tendency to avoid 40 versus 35 °C was observed but it was still impaired as compared to the untreated controls (Szolcsányi 1983b).

In respect of physiological thermoregulation of capsaicin pretreated rats there was differential upward shift in threshold for activation various heat-loss mechanisms. It was striking that rats with complete loss of heat avoidance behaviour at 35 °C ambient temperature responded with cutaneous vasodilatation in the tail when their body temperature was increased only by 1 °C or their skin temperature by 4.4 °C (Szolcsányi 1983). Nevertheless when the ambient temperature was raised from 25 to 35 °C cutaneous vasodilatation started later at higher cutaneous and body temperatures than those of the controls. Furthermore, in contrast to the abrupt marked tail vasodilatation of the controls, the pretreated rats responded with slowly developing vasodilatation which were often interrupted with vasoconstrictor periods in an oscillatory manner. Heat-loss grooming was rare and appeared at higher body temperatures. Thus the thermoneutral zone shifted upwards, but various effector mechanisms switched on at highly different levels which seems to be in accordance with the multiple thermostat theory (Satinoff 1978).

The role of central warmth sensors of the preoptic area as site of action of capsaicin are indicated by the following data:

1. In rats localized heating the preoptic area induces fall in body temperature with vasodilatation and interruption of shivering. These responses are significantly inhibited for days after systemic capsaicin pretreatment (Jancsó-Gábor et al. 1970a).
2. Microinjection of capsaicin into the *preoptic/anterior hypothalamus* (POAH) (rat, rabbit) elicits coordinated heat-loss responses. After repeated capsaicin application the responses are desensitized and these animals afterwards show impaired heat-loss regulation (Szolcsányi 1982; Jancsó-Gábor et al. 1970a; Urbán et al. 1985).
3. Microiontoforetic application of capsaicin into POAH cells excited most of the warm-sensitive neurons and decreased the firing rate of the cold ones (Hori 1984).
4. After systemic capsaicin desensitization by s.c. administration (a) the heat-loss responses to preoptic heating are inhibited (b) preoptic microinjection of capsaicin induces only slight fall in body temperature (Jancsó-Gábor et al. 1970a; Pierau et al. 1986) (c) proportion of thermoresponsive neurons in POAH are significantly diminished (Hori 1981) (d) long-lasting ultrastructural changes in some small type neurons of POAH were observed (Szolcsányi et al. 1971).
5. After preoptic lesions heat loss response to s.c. injection of capsaicin injection is diminished, shortened but not abolished (Szolcsányi and Jancsó-Gábor 1975b).

Detailed description of the characteristics of POAH warm-sensitive units and their responses to capsaicin and preoptic heating have been summarized in a thorough review of Tetsuro Hori (1984).

Thus, presence of POAH warmth sensitive neurons and their sensitivity to capsaicin is well established (Caterina 2007; Hori 1984) their integrative function in thermoregulation support the Hammel's model (Boulant 2006) although in this field neural pathways and hypothalamic circuitry is still under investigation (Morrison and Nakamura 2011). Particularly important is that capsaicin elicits a species-specific coordinated heat-loss response either when applied into the POAH area or when it is applied subcutaneously. TRPV1 knockout (Szelényi et al. 2004; Garami et al. 2011) and TRPV1 knockdown (Tóth et al. 2011) mice have no profound alteration in basal body temperature except that in TRPV1 knockout mice a slightly higher circadian fluctuation (Szelényi et al. 2004), preference for a cooler floor temperature and their slightly higher thermoneutral zone for evoking tail vasodilatation and lower oxygen consumption were described (Garami et al. 2011). It is worthy to mention, however, that in TRPV1 reporter mice TRPV1 expression was also detected in the arterial walls which could participate in the vascular effects (Caterina 2007). The most pronounced effect of capsaicin is on the thermoregulatory behaviour against overheating is not coupled with impaired regulation against cold. Temperature difference limen on the human tongue is also impaired in warm temperature range but not in the cold one (Szolcsányi 1977). Certainly several important aspects of actions of capsaicin on thermosensation remained unanswered. The tempting hypothesis about the tonic not thermal influence of TRPV1-expressing neural input into the thermoregulatory network (Garami et al. 2010) still is not supported by convincing evidence, but I agree that the TRPV1 channel itself "it is not" the principal transducer molecule for signaling warmth in thermoregulation (Romanovsky et al. 2009).

1.7 Perspectives and General Comments

The highly selective action of capsaicin on the major subgroup of nociceptive primary afferent neurons and several lines of evidence for the existence of capsaicin receptors supplied the clues for a successful functional genomic screening strategy to isolate an unknown cDNA clone from dorsal root ganglia that reconstitutes a nociceptive responsiveness in non-neural cells (Caterina et al. 1997). Thus, cloning the capsaicin receptor has been a real breakthrough from several aspects for basic neuroscience and particularly for drug development to open a new chapter which could be denoted as the nociceptor blocking analgesics.

1. The receptor of capsaicin renamed to Transient Receptor Potential Vanilloid-1 (TRPV1) turned out to be a cation channel with integrative function (Tominaga et al. 1998) directly gated by noxious heat (Cao et al. 2013), protons, capsaicin, RTX and several endogenous ligands as anandamide, lipoxygenase metabolites, oleoyldopamine, lysophosphatidic acid, arachydonyl dopamine, 9-hydroxyoctadecadienoic acid (Szolcsányi and Pintér 2013; Szolcsányi and Sándor 2012) Fig. 1.1.
2. It is a nocisensor transducer molecule of the plasma membrane which can be activated not only by a variety of pain producing chemical agents but indirectly it is stimulated or sensitized by activation other endogenous pain producing mediators released in the tissues under acute or chronic inflammatory conditions as bradykinin, prostanoids, nerve growth factor, chemokines, serotonin, proteinase, ATP etc. (Huang et al. 2006; Szolcsányi and Pintér 2013).
3. The structure of capsaicin receptor with six transmembrane domains and a pore loop region between TM5 and TM6 segments is similar to a previously described cation channel in the retina of the mutant Drosophila fruit flye (Montell 2011). Hence its present name of TRPV1 was given on this ground. After cloning TRPV1 a large group of TRP channels with at least 28 members were cloned in mammalian species. Nine of them are gated by thermal stimuli (six by heating, three by cooling) and they are often denoted as thermo-TRP channels (Nilius and Owsianik 2011; Vay et al. 2012).
4. Gating function of TRPV1 channel is in several aspect different from the canonical ligand-gated and voltage-gated channels (Szolcsányi and Sándor 2012).

The large-scale of chemical structures subserve the role for signaling noxious events and opens the TRPV1 cation channel by acting on different parts of the protein in a "multisteric" way (Szolcsányi and Sándor 2012). It is not dedicated to convey specific chemical messages in cell to cell communication as the ligand-gated channels do. Although its chemical structure is similar to the K^+ channels and TRPV1 can be activated by depolarization and particularly sensitized the gating effects of thermal or capsaicin stimuli, its voltage-sensitivity is in the non-physiological range which makes its role not primary importance in function (Szolcsányi and Sándor 2012).

5. TRPV1 was the first channel which could be opened by thermal stimuli with high Q_{10}, large enthalpy changes. Structural basis of conformational changes in molecular rearrangement in noxious heat range is challenging for further research (Szolcsányi and Sándor 2012; Clapham and Miller 2011; Baez-Nieto et al. 2011).
6. TRPV1 is expressed in most cases in homotrameric form but could be coupled to a heterotetrameric arrangement with another nocisensor TRP channel, the noxious cold and chemoceptive channel of Transient Receptor Potential Ankyrin 1 (TRPA1) (Vay et al. 2012). In this way further possible tissue selective analgesic drug targets are emerging (Szolcsányi and Pintér 2013).
7. Highly interesting feature of gating the TRPV1 and TRPA1 channels is that they show a phenomenon of "pore dilation" after prolonged chemical activation (Szolcsányi and Pintér 2013; Chung et al. 2008; Banke 2011). In other words after high capsaicin concentration larger cations up to 500 Da could enter into the nerve terminal. Uptake of a quaternary lidocaine analogue molecule of QX-314 induced selective local anesthetic blockade of TRPV1-expressing nociceptors (Vay et al. 2012; Binshtok et al. 2007).
8. "Pore dilation", calcium overload, intracellular acidosis might contribute to the surprisingly selective mitochondrial swelling lasting for months (Szolcsányi and Pintér 2013; Chung et al. 2008; Szolcsányi et al. 1971) which seems to have primary importance to induce different severities of impairment of nociceptor functions from functional desensitization to complete elimination of the central and peripheral terminals of the TRPV1-expressing nociceptive neurons which subserve not only pain, but itch, cough, and sneezing (Szolcsányi and Pintér 2013).
9. The selective site of action of capsaicin on nociceptors has been and will be utilized as a powerful tool in clinical trials for testing analgesic, (Andresen et al. 2011) antitussive drugs. Furthermore, in human settings important insights in neural circuitry for central sensitization were revealed with the help of capsaicin (LaMotte et al. 1991; Woolf 2011).
10. The exciting new horizons appeared with cloning the capsaicin receptor TRPV1 cation channel is in development of new analgesics with a target on nociceptors. It is inevitable for the target-oriented drug industry to have a transfected cell line for high throughput screening for TRPV1 antagonists. First generation of compounds led to potent agents but some drug candidates

had powerful effect of blocking also noxious heat sensation which induced burn risk and some others induced either in preclinical or clinical studies hyperthermia (Szolcsányi and Sándor 2012; Vay et al. 2012; Kort and Kym 2012; Gunthorpe and Chizh 2012). Second generation of TRPV1 antagonists seems to overcome these obstacles (Szolcsányi and Sándor 2012; Kort and Kym 2012; Gunthorpe and Chizh 2012).

Utilization of the nociceptor blocking/damaging effect of high concentration of capsaicin applied topically, however, already resulted in the introduction the first nociceptor-targeted analgesic drug in therapy of neuropathic pain. On the basis of recent Cochrane Database, topically applied high-concentration (8 %) capsaicin in chronic neuropathic pain patients (involving 2,073 participants including 1,272 with postherpetic neuralgia) established the efficacy which lasted at both eight and 12 weeks (Derry et al. 2013). On the other hand, low concentration of capsaicin (0.075 %) applied several times daily over several weeks was "without meaningful effect" on neuropathic pain patients (Derry and Moore 2012). More recent results with the 8 % dermal patch from German pain centers revealed high level of pain relief in HIV-associated neuropathy, postherpetic neuralgia, cervical spinal radiculopathy and back pain (Treede et al. 2013).

These clinical data provide not only further step in treatment of patients with severe persistent pain states but provide a conceptual message about the significance of nociceptors in triggering neuropathic pain which certainly mediate also chronic inflammatory pain. Revision of common view is needed which suggests that "nociceptor pain" is a physiological signal in acute pain stages to injury but play no role in pathological pain in which action potentials conducted in nociceptive afferents was assumed to have negligible role. Owing to technical and ethical burdens there are few microneurography studies which were against this traditional view. These details will be summarized in another chapter of this book. I refer here only to one recent study which documented by recording from C-fiber nociceptors spontaneous activity in patients having painful polyneuropathy (Kleggetveit et al. 2012).

Acknowledgments This work was supported by the grants of OTKA NK-78059 and SROP 4.2.2.A-11/1/KONV-2012-0024.

References

Abelli L, Geppetti P, Maggi CA (1993) Relative contribution of sympathetic and sensory nerves to thermal nociception and tissue trophism in rats. Neuroscience 57:739–745

Akagi H, Konishi S, Otsuka M, Yanagisava M (1985) The role of substance P as a neurotransmitter in the reflexes of slow time courses in the neonatal rat spinal cord. Br J Pharmacol 84:663–673

Andresen T, Staahl C, Oksche A, Mansikka H, Arendt-Nielsen L, Drewes AM (2011) Effect of transdermal opioids in experimentally induced superficial, deep and hyperalgesic pain. Br J Pharmacol 164:934–945

Baccaglini PJ, Hogan PG (1983) Some rat sensory neurons in culture express characteristics of differentiated pain sensory cells. Proc Natl Acad Sci 80:594–598

Baez-Nieto D, Castillo JP, Dragicevic C, Alvarez O, Latorre R (2011) Thermo-TRP channels: biophysics of polymodal receptors. In: Islam MS (ed) Transient receptor potential channels. Advances in experimental medicine and biology. Springer, Berlin
Banke TG (2011) The dilated TRPA1 channel pore state is blocked by amiloride and analogues. Brain Res 1381:21–30
Barthó L, Szolcsányi J (1978) The site of action of capsaicin on the guinea-pig isolated ileum. Naunyn-Schmiedeberg's Arch Pharmacol 305:75–81
Barthó L, Stein C, Herz A (1990) Involvement of capsaicin-sensitive neurons in hyperalgesia and enhanced opioid antinociception in inflammation. Naunyn-Schmiedeberg's Arch Pharmacol 342:666–670
Bauman TK, Simone DA, Shain CN, LaMotte RH (1991) Neurogenic hyperalgesia the search for the primary cutaneous affeent fibers that contribute to capsaicin-induced pain and hyperalgesia. J Neurophysiol 66:212–227
Bayliss WM (1901) On the origin from the spinal cord of vaso-dilator fibres of the hindlimb and on the nature of these fibres. J Physiol 26:173–209
Bessou P, Perl ER (1969) Response of cutaneous sensory units with unmyelinated fibers to noxious stimuli. J Neurophysiol 32:1025–1043
Bevan S, Docherty RJ (1993) Cellular mechanisms of the action of capsaicin. In: Wood JN (ed) Capsaicin in the study of pain. Academic Press, New York, pp 27–44
Bevan S, Szolcsányi J (1990) Sensory neuron-specific actions of capsaicin: mechanisms and applications. Trends Pharmacol Sci 11:330–333
Binshtok AM, Bean BP, Woolf CJ (2007) Inhibition of nociceptors by TRPV1-mediated entry of impermeant sodium channel blockers. Nature 449:607–610
Bölcskei K, Tékus V, Dézsi L, Szolcsányi J, Pethő G (2010) Antinociceptive desensitizing actions of TRPV1 receptor agonists capsaicin, resiniferatoxin and N-oleoyldopamine as measured by determination of the noxious heat and cold thresholds in the rat. Eur J Pain 14:480–486
Boulant JA (2006) Neuronal basis of Hammel's model for set-point thermoregulation. J Appl Physiol 100:1347–1350
Browning KN, Babic T, Holmes GM, Swartz E, Travagli RA (2013) A critical re-evaluation of the specificity of action of perivagal capsaicin. J Physiol 591:1563–1580
Buck SH, Burks TF (1986) The neuropharmacology of capsaicin: a review of some recent observations. Pharmacol Rev 38:179–226
Buck SH, Deskmukh PP, Yamamura HI, Burks TF (1981) Thermal analgesia and substance P depletion induced by capsaicin in guinea-pigs. Neuroscience 6:2217–2222
Cao E, Cordero-Morales JF, Liu B, Qin F, Julius D (2013) TRPV1 channels are intrinsically heat sensitive and negatively regulated by phosphoinositide lipids. Neuron 77:667–679
Caterina MJ (2007) Transient receptor potential ion channels as participants in thermosensation and thermoregulation. Am J Physiol Regul Integr Comp Physiol 292:R64–R76
Caterina MJ, Schumacher MA, Tominaga M, Rosen TA, Levine JD, Julius D (1997) The capsaicin receptor: a heat-activated ion channel in the pain pathway. Nature 389:816–824
Cavanaugh DJ, Chesler AT, Jackson AC, Sigal YM, Yamanaka H, Grant R, O'Donnell D, Nicoll RA, Shah NM, Julius D, Basbaum AI (2011) Trpv1 reporter mice reveal highly restricted brain distribution and functional expression in arteriolar smooth muscle cells. J Neurosci 31:5067–5077
Cervero F, McRitchie HA (1981) Neonatal capsaicin and thermal nociception: a paradox. Brain Res 215:414–418
Chiba T, Masuko S, Kavano H (1986) Correlation of mitochondrial swelling after capsaicin treatment and substance P and somatostatin immunoreactivity in small neurons of dorsal root ganglion in the rat. Neurosci Lett 64:311–316
Chiu IM, von Hehn CA, Woolf CJ (2012) Neurogenic inflammation and the peripheral nervous system in host defense and immunopathology. Nat Neurosci 15:1063–1067
Chung K, Schwen RJ, Coggeshall RE (1985) Ureteral axon damage following subcutaneous administration of capsaicin in adult rats. Neurosci Lett 53:221–226

Chung K, Klein CM, Coggeshall RE (1990) The receptive part of the primary afferent axon is most vulnerable to systemic capsaicin in adult rats. Brain Res 511:222–226

Chung MK, Güler AD, Caterina MJ (2008) TRPV1 shows dynamic ionic selectivity during agonist stimulation. Nat Neurosci 11:555–564

Clapham DE, Miller C (2011) A thermodynamic framework for understanding temperature sensing by transient receptor potential (TRP) channels. Proc Natl Acad Sci 108:19492–19497

De Vries DJ, Blumberg PM (1989) Thermoregulatory effects of resiniferatoxin in the mouse: comparison with capsaicin. Life Sci 44:711–715

Derry S, Moore RA (2012) Topical capsaicin (low concentration) for chronic neuropathic pain in adults. Cochrane Database Syst Rev 9:CD010111

Derry S, Sven-Rice A, Cole P, Tan T, Moore RA (2013) Topical capsaicin (high concentration) for chronic neuropathic pain in adults. Cochrane Database Syst Rev. doi:10.1002/14651858.CD007393.pub3

Dickenson A, Hughes C, Fueff A, Dray A (1990) A spinal mechanism of action is involved in the antinociception produced by the capsaicin analogue NE 19550 (olvanil). Pain 43:353–362

Du Mez AG (1917) A century of the United States Pharmacopoeia (1820–1920). Ph.D. Thesis, University of Wisconsin cf. Capsaicin Wikipedia, the free encyclopedia

Dux M, Sann H, Schemann M, Jancsó G (1999) Changes in fibre populations of the rat hairy skin following selective chemodenervation by capsaicin. Cell Tissue Res 296:471–477

Foster RW, Ramage AG (1981) The action of some chemical irritants on somatosensory receptors of the cat. Neuropharmacology 20:191–198

Fr-K Pierau, Szolcsányi J (1989) Neurogenic inflammation; axon reflex in pigs. Agents Actions 26:231–232

Fr-K Pierau, Szolcsányi J, Sann H (1986) The effect of capsaicin on afferent nerves and temperature regulation of mammals and birds. J Therm Biol 11:95–100

Gamse R (1982) Capsaicin and nociception in the rat and mouse: possible role of substance P. Naunyn-Schmiedeberg's Arch Pharmacol 320:205–216

Garami A, Almeida MC, Nucci TB, Hew-Butler T, Soriano RN, Pakai E, Nakamura K, Morrison SF, Romanovsky AA (2010) The TRPV1 channel in normal thermoregulation: what thave we learned from experiments using different tools? In: Gomtsyan A, Faltynek CR (eds) Vanilloid receptor TRPV1 in drug discovery. Wiley, Hoboken, pp 351–402

Garami A, Pakai E, Oliveira DL, Steiner AA, Wanner SP, Almeida MC, Lesnikov VA, Gavva NR, Romanovsky AA (2011) Thermoregulatory phenotype of the Trpv1 knockout mouse: thermoeffector dysbalance with hyperkinesis. J Neurosci 31:1721–1733

Geissler E, Moeller J (1887) Real-Encyclopadie der gesamten Pharmacie, vol 2. Urban and Co, Leipzig

Guenther S, Reeh PW, Kress M (1999) Rises in [Ca^{2+}]i mediate capsaicin- and proton-induced heat sensitization of rat primary nociceptive neurons. Eur J Neurosci 11:3143–3150

Gunthorpe MJ, Chizh BA (2012) Clinical development of TRPV1 antagonists: targeting a pivotal point in the pain pathway. Drug Discov Today 14:56–57

Hamalainen MM, Subieta A, Arpey C, Brennan TJ (2009) Differential effect of capsaicin treatment of pain-related behaviors after plantar incision. J Pain 10:637–645

Han L, Ma C, Liu Q, Weng HJ, Cui Y, Tang Z, Kim Y, Nie H, Qu L, Patel KN, Li Z, McNeil B, He S, Guan Y, Xiao B, LaMotte RH, Dong X (2013) A subpopulation of nociceptors specifically linked to itch. Nat Neurosci 16:174–182

Heyman I, Rang HP (1985) Depolarizing responses to capsaicin in a subpopulation of rat dorsal root ganglion cells. Neurosci Lett 56:69–75

Hőgyes A (1878) Beitrage zur physiologischen Wirkung der Bestandteile des Capsicum annuum. Arch Exp Pathol Pharmakol 9:117–130

Holzer P (1991) Capsaicin: cellular targets, mechanism of action, and selectivity for thin sensory neurons. Pharmacol Rev 43:143–201

Holzer P (2007) Role of visceral afferent neurons in mucosal inflammation and defense. Curr Opin Pharmacol 7:563–569

Holzer P, Sametz W (1986) Gastric mucosal protection against ulcerogenic factors in the rat mediated by capsaicin-sensitive afferent neurons. Gastroenterology 91:975–981

Hori T (1981) Thermosensitivity of preoptic and anterior hypothalamic neurons in the capsaicin-desensitized rat. Pfügers Arch 389:297–299

Hori T (1984) Capsaicin and central control of thermoregulation. Pharm Ther 26:389–416

Huang J, Zhang X, McNaughton PA (2006) Inflammatory pain: the cellular basis of heat hyperalgesia. Curr Neuropharmacol 4:197–206

Jancsó N (1955) Speicherung Stoffanreicherung im Retikuloendothel und in der Niere. Akadémiai Kiadó, Budapest

Jancsó N (1964) Neurogenic inflammatory response. Acta Physiol Hung Suppl 24:3–4

Jancsó N (the late), Jancsó-Gábor A, Szolcsányi J (1967) Direct evidence for neurogenic inflammation and its prevention by denervation and by pretreatment with capsaicin. Br J Pharmacol 31:138–151

Jancsó N (the late), Jancsó-Gábor A, Szolcsányi J (1968) The role of sensory nerve endings in neurogenic inflammation induced in human skin and in the eye and paw of the rat. Br J Pharmac 33:32–41

Jancsó G, Király E, Jancsó-Gábor A (1977) Pharmacologically induced selective degeneration of chemosensitive primary sensory neurons. Nature 270:741–743

Jancsó G, Király E, Jancsó-Gábor A (1980) Direct evidence for an axonal site of action of capsaicin. Naunyn Schmiedebergs Arch Pharmacol 313:91–94

Jancsó G, Király E, Such G, Joó F, Nagy A (1987) Neurotoxic effect of capsaicin in mammals. Acta Physiol Hung 69:295–313

Jancsó-Gábor A, Szolcsányi J (1972) Neurogenic inflammatory responses. J Dental Res 41:264–269

Jancsó-Gábor A, Szolcsányi J, Jancsó N (1970a) Stimulation and desensitization of the hypothalamic heat-sensitive structures by capsaicin in rats. J Physiol 208:449–459

Jancsó-Gábor A, Szolcsányi J, Jancsó N (1970b) Irreversible impairment of thermoregulation induced by capsaicin and similar pungent substances in rats and guinea-pigs. J Physiol 206:495–507

Jessell TM, Iversen LL, Cuello AC (1978) Capsaicin-induced depletion of substance P from primary sensory neurones. Brain Res 152:183–188

Jhamandas K, Yaksh TL, Harty G, Szolcsányi J, Go VL (1984) Action of intrathecal capsaicin and its structural analogues on the content and release of spinal substance P: selectivity of action and relationship to analgesia. Brain Res 306:215–225

Johanek LM, Meyer RA, Friedman RM, Greenquist KW, Shim B, Borzan J, Hartke T, LaMotte RH, Ringkamp M (2008) A role for polymodal C-fiber afferents in nonhistaminergic itch. J Neurosci 28:7659–7669

Joó F, Szolcsányi J, Jancsó-Gábor A (1969) Mitochondrial alterations in the spinal ganglion cells of the rat accompanying the long-lasting sensory disturbance induced by capsaicin. Life Sci 8:621–626

Kauer JA, Gibson HE (2009) Hot flash: TRPV channels in the brain. Trends Neurosci 32:215–224

Kenins P (1982) Responses of single nerve fibres to capsaicin applied to the skin. Neurosci Lett 29:83–88

Kim H, Cui L, Kim J, Kim SJ (2009) Transient receptor potential vanilloid type 1 receptor regulates glutamatergic synaptic inputs to the spinothalamic tract neurons of the spinal cord deep dorsal horn. Neuroscience 160:508–516

Kissin I (2008) Vanilloid-induced conduction analgesia: selective, dose-dependent, long-lasting, with a low level of potential neurotoxicity. Anesth Analg 107:271–281

Kleggetveit IP, Namer B, Schmidt R, Helas T, Rückel M, Orstavik K, Schmelz M, Jorum E (2012) High spontaneous activity of C-nociceptors in painful polyneuropathy. Pain 153:2040–2047

Konietzny F, Hensel H (1983) The effect of capsaicin on the response characteristics of human C-polymodal nociceptors. J Therm Biol 8:213–215

Kort ME, Kym PR (2012) TRPV1 antagonists: clinical setbacks and prospects for future development. Prog Med Chem 51:57–70

LaMotte RH, Shain CN, Simone DA, Tsai EF (1991) Neurogenic hyperalgesia: psychophysical studies of undrlying mehcanisms. J Neurophysiol 66:190–211
LaMotte RH, Lundberg LE, Torebjörk HE (1992) Pain, hyperalgesia and activity in nociceptive C units in humans after intradermal injection of capsaicin. J Physiol 448:749–764
Lawson SN, Harper AA (1984) Neonatal capsaicin is not a specific neurotoxin for sensory C-fibres or small dark cells of rat dorsal root ganglia. In: Chahl LA, Szolcsányi J, Lembeck F (eds) Antidromic Vasodilatation and Neurogenic Inflammation. Akadémiai Kiadó, Budapest, pp 111–116
Lee TS (1954) Physiological gustatory sweating in a warm climate. J Physiol 124:528–542
Lembeck F (1987) Columbus, capsicum and capsaicin: past, present and future. Acta Physiol Hung 69:263–273
Lewis T (1927) The blood vessels of the human skin and their responses. Shaw, London
Lewis T (1937) The nocifensor system of nerves and its reactions. Br Med J 194:431–435
Lundberg JM (1996) Pharmacology of cotransmission in the autonomic nervous system: integrative aspects on amines, neuropeptides, adenosin triphosphate, amino acids and nitric oxid. Pharmacol Rev 48:113–178
Lynn B, Schütterle S, Pierau Fr-K (1996) The vasodilator component of neurogenic inflammation is caused by a special subclass of heat-sensitive nociceptors in the skin of the pig. J Physiol 494:587–593
Mac Neish RS (1964) Ancient mesoamerican civilization. Science 143:531–553
Maggi CA (1995) Tachykinins and calcitonin gene-related peptide (CGRP) as co-transmitters released from peripheral endings of sensory nerves. Prog Neurobiol 45:1–98
Maggi CA, Borsini F, Santicioli P, Geppetti P, Abelli L, Evangelista S, Manzini S, Theodorsson-Norheim E, Somma V, Amenta F (1987) Cutaneous lesions in capsaicin-pretreated rats. A trophic role of capsaicin-sensitive afferents? Naunyn Schmiedebergs Arch Pharmacol 336:538–545
Maggi CA, Patacchini R, Giuliani S, Santicioli P, Meli A (1988) Evidence for two independent modes of activation of the "efferent" function of capsaicin-sensitive nerves. Eur J Pharmacol 156:367–373
Majno G, Palade GE, Schoefl GS (1961) Studies on inflammation. II. The site of action of histamine and serotonin along the vascular tree: a topographic study. J Biophys Biochem Cytol 11:607–626
Makara GB, Stark E, Mihály K (1967) Sites at which formalin and capsaicin act to stimulate corticotropin secretion. Can J Physiol Pharmacol 45:669–674
Marsh SJ, Stansfeld CE, Brown DA, Davey R, McCarthy D (1987) The mechanism of action of capsaicin on sensory C-type neurons and their axon in vitro. Neuroscience 23:275–290
Martin HA, Basbaum AJ, Kwiat GC, Goetzl EJ, Levine JD (1987) Leukotriene and prostaglandin sensitization of cutaneous high-threshold C- and A-delta mechanoreceptors in the hairy skin of rat hindlimbs. Neurosci 22:651–659
McDonald DM (1988) Neurogenic inflammation in the rat trachea I. Changes in venules, leucocytes and epithelial cells. J Neurocytol 17:583–603
Melzack R, Wall PD (1965) Pain mechanisms: a new theory. Science 150:971–979
Micevych PE, Yaksh TL, Szolcsányi J (1983) Effect of intrathecal capsaicin analogues on the immunofluorescence of peptides and serotonin in the dorsal horn in rats. Neuroscience 8:123–131
Molnár J (1965) Pharmacologic effect of capsaicin the sharp tasting principle in paprika (in German). Arzneimittel Forschung 15:718–727
Montell C (2011) The history of TRP channels, a commentary and reflection. Pfügers Arch 461:499–506
Morrison SF, Nakamura K (2011) Central neural pathways for thermoregulation. Front Biosci 16:74–104
Mózsik Gy, Dömötör A, Past T, Vas V, Perjési P, Kuzma M, Blázich Gy, Szolcsányi J (2009) Capsaicinoids from the plant cultivation to the production of the human medical drug. Akadémiai Kiadó, Budapest

Nagy JI, Iversen LL, Goedert M, Chapman D, Hunt SP (1983) Dose-dependent effects of capsaicin on primary sensory neurons in the neonatal rat. J Neurosci 3:399–406
Nelson EK (1919) The constitution of capsaicin, the pungent principle of capsicum. J Am Chem Soc 41:1115–1121
Németh J, Zs Helyes, Oroszi G, Jakab B, Pintér E, Szilvássy Z, Szolcsányi J (2003) Role of voltage-gated cation channels and axon reflexes in the release of sensory neuropeptides by capsaicin from isolated rat trachea. Eur J Pharmacol 458:313–318
Nilius B, Owsianik G (2011) The transient receptor potential family of ion channels. Genome Biol 12:218–228
Nothnagel H (1870) Handbuch der Arzneimittellehre. Hirschwald A Verlag, Berlin
Palazzo E, Rossi F, Maione S (2008) Role of TRPV1 receptors in descending modulation of pain. Mol Cell Endocrinol 286:S79–S83
Palermo NN, Brown HK, Smith DL (1981) Selective neurotoxic action of capsaicin on glomerular C-type terminals in rat substantia gelatinosa. Brain Res 208:506–510
Pan YZ, Pan HL (2004) Primary afferent stimulation differentially potentiates excitatory and inhibitory inputs to spinal lamina II outer and inner neurons. 91:2413–2421
Pethő G, Szolcsányi J (1996) Excitation of central and peripheral terminals of primary afferent neurons by capsaicin in vivo. Life Sci 58:47–53
Petsche U, Fleischer E, Lembeck F, Handwerker HO (1983) The effect of capsaicin application to a peripheral nerve on impulse conduction in functionally identified afferent nerve fibres. Brain Res 265:233–240
Pini A, Baranowski R, Lynn B (1990) Long-term reduction in the number of C-fibre nociceptors following capsaicin treatment of a cutaneous nerve in adult rats. Eur J Neurosci 2:89–97
Pintér E, Szolcsányi J (1995) Plasma extravasation in the skin and pelvic organs evoked by antidromic stimulation of the lumbosacral dorsal roots of the rat. Neuroscience 68:603–614
Pintér E, Zs Helyes, Szolcsányi J (2006) Inhibitory effect of somatostatin on inflammation and nociception. Pharmacol Ther 112:440–456
Planells-Cases R, Valente P, Ferrer-Montiel A, Qin F, Szállási Á (2011) Complex regulation of TRPV1 and related thermo-TRPs: implications for therapeutic intervention. Adv Exp Med Biol 704:491–515
Pórszász R, Szolcsányi J (1994) Antidromic vasodilatation in the striated muscle and its sensitivity to resiniferatoxin in the rat. Neurosci Lett 182:267–270
Romanovsky AA, Almeida MC, Garami A, Steiner AA, Norman MH, Morrison SF, Nakamura K, Burmeister JJ, Nucci TB (2009) The transient receptor potential vanilloid-1 channel in thermoregulation: a thermosensor it is not. Pharmacol Rev 61:228–261
Rukwied R, Dush M, Schley M, Forsh E, Schmelz M (2008) Nociceptor sensitization to mechanical and thermal stimuli in pig skin in vivo. Eur J Pain 12:242–250
Satinoff E (1978) Neural organization and evolution of thermal regulation in mammals. Science 201:16–22
Schmelz M, Schmidt R, Ringkamp M, Handwerker HO, Torebjörk HE (1994) Sensitization of insensitive branches of C nociceptors in human skin. J Physiol 480:389–394
Schmelz M, Schmidt R, Handwerker HO, Torebjörk HE (2000a) Enconding of burning pain from capsaicin-treated human skin in two categories of unmyelinated nerve fibres. Brain 3:560–571
Schmelz M, Michael K, Weidner C, Schmidt R, Torebjörk HE, Handwerker HO (2000b) Which nerve fibers mediate the axon reflex flare in human skin. NeuroReport 11:645–648
Schmidt R, Schmelz M, Torebjörk HE, Handwerker HO (2000) Mechano-insensitive nociceptors encode pain evoked by tonic pressure to human skin 98:793–800
Seno N, Dray A (1993) Capsaicin-induced activation of fine afferent fibres from rat skin in vitro. Neuroscience 55:563–569
Sherrington CS (1906) The integrative action of the nervous system. Scribner, New York
Steenland HVV, Ko SW, Wu LJ, Zhuo M (2006) Hot receptors in the brain. Mol Pain 8:2–34
Suzuki T, Iwai K (1984) Constituents of red pepper species: chemistry, biochemistry, pharmacology and food science of the pungent principle of Capsicum species. In: Brossi A (ed) The alkaloids, vol 23. Academic Press, Orlando, pp 227–299

Szállási Á, Blumberg PM (1989) Resiniferatoxin, a phorbol-related diterpene, acts as an ultrapotent analog of capsaicin, the irritant constituent in red pepper. Neuroscience 30:515–520
Szállási Á, Blumberg PM (1990) Specific binding of resiniferatoxin, an ultrapotent capsaicin analog, by dorsal root ganglion membranes. Brain Res 524:106–111
Szállási Á, Blumberg PM (1999) Vanilloid (capsaicin) receptors and mechanism. Pharmacol Rev 51:159–211
Szelényi Z, Hummel Z, Szolcsányi J, Davis JB (2004) Daily body temperature rhythm and heat tolerance in TRPV1 knockout and capsaicin pretreated mice. Eur J Neurosci 19:142–144
Szikszay M, Obál F, Obál F (1982) Dose-response relationships in the thermoregulatory effects of capsaicin. Naunyn-Schmiedeberg's Arch Pharmacol 320:97–100
Szőke É, Seress L, Szolcsányi J (2002a) Neonatal capsaicin treatment results in prolonged mitochondrial damage and delayed cell death of B cells in the rat trigeminal ganglia. Neuroscience 113:925–937
Szőke É, Czéh G, Szolcsányi J, Seress L (2002b) Neonatal anandamide treatment results in prolonged mitochondrial damage in the vanilloid receptor type 1-immunoreactive B-type neurons of the rat trigeminal ganglion. Neuroscience 115:805–814
Szolcsányi J (1977) A pharmacological approach to elucidate the role of different nerve fibres and receptor endings in mediation of pain. J Physiol (Paris) 73:251–259
Szolcsányi J (1980) Role of polymodal nociceptors in mediation of chemogenic pain and inflammatory hyperalgesia. In: Proceedings of the international congress of physiological science, vol 14, Budapest, p 734
Szolcsányi J (1982) Capsaicin type pungent agents producing pyrexia. In: Milton AS (ed) Handbook of experimental pharmacology, pyretics and antipyretics, vol 60. Springer, Berlin, pp 437–478
Szolcsányi J (1983a) Tetrodotoxin-resistant non-cholinergic neurogenic contraction evoked by capsaicinoids and piperine on the guinea-pig trachea. Neurosci Lett 42:83–88
Szolcsányi J (1983b) Disturbances of thermoregulation induced by capsaicin. J Therm Biol 8:207–212
Szolcsányi J (1984) Capsaicin-sensitive chemoceptive neural system with dual sensory-efferent function. In: Chahl LA, Szolcsányi J, Lembeck F (eds) Antidromic vasodilatation and neurogenic inflammation. Akadémiai Kiadó, Budapest, pp 27–56
Szolcsányi J (1987a) Selective responsiveness of polymodal nociceptors of the rabbit ear to capsaicin, bradykinin and ultra-violet irradiation. J Physiol 388:9–23
Szolcsányi J (1987b) Capsaicin and nociception. Acta Physiol Hung 69:323–332
Szolcsányi J (1988) Antidromic vasodilatation and neurogenic inflammation. Agents Actions 23:4–11
Szolcsányi J (1990) Capsaicin, irritation and desensitization. Neurophysiological basis and future perspectives. In: Green BR, Mason JR, Kare MR (eds) Chemical senses: irritation, vol 2. Marcel Dekker, New York, pp 141–168
Szolcsányi J (1993) Actions of capsaicin on sensory receptors. In: Wood JN (ed) Capsaicin in the study of pain. Academic Press, London, pp 1–26
Szolcsányi J (1996) Capsaicin-sensitive sensory nerve terminals with local and systemic efferent functions: facts and scopes of an unorthodox neuroregulatory mechanism. Prog Brain Res 113:343–359
Szolcsányi J (2004) Forty years in capsaicin research for sensory pharmacology and physiology. Neuropeptides 38:377–384
Szolcsányi J (2005) Hot peppers, pain and analgesics. In: Malmberg AB, Bley KR (eds) Turning up to heat on pain: TRPV1 receptors in pain and inflammation. Birkhäuser Verlag, Basel, pp 3–22
Szolcsányi J, Barthó L (1978) New type of nerve-mediated cholinergic contractions of the guinea-pig small intestine and its selective blockade by capsaicin. Naunyn-Schmiedeberg's Arch Pharmacol 305:83–90
Szolcsányi J, Barthó L (1979) Capsaicin-sensitive innervation of the guinea-pig taenia caeci. Naunyn-Schmiedebergs Arch Pharmacol 309:77–82

Szolcsányi J, Barthó L (1981) Impaired defense mechanism to peptic ulcer in the capsaicin-desensitized rat. In: Mózsik G, Hänninen O, Jávor T (eds) Gastrointestinal defense mechanisms. Advances in Physiological Sciences, vol 29. Akadémiai Kiadó, Pergamon Press, Oxford, pp 39–51

Szolcsányi J, Barthó L (2001) Capsaicin-sensitive afferents and their role in gastroprotection: an update. J Physiol (Paris) 95:181–188

Szolcsányi J, Jancsó-Gábor A (1973) Capsaicin and other pungent agents as pharmacological tools in studies on thermoregulation. In: Schönbaum E, Lomax P (eds) The pharmacology of thermoregulation. Karger, Basel, pp 395–409

Szolcsányi J, Jancsó-Gábor A (1975a) Sensory effects of capsaicin congeners I. Relationship between chemical structure and pain-producing potency. Arzneim Forsch (Drug Res) 25:1877–1881

Szolcsányi J, Jancsó-Gábor A (1975b) Analysis of the role warmth detectors by means of capsaicin under different conditions. In: Lomax P, Schönbaum E, Jacob J (eds). Karger, Basel, pp 331–338

Szolcsányi J, Jancsó-Gábor A (1976) Sensory effects of capsaicin congeners II. Importance of chemical structure and pungency in desensitizing activity of capsaicin-type compounds. Arzneim Forsch (Drug Res) 26:33–37

Szolcsányi J, Pintér E (2013) Transient receptor potential vanilloid 1 as a therapeutic target in analgesia. Expert Opin Ther Targets 17(6):641–657

Szolcsányi J, Sándor Z (2012) Multisteric TRPV1 nocisensor: a target for analgesics. Trends Pharmacol Sci 33:646–655

Szolcsányi J, Joó F, Jancsó-Gábor A (1971) Mitochondrial changes in preoptic neurones after capsaicin desensitization of the hypothalamic thermodetectors in rats. Nature 229:116–117

Szolcsányi J, Jancsó-Gábor A, Joó F (1975) Functional and fine structural characteristics of the sensory neuron blocking effect of capsaicin. Naunyn-Schmiedeberg's Arch Pharmacol 287:157–169

Szolcsányi J, Sann H, Pierau Fr-K (1986) Nociception in pigeon is not impaired by capsaicin. Pain 27:247–260

Szolcsányi J, Anton F, Reeh P, Handwerker HO (1988) Selective excitation by capsaicin of mechano-heat sensitive nociceptors in rat skin. Brain Res 446:262–268

Szolcsányi J, Szállási Á, Szállási Z, Joó F, Blumberg PM (1990) Resiniferatoxin: an ultrapotent selective modulator of capsaicin-sensitive primary afferent neurons. J Pharmacol Exp Ther 255:923–928

Szolcsányi J, Nagy J, Pethő G (1993) Effect of CP-96,345 a non-peptide substance P antagonist, capsaicin, resiniferatoxin and ruthenium red on nociception. Regul Pept 46:437–439

Szolcsányi J, Pórszász R, Pethő G (1994) Capsaicin and pharmacology of nociceptors. In: Besson JM, Guilbaud G, Ollat H (eds) Peripheral neurons in nociception: physio-pharmacological aspects. Elsevier, Amsterdam, pp 109–124

Szolcsányi J, Pintér E, Helyes Zs (2011) Inhibition of the function of TRPV1-expressing nociceptive sensory neurons by somatostatin 4 receptor agonism: mechanism and therapeutical implications. Curr Top Med Chem 11:2253–2263

Thresh J, JC (1876) Capsaicin the active principle in Capsicum fruits. Pharm J Transact 7:21

Tominaga M, Caterina MJ, Malmberg AB, Rosen TA, Gilbert H, Skinner K, Raumann BE, Basbaum AI, Julius D (1998) The cloned capsaicin receptor integrates multiple pain-producing stimuli. Neuron 21:531–543

Tóth DM, Szőke É, Bölcskei K, Kvell K, Bender B, Bosze Z, Szolcsányi J, Sándor Z (2011) Nociception, neurogenic inflammation and thermoregulation in TRPV1 knockdown transgenic mice. Cell Mol Life Sci 68:2589–2601

Tóth-Kása I, Jancsó G, Bognár A, Husz S, Obál F (1986) Capsaicin prevents histamine-induced itching. Int J Clin Pharmacol Res 6:163–170

Touska F, Marsakova L, Teisinger J, Vlachova V (2011) A "cute" desensitization of TRPV1. Curr Pharm Biotechnol 12:122–129

Treede RD, Wagner T, Kern KU, Husstedt IVV, Arendt G, Birklein F, Cegla T, Freynhagen R, Gockel HH, Heskamp ML, Jager H, Joppich R, Maier C, Leffler A, Nagelein HH, Rolke R, Seddigh S, Sommer C, Stander S, Wasner G, Baron R (2013) Mechanism- and experience-based strategies to optimize treatment response to the capsaicin 8% cutaneous patch in patients with localized neuropathic pain. Curr Med Res Opin 29:527–538

Urbán L, Willetts J, Randic M, Papka RE (1985) The acute and chronic effects of capsaicin on slow excitatory transmission in rat dorsal horn. Brain Res 330:39–396

Vay L, Gu C, McNaughton PA (2012) The thermo-TRP ion channel family: properties and therapeutic implications. Br J Pharmacol 165:787–801

Wall PD (1987) The central consequences of the application of capsaicin to one peripheral nerve in adult rat. Acta Physiol Hung 69:275–286

Wallengren J, Chen D, Sundler F (1999) Neuropeptide-containing C-fibers and wound healing in rat skin. Neither capsaicin nor peripheral neurotomy affect the rate of healing. Br J Dermatol 140:400–408

Weidner C, Schmelz M, Schmidt R, Hansson B, Handwerker HO, Torebjörk HE (1999) Functional attributes discriminating mechano-insensitive and mechano-responsive C nociceptors in human skin. J Neurosci 19:10184–10190

Welk E, Fleischer E, Petsche U, Handwerker HO (1984) Afferent C-fibers in rats after neonatal capsaicin treatment. Pflügers Arch 400:66–71

Winter J, Dray A, Wood JN, Yeats JC, Bevan S (1990) Cellular mechanism of action of resiniferatoxin: a potent sensory neuron excitotoxin. Brain Res 520:131–140

Wood JN, Winter J, James IF, Rang HP, Yeats J, Bevan S (1988) Capsaicin-induced ion fluxes in dorsal root ganglion cells in culture. J Neurosci 8:3208–3220

Woolf CJ (2011) Central sensitization: Implications for the diagnosis and treatment of pain. Pain 152:S2–S15

Xia R, Samad TA, Btesh J, Jiang LH, Kays I, Stjernborg L, Dekker N (2011) TRPV1 signaling: mechanistic understanding and therapeutic potential. Curr Top Med Chem 11:2180–2189

Yaks TL, Farb DH, Leeman SE, Jessell TM (1979) Intrathecal capsaicin depletes substance P in the rat spinal cord and produces prolonged thermal analgesia. Science 206:481–483

Chapter 2
Pharmacology of the Capsaicin Receptor, Transient Receptor Potential Vanilloid Type-1 Ion Channel

Istvan Nagy, Dominic Friston, João Sousa Valente, Jose Vicente Torres Perez and Anna P. Andreou

Abstract The capsaicin receptor, transient receptor potential vanilloid type 1 ion channel (TRPV1), has been identified as a polymodal transducer molecule on a sub-set of primary sensory neurons which responds to various stimuli including noxious heat (>~42 °C), protons and vanilloids such as capsaicin, the hot ingredient of chilli peppers. Subsequently, TRPV1 has been found indispensable for the development of burning pain and reflex hyperactivity associated with inflammation of peripheral tissues and viscera, respectively. Therefore, TRPV1 is regarded as a major target for the development of novel agents for the control of pain and visceral hyperreflexia in inflammatory conditions. Initial efforts to introduce agents acting on TRPV1 into clinics have been hampered by unexpected side-effects due to wider than expected expression in various tissues, as well as by the complex pharmacology, of TRPV1. However, it is believed that better understanding of the pharmacological properties of TRPV1 and specific targeting of tissues may eventually lead to the development of clinically useful agents. In order to assist better understanding of TRPV1 pharmacology, here we are giving a comprehensive account on the activation and inactivation mechanisms and the structure–function relationship of TRPV1.

2.1 Introduction

The biological effects of chilli peppers, which are produced by capsaicin, the archetypical exogenous activator of the transient receptor potential vanilloid type 1 ion channel (TRPV1) (Caterina et al. 1997; Thresh 1876a, b), have been known

I. Nagy (✉) · D. Friston · J. S. Valente · J. V. T. Perez · A. P. Andreou
Department of Surgery and Cancer, Section of Anaesthetics, Pain Medicine and Intensive Care, Imperial College London, Chelsea and Westminster Hospital, 369 Fulham Road, London SW10 9NH, UK
e-mail: i.nagy@imperial.ac.uk

O. M. E. Abdel-Salam (ed.), *Capsaicin as a Therapeutic Molecule*, Progress in Drug Research 68, DOI: 10.1007/978-3-0348-0828-6_2, © Springer Basel 2014

for several thousands of years. When applied through the oral rout (e.g. eating spicy dishes), these effects include burning pain in the mouth, heavy perspiration and increased bowel movements. It is rather perplexing why, in spite of the pain and discomfort, the majority of people still enjoy eating hot dishes. Nevertheless, the biological effects through topical application (e.g. accidental application on mucous membranes) which include erythema in addition to a burning pain sensation are also well known. It is also an everyday experience that repeated consumption of, or contact with, hot peppers results in reduced sensitivity to chilli pepper and even to other stimuli. This desensitizing effect was widely used by native Americans, and later in Europe, for analgesia.

The first animal and human experiments to find out the physiological effects of capsaicin were conducted by a Hungarian doctor, Hőgyes (1878a, b). He noted that oral application of capsaicin reduced the respiratory and heart rate and body temperature in dogs. Topical application onto his own or his assistant's arm produced the well-known hyperaemia and burning pain. When Hőgyes put capsaicin onto his tongue he felt a sharp burning pain. When he consumed capsaicin in a capsule, he first felt warmth in the epigastrium, then experienced belching and flatulence (Hőgyes 1878b).

Following more than 60 years of dormancy, pharmacological studies with capsaicin were revitalized by three, again Hungarian, scientists Nicolas Jancsó, Aurelia Jancsó-Gábor and János Pórszász (Jancsó and Jancsóné 1949; Pórszász and Jancsó 1959). They noted that capsaicin activated a subpopulation of sensory nerve fibres, which belonged to the so-called nociceptive sensory nerves. They also noted that following capsaicin application, the responsiveness of the nerves was reduced not only to capsaicin but also to other chemical activators, such as mustard oil (Pórszász and Jancsó 1959). These authors then noted that topical capsaicin application increased mechanical responsiveness, a phenomenon which was recreated and analysed in humans by Simone et al. 30 years later (Pórszász and Jancsó 1959; Simone et al. 1989). Jancsó et al. later found evidence that capsaicin, through activating a group of sensory nerve fibres, induced neurogenic inflammation (Jancsó et al. 1967) and that capsaicin impaired thermoregulation through an action in the hypothalamus (Jancsó-Gábor et al. 1970). Another major step in studying the biological actions of capsaicin was when Nicolas Jancsó's son, Gábor Jancsó showed that capsaicin activated, and was able to induce degeneration in, a subset of chemosensitive primary sensory neurons (Jancsó et al. 1977). An undisputable evidence for the presence of a specific and selective receptor for capsaicin on a sub-set of small diameter (nociceptive) primary sensory neurons was finally showed by Szallasi and Blumberg (1990). Although many laboratories had tried to find the capsaicin receptor, particularly after Jancsó et al. and Szallasi and Blumberg's findings (Jancsó et al. 1977; Szallasi and Blumberg 1990), the capsaicin receptor, then called as vanilloid type 1 receptor, was cloned only in 1997 (Caterina et al. 1997). Since then, the number of papers dealing with the pharmacology of capsaicin and its receptor the transient receptor potential vanilloid type 1 ion channel (TRPV1) has grown at an exponential rate. This is because it became clear that TRPV1, in addition to some physiological functions, also plays a pivotal role in the development of various pathological processes; most prominently, in the development of inflammatory pain (for further references see: White et al. 2011; Nagy et al. 2004). Here, we give an account of our current knowledge of the pharmacology of the capsaicin receptor, TRPV1.

2.2 Exogenous Activators of TRPV1

As a polymodal nocisensor, TRPV1 is responsive to different exogenous activators including various toxins and other painful agents, heat above 42 °C, protons and membrane depolarisation.

2.2.1 Chemical Activators

Of TRPV1's activating agents, the prototypical activator is capsaicin (trans-8-methyl-N-vanillyl-6-nonenamide), the main pungent ingredient of the hot chilli pepper (*Capsicum* peppers; Thresh 1876a). Capsaicin, which is believed to be a selective and specific TRPV1 activator, has a half-maximal effective concentration (EC_{50}) of ~700 nM on this ion channel, though the efficacy of capsaicin on TRPV1 slightly varies depending on the species, expression system and read out (Oh et al. 1996; Caterina et al. 1997). Activation of TRPV1 by capsaicin (and by other activators as well, see below) results in increased open probability of the ion channel and subsequent increase in cationic flux (Liu et al. 2006a; Wood et al. 1988; Dray 1992; Caterina et al. 1997).

TRPV1 is a non-selective cationic channel; hence it is permeable to all the major cations found extracellularly and intracellularly (Caterina et al. 1997). Therefore, when TRPV1 is expressed by cells with excitable membranes such as neurons, its activation results in a net cationic influx and subsequent depolarisation upon which neurons are capable of generating and propagating action potentials (Caterina et al. 1997). In the case of nociceptive primary sensory neurons, which are believed to be the main type of neurons expressing TRPV1 (Cavanaugh et al. 2011), the initial excitation in vivo is accompanied by a local increase of inflammatory mediators and the development of a burning pain sensation. However, the initial excitation is followed by a refractory state in which the neurons do not respond to capsaicin (Pórszász and Jancsó 1959). This process is known as nociceptor desensitization (Caterina et al. 1997) (for details see below).

Nociceptive primary sensory neurons play a pivotal role in the development and maintenance of various pain conditions (Nagy 2004). Hence, the capsaicin-induced desensitisation explains the paradoxical use of capsaicin as an analgesic agent to treat different pain disorders (Ueda et al. 2013b; Noto et al. 2009; Webster et al. 2011). Importantly, when capsaicin is applied in sufficiently high concentration and duration, it induces degeneration due to excessive Ca^{2+} influx (Jancsó et al. 1977).

Capsaicin possesses a vanillyl moiety (Fujiwake et al. 1980). A large series of other plant-derived molecules, including piperine and piperinoyl-piperidine, the alkaloids present in black or white pepper (Izzo et al. 2001; Mandadi and Roufogalis 2008), eugenol, a phenol derived from clove and cinnamon leaf oil and gingerols, which are phenol compounds in ginger (Holzer 2008; Mandadi and Roufogalis 2008), also have this moiety, and they can activate TRPV1 with various efficacies and potencies. Still, perhaps the best-known vanilloid is resiniferatoxin (RTX) from *Euphorbia resinifera.*

RTX is an unusual phorbol-related diterpene which is more potent (with an EC_{50} of ~40 nM) than capsaicin in producing TRPV1-mediated biological effects (Caterina et al. 1997). The acute excitatory response of TRPV1 evoked by RTX is also followed by desensitization, and these two agents produce cross-desensitization. However, RTX produces prolonged depolarisation. Further, the depolarisation produced by a given concentration of RTX results in a significantly lower number of action potentials than the same extent of depolarisation produced by capsaicin. This could be due to the slower kinetics of RTX than of capsaicin in activating TRPV1. The subsequent slow depolarisation during RTX application then induces fewer simultaneous activation of sodium channels than the fast depolarisation during capsaicin application. Based on these properties, RTX may be useful for clinical treatments as it produces less pain than capsaicin (Raisinghani et al. 2005).

In addition to vanilloids, other plant-derived molecules also activate TRPV1. Allicin can be found in garlic and activates TRPV1 in addition to the ankyrin type 1 ion channel (TRPA1), another transient receptor potential (TRP) molecule (Macpherson et al. 2005). The EC_{50} of allicin-containing garlic extract in TRPV1-expressing CHO cells is ~1:3500 dilution (Macpherson et al. 2005), whereas it is 1:500 dilution in TRPV1-expressing *Xenopus* oocytes (Macpherson et al. 2005). The specific EC_{50} of allicin in TRPV1-expressing CHO cells is ~50 μM (Macpherson et al. 2005). Allicin activates TRPV1 differently from capsaicin as it acts by covalent modification of a single cysteine residue in the N-terminus of the channel, C157 (see below) (Salazar et al. 2008).

Allyl isothiocyanate is another plant-derived agent which activates TRPV1 (Ohta et al. 2007). Allyl isothiocyanate, which can be found in the genus *Brassica*, is an agent we consume in mustard and wasabi. Similarly to allicin, allyl isothiocyanate also activates both TRPV1 and TRPA1 (Everaerts et al. 2011). Mustard oil causes a concentration-dependent increase in TRPV1-mediated currents above ~100 μM (Everaerts et al. 2011). The TRPV1-mediated response induced by allyl isothiocyanate is significantly smaller than that of 1 μM capsaicin suggesting that it is a weak partial agonist of TRPV1 (Everaerts et al. 2011). It is assumed that the residue S513 (see below) may have a role in allyl isothiocyanate-induced activation of TRPV1 (Gees et al. 2013).

Camphor (1,7,7-Trimethylbicyclo[2.2.1]heptan-2-one) is isolated from the plant *Cinnamomum camphora* and activates TRPV1, as well as another vanilloid type TRP molecule, TRPV3. The camphor-induced TRPV1 activation is followed by desensitization of the ion channel, which is more complete than that induced by capsaicin (Xu et al. 2005). Hence, the camphor-induced TRPV1 desensitisation together with the inhibitory effect on TRPA1 (Fajardo et al. 2008), which also plays a pivotal role in the development of pain associated with inflammation of tissues, might be responsible for the well-known and widely used antinociceptive effect of this agent (Xu et al. 2005; Fajardo et al. 2008). The molecular basis of camphor-sensitivity of TRPV1 is separate from its capsaicin-sensitivity but, similarly to capsaicin, camphor fails to activate chicken TRPV1 (Xu et al. 2005). Hence, camphor may activate TRPV1 by a novel mechanism, which is distinct from vanilloid-induced activation.

In addition to plant-derived TRPV1 activators, some molecules synthesised and excreted by animals can also activate TRPV1. For example, the peptides vanillotoxins (VaTxs) are present in tarantula venom (*Psalmopoeus cambridgei* and *Ornithoctonus huwena*). In addition to TRPV1, some VaTxs (VaTx1-3) act on voltage-gated potassium channels, which supports the close relationship suggested between TRP and voltage-gated potassium channels (Siemens et al. 2006). Interestingly, while the great majority of molecules acting on TRPV1 are hydrophobic and act at the intracellular side of the channel, VaTxs are amphiphilic and activate TRPV1 at its extracellular side (Cromer and McIntyre 2008).

Several widely used synthetic compounds including four of the most commonly used artificial sweeteners (saccharin, aspartame, acesulfame-K and sodium cyclamate) have been shown to activate TRPV1 in a dose-dependent manner (Riera et al. 2007). Interestingly, there is a shift from pleasant to unpleasant (bitter/metallic) taste perception when the concentration of these agents is increased (Vincent et al. 1955; Helgren et al. 1955; Schiffman et al. 1995). In addition to activating TRPV1, artificial sweeteners also sensitize this ion channel to acids and thermal stimuli (Riera et al. 2007).

Electrophysiological recordings demonstrated that extracellular Na^{+}, Mg^{2+} and Ca^{2+} ions sensitize and activate TRPV1 via electrostatic interactions with the residues E600 and E648 (see below) (Ahern et al. 2005b). Mg^{2+} is even capable of reducing capsaicin's EC_{50} by about 50 % (Ahern et al. 2005b). Three other salts ($CySO_4$, $ZnSO_4$ and $FeSO_4$), which produce a metallic taste sensation, have also been shown to activate TRPV1 (Riera et al. 2007). It is still not clear how these salts activate TRPV1, although they have been suggested to act through intracellular binding sites (Riera et al. 2007). The activation of TRPV1 by these sulphuric salts could be explained by the potential harmfulness of the sulphate group and the function of TRPV1 as a sensor for potentially dangerous stimuli. This view is supported by the difficulty to distinguish between bitter/metallic taste and burning sensation (Green and Hayes 2003; Lim and Green 2007).

Ethanol, between 0.1 and 3 %, potentiates TRPV1 responses evoked by other activators (Trevisani et al. 2002), including capsaicin, protons and heat (Trevisani et al. 2002). The ethanol-induced sensitisation, at least to heat stimuli, is mediated through lowering the heat threshold of the ion channel (from approx. 42 °C to approx. 34 °C) (Trevisani et al. 2002). Hence, TRPV1-expressing sensory nerve fibres become activated by the body temperature following exposure to ethanol. The ethanol-induced sensitisation of TRPV1 explains why high alcohol content drinks induce burning sensation and why those drinks do not produce the burning sensation when they are consumed with ice.

TRPV1 also seems to be important for specific behavioural actions induced by ethanol (Blednov and Harris 2009; Glendinning et al. 2012). For example, attenuation of ethanol's capsaicin-like burning sensation could at least partially explain why adolescent ethanol use and abuse behaviour in humans is associated with foetal ethanol exposure (Glendinning et al. 2012). Further, given the role of TRPV1 in thermoregulation (Gavva et al. 2007), ethanol's effects on TRPV1 also underlay its effects on body temperature (Trevisani et al. 2002) and the lethal hypothermia commonly observed following alcohol intoxication.

2.2.2 Protons

Acidic pH also activates TRPV1 (Tominaga et al. 1998; Jordt et al. 2000; Baumann and Martenson 2000; McLatchie and Bevan 2001). Extracellular protons are considered to be TRPV1 modulators as they increase the potency of heat and capsaicin by lowering the threshold of channel activation (Jordt et al. 2000; Tominaga et al. 1998). However, protons also directly activate TRPV1 ($pH < 6.0$) (Tominaga et al. 1998). Remarkably, in addition to protonation, deprotonation also activates TRPV1 (Dhaka et al. 2009). In contrast to the extracellular sites for protonation, the site for deprotonation is located intracellularly (see below). Hence TRPV1 must play an important role in sensing and maintaining extracellular and intracellular pH.

2.2.3 Heat

The great majority of TRP channels respond to changes in various physical stimuli such as heat or pressure (Nilius and Appendino 2011). TRPV1 was the first TRP channel, and indeed molecule, shown to respond specifically to increased temperatures (Caterina et al. 1997). Interestingly, TRPV1 seems to be tonically active in vivo, hence it acts as a molecular thermometer (Gavva et al. 2007). Accordingly, it has been proposed that the main function of TRPV1 is to maintain body temperature (Gavva et al. 2007). This putative function explains why some TRPV1 agonist, e.g. capsaicin and RTX, cause a reduction in body temperature, and also why TRPV1 antagonists induce considerable hyperthermia in several species (Holzer 2008). The role of TRPV1 in thermoregulation may hamper the use of TRPV1 antagonists in treating pain conditions.

The heat sensor of TRPV1 allows the receptor to detect noxious heat. It is a specific heat-induced signalling-event with a temperature coefficient of about 26 (Liu et al. 2003). In comparison, the temperature coefficient of molecules which do not specifically respond to heat is about 2 (Liu et al. 2003). An increase from the ambient temperature to about 45 °C leads to a pronounced increase in the intracellular calcium concentration in TRPV1-expressing cells (Caterina et al. 1997). Studies of chimeric thermo-sensitive TRP channels show that a segment in the C-terminus of TRPV1 confers heat-sensitivity to the channel ((Brauchi et al. 2006), see details below). Apparently, heat acts by prolonging the burst of TRPV1 channel opening and the sensitivity of the channel to heat can be modulated by environmental agents such as ethanol (Trevisani et al. 2002).

It seems puzzling that TRPV1 could be involved both in thermoregulation with maintaining the body's core temperature at ~37 °C, and in the detection of noxious heat above ~42 °C. Little is known about the mechanism of molecular thermo-thresholding of TRPV1 and further studies must be done to determine them. There are multiple putative mechanisms which could explain how TRPV1 plays a role both in maintaining the body temperature and in the detection of noxious heat stimuli. These include the presence of different splice variants of TRPV1, post-translational modification (e.g. specific phosphorylation sites), or tetrameric combinations of TRP channels (see below) in various tissues. Alternatively tissue-specific agents may regulate the gating properties of TRPV1.

Ectotherm animals such as fish, amphibians or reptiles, which use external source of heat to regulate their body temperature, also require a temperature sensor since the ability to sense environmental temperature is necessary for survival, to maintain homeostasis and to avoid tissue damage. Zebrafish (*Danio rerio*) express a single TRPV1/2-like orthologue, which could be derived from an evolutionary precursor of tetrapod TRPV1 and another vanilloid type TRP molecule, TRPV2 (Saito and Shingai 2006). Based on the expression of this zebrafish TRPV1 in nearly all early-born trigeminal neurons (Gau et al. 2013), and the fact that environmental hot temperatures activate TRPV1-expressing neurons in zebrafish (Gau et al. 2013), it has been suggested that TRPV1 has been involved in heat sensation for at least 360–450 million years, when fish diverged from tetrapods (Volff 2005).

2.3 Endogenous Activators

TRPV1 is activated by two major types of endogenous molecules. The first group of endogenous activators comprise of ligands which, similarly to exogenous ligands, bind to TRPV1 and increase the open probability of the ion channel. The second group of endogenous TRPV1 activators includes intracellular signaling molecules which, mainly through phosphorylation of discrete amino acid residues, increase either the open probability of TRPV1 or the efficacy or potency of TRPV1-activating ligands (sensitization). The separation between these molecules is not entirely unambiguous. For example, while anandamide (see below) has previously been considered as a ligand (i.e. endovanilloid), recent evidence suggests that it is also an intracellular signaling molecule. Nevertheless, while ligand binding results in transient activation (i.e. while the ligand is present), sensitization induced by intracellular signaling molecules may last longer.

2.3.1 Ligands from the Inside (Autocrine Signalling)

A series of putative endovanilloids, containing unsaturated fatty acids with 18 or 20 carbon atoms, have been identified in recent years. In these molecules, arachidonic or oleic acids bind to various moieties, such as glycerol, ethanolamine or dopamine.

Arachidonylethanolamide (anandamide), which was established as an endogenous ligand for the G protein-coupled cannabinoid 1 (CB1) receptor (Matsuda et al. 1990; Devane et al. 1992), was the first endogenous molecule to be identified as a putative endogenous TRPV1 activator (Zygmunt et al. 1999). Although a series of other target molecules for anandamide has recently been found (Goodfellow and Glass 2009), the CB1 receptor and TRPV1 are still considered to be the main targets for anandamide.

Anandamide is synthesized by various cells including primary sensory neurons (Carrier et al. 2004; Di Marzo et al. 1996; Di Marzo et al. 1994; van der Stelt and Di Marzo 2005; Vellani et al. 2001). Multiple enzymatic pathways are involved in anandamide synthesis, which produce this ligand either in a Ca^{2+} dependent or Ca^{2+} independent manner (Okamoto et al. 2004; Sun et al. 2004; Liu et al. 2008; Simon and Cravatt 2008; Vellani et al. 2008). In primary sensory neurons, both increased intracellular Ca^{2+} concentration, which, for example, occurs following TRPV1 activation (Caterina et al. 1997), and activation of protein kinase A (PKA) and protein kinase C (PKC) result in anandamide synthesis (van der Stelt et al. 2005). Accordingly, TRPV1-expressing primary sensory neurons express several enzymes which have been implicated in anandamide-synthesis, and those enzymes seem to form functional anandamide synthesising pathways (Nagy et al. 2009; Varga et al. 2013). It has consistently been shown that anandamide produced by primary sensory neurons activate TRPV1 (van der Stelt et al. 2005; Varga et al. 2013). Based on the expression pattern of anandamide-synthesising enzymes and TRPV1, the trigger for anandamide production and the effect of anandamide of primary sensory neuron origin, Di Marzo et al. suggested that anandamide acts as a signal amplifier for TRPV1 (van der Stelt and Di Marzo 2005). Anandamide is believed to bind to the same site as capsaicin in TRPV1 (Jordt and Julius 2002).

Another ethanolamide, which instead of arachidonic acid contains oleic acid, also activates TRPV1 (Ahern 2003; Movahed et al. 2005). Oleoylethanolamide has been identified as a peripheral satiety factor whose actions are mediated primarily through peroxisome proliferator-activated receptor alpha (Fu et al. 2003). Oleoylethanolamide activates TRPV1 with a potency similar to that of anandamide (Ahern 2003; Movahed et al. 2005). However, phosphorylation of TRPV1 by PKC is essential for TRPV1 to respond to oleoylethanolamide (Ahern 2003). Consistently with oleoylethanolamide being an endogenous TRPV1 ligand, intraperitoneal oleoylethanolamide administration induces visceral -related behavior, which is absent in TRPV1$^{-/-}$ mice (Wang et al. 2005). These data suggest that oleoylethanolamide has a physiological role in modulating TRPV1 in pathological conditions (Almasi et al. 2008).

N-arachidonyldopamine (NADA) is an endogenous molecule identified in several brain regions with particularly high concentrations in the striatum (Huang et al. 2002b). Administration of NADA to cultured primary sensory neurons results in TRPV1-mediated calcium influx and neuropeptide release (Huang et al. 2002a). Further, intradermal injection of NADA into the hind paw of mice induces thermal hyperalgesia in a TRPV1-dependent manner (Huang et al. 2002a). As with oleoylethanolamide, TRPV1's sensitivity to NADA is greatly increased by PKC-mediated phosphorylation at Ser502 and 800 (Premkumar et al. 2004).

Lipoxygenases (LOX) produce molecules which are capable of activating heterologously expressed, as well as native, TRPV1 (Hwang 2000). These products include some hydroperoxy eicosatetraenoic acids (HPETEs) and leukotrienes which are derivatives of fatty acids (Samuelsson 1983). Among the LOX products, 12-(S)-, 15-(S)- and 5-(S)-HPETE and leukotriene B4 exhibit high potency in activating TRPV1 (Hwang 2000). LOX products are produced during inflammation, and their intradermal injection has been shown to produce hyperalgesia (Levine et al. 1986). A link between inflammation, LOX products and TRPV1 activity has been established by Shin et al. (2002). They found that 12- HPETE, which has the highest potency in activating TRPV1, is produced by primary sensory neurons following activation of the bradykinin 2 (B2) receptor by one of the most important inflammatory mediators, bradykinin, and subsequent production of arachidonic acid by B2 receptor-evoked phospholipase A2 activity (Shin et al. 2002).

Lysophosphatidic acid (1-acyl-glycerol-3-phosphate, LPA) is a precursor of phospholipid biosynthesis but also functions as an intercellular signaling molecule participating in cell survival, neurite retraction, cancer cell migration and invasion, fertilization, embryonic implantation, spermatogenesis, vasculogenesis, angiogenesis, proliferation and differentiation of neural progenitor cells (Ueda et al. 2013a). These biological functions have been linked to a specific class of receptor, called LPA receptors 1-6 (Noguchi et al. 2009). Most recently, TRPV1 has also been shown to be activated by LPA (Nieto-Posadas et al. 2012). Hence, intracellular application of LPA results in TRPV1 activation via a direct interaction with the proximal C terminus of TRPV1, specifically with K710, which is also a binding site for phosphatidylinositol 4,5-bisphosphate (PIP2; see below) (Brauchi et al. 2007). In agreement with the cellular response, LPA injection into the paw induces significantly less acute pain-related behavior in TRPV1$^{-/-}$ mice than in wild-type mice (Nieto-Posadas et al. 2012).

The group of putative endovanilloids, in addition to some lipophylic compounds, also include some hydrophylic molecules which bind to and activate TRPV1. ATP is an important mediator of pain because it is released from tissues during inflammation and/or tissue damage (Bours et al. 2006). While ATP primarily activates P2X and P2Y receptors (Burnstock and Kennedy 2011; Burnstock 2008, 2009), it can also bind directly to TRPV1 in a region between the ankyrin repeats in the N-terminus (Lishko et al. 2007) as well as at the C terminus (Kwak et al. 2000). ATP interacts with calmodulin (CaM; see below) at these binding sites.

Calcium overload induces cells death (Kass and Orrenius 1999; Caterina et al. 1997). Hence, maintaining Ca^{2+} homeostasis is crucial. One way to maintain Ca^{2+} homeostasis is to regulate Ca^{2+}-permeable channels such as TRPV1 (Caterina et al. 1997). Several molecules seem to be involved in the modulation of TRPV1 activity based on the Ca^{2+} influx. One such molecule is calmodulin (CaM), which binds four Ca^{2+} (Vetter and Leclerc 2003). The Ca^{2+}-CaM complex has been implicated in one of the most characteristic features of TRPV1, Ca^{2+}-dependent desensitization (Koplas et al. 1997) (more details on desensitisation is presented later in this Chapter). TRPV1 has two putative CaM-binding sites. One of them is present in the NH_2-terminus, in a region including amino acids 189-222 (Rosenbaum et al. 2004), a site that can also bind triphosphate nucleotides such as ATP. Here, CaM and ATP are believed to compete for binding. While binding of the Ca^{2+}-CaM complex reduces responses of TRPV1 to its activators (desensitization/tachyphylaxis), ATP binding prevents desensitization (Lishko et al. 2007). It is proposed that this effect is mediated by modulating the channels sensitivity to calcium fluctuations and possibly metabolic state (Phelps et al. 2010). Mutation on this shared binding site eliminates desensitization (Lishko et al. 2007). A second putative CaM-binding site is located in the C terminus (Numazaki et al. 2003). Mutation at this site does not eliminate desensitization, though its kinetics are altered (Rosenbaum et al. 2004). Hence, this CaM-binding site could also be involved in TRPV1 desensitization.

Although the Ca^{2+}-calmodulin dependent kinase II (CaMKII) does not bind to TRPV1, we discuss its function here due to its role in Ca^{2+}-dependent modulation of TRPV1 activity. CaMKII-mediated phosphorylation of TRPV1 is fundamental for TRPV1 responsiveness to capsaicin (Jung et al. 2004). In contrast, the dephosphorylation of TRPV1 by the Ca^{2+}-dependent phosphatase calcineurin leads to a desensitization of the receptor (Docherty et al. 1996). Hence, it is believed that there is a dynamic balance between the phosphorylation and dephosphorylation of the TRPV1 channel by CaMKII and calcineurin respectively, which controls the responsiveness/desensitization states of the channel. In addition, Ca^{2+} has also been shown to stimulate phospholipase C (PLC)-mediated cleavage of the sensitizing agent phosphatidylinositol-4,5-bisphosphate (PIP2) (Liu et al. 2005; Stein et al. 2006; Lishko et al. 2007; Lukacs et al. 2007; Mercado et al. 2010; Lau et al. 2012).

Phosphatidylinositol-4,5-bisphosphate (PIP2) is a minor component of the plasma membrane that can serve multiple roles in cell physiology. It is involved in the regulation of many proteins and can also anchor proteins to the plasma membrane through pleckstrin homology and other domains (DiNitto et al. 2003; Lemmon 2003; Cho and Stahelin 2005). One of the most important roles of PIP2, however, is acting as a source of intracellular second messengers (Dietrich et al. 2005) as it is cleaved by PLC to generate diacylglycerol (DAG) (Woo et al. 2008b) and inositol 1,4,5-trisphosphate (IP3).

Phosphatidylinositol-4,5-bisphosphate is involved in the regulation of TRPV1 activity via at least three mechanisms: by direct binding (Prescott and Julius 2003;

Chuang et al. 2001; Brauchi et al. 2007), through the generation of DAG (Woo et al. 2008b) and IP3 (Ahern et al. 2005a) and by activating the accessory membrane protein phosphoinositide interacting regulator of TRP (Kim et al. 2008).

Although the role of direct binding has been studied extensively, its role still remains controversial. Early reports suggested that PIP2 is an inhibitor of TRPV1 activity (Chuang et al. 2001). More recently, several groups reported that PIP2 binding and depletion sensitizes and desensitizes the channel, respectively, in mammalian cells (Liu et al. 2005; Stein et al. 2006). In agreement with the latter findings, the presence of PIP2 appears to prevent TRPV1 desensitization (Lishko et al. 2007).

Regarding PLC-mediated PIP2 cleavage, DAG activates PKC, which then phosphorylates TRPV1 (Bhave et al. 2003) (see below). In addition, DAG is also a partial agonist of heterologously-expressed TRPV1 (Woo et al. 2008a).

Nitric oxide (NO) is an important cellular signaling molecule, participating in many physiological and pathological processes such as vasodilation (Culotta and Koshland 1992). NO can induce calcium entry into cells via TRP channels, including TRPV1, through an activation mechanism mediated by S-nitrosilation of cysteine residues (Yoshida et al. 2006). S-nitrosilation involves covalent incorporation of the nitric oxide moiety into the thiol group of cysteine to form S-nitrosothiol. This is a reversible post-translational modification analogous to phosphorylation.

A-kinase anchoring proteins (AKAPs) are well known for their ability to scaffold PKA, PKC, or calcineurin to a large number of different ion channels, promoting fast and precise phosphorylation. AKAP79 was found to be able to bind TRPV1 (Zhang et al. 2008). Interestingly ablation of this protein, by genetic manipulation, resulted in a strong reduction of PKC-mediated sensitization of TRPV1 (see below; (Jeske et al. 2009)). More recently, an antagonist of TRPV1-AKAP79 binding has been developed and shown to potently block TRPV1 sensitization (Fischer et al. 2013).

Another scaffolding protein, β-arrestin-2, has also been recently implicated in the desensitization of TRPV1 (Por et al. 2012) by linking the phosphodiesterase PDE4D5 to the receptor and limiting its PKA-phosphorylation status (for details of PKA-mediated phosphorylation see below). Further, knocking down β-arrestin-2 using small interfering RNA resulted in an increase of TRPV1-mediated cellular responses to capsaicin both to initial and repeated administrations (Por et al. 2012).

In addition to their interaction with polymerized microtubules, tubulin dimers can interact with the C-terminus region of TRPV1 in vitro (Goswami et al. 2004). Recently, a region in the N-terminus of TRPV1 has also been shown to bind tubulin independently (Lainez et al. 2010). Hence, TRPV1 may have multiple tubulin-binding sites. Storti et al. have demonstrated that the microtubule cytoskeleton helps to form the TRPV1 tetramer (see below) in the membrane (Storti et al. 2012). Therefore, it is possible that tubulin interaction with TRPV1 is a dynamic process and helps to modulate TRPV1 function.

2.3.2 Second Messenger Interactions

TRPV1 activity which is induced by heat or/and ligands can be modified by the activation of other receptors including those coupled to tyrosine kinase (trk) or G proteins (Nagy et al. 2004). Activation of tyrosine kinase (trk)-coupled or Gq/s protein-coupled receptors results in reducing the molecule's heat threshold and/or increasing the efficacy and potency of ligands (Tominaga et al. 2001; Vellani et al. 2001; Cesare and McNaughton 1996; Moriyama et al. 2005b; Lopshire and Nicol 1998). This type of modulation appears to be crucial in inflammation, where inflammatory mediators including nerve growth factor, bradykinin, serotonin, histamine and prostaglandins accumulate, activate their cognate receptors on TRPV1-expressing neurons and induce TRPV1 sensitisation. The downstream effectors of inflammatory mediators on TRPV1 include molecules belonging to trk-, protein kinase A (PKA)- or protein kinase C (PKC)-dependent pathways (Cesare et al. 1999; Premkumar and Ahern 2000; Vellani et al. 2001) and various endogenous activators such as anandamide or 12-HPETE (Shin et al. 2002; Vellani et al. 2008).

PKA within primary sensory neurons plays a major role in producing inflammatory hyperalgesia (Levine and Taiwo 1990). Prostaglandins, such as prostaglandin E2 (PGE2), produce hyperalgesia by elevating intracellular cAMP levels and hence activating PKA in sensory neurons (Taiwo et al. 1989; Taiwo and Levine 1990). PKA's action on TRPV1 depends on the phosphorylation of residues implicated in the sensitisation of heat-evoked responses (Rathee et al. 2002). It appears that PKA-mediated phosphorylation is essential to keep TRPV1 in a responsive state (Bhave et al. 2002; Mahmud et al. 2009).

The PKC pathway can be activated following activation of Gq-coupled receptors by several inflammatory mediators including ATP, bradykinin, prostaglandins and trypsin or tryptase (Moriyama et al. 2003, 2005a; Tominaga et al. 1998; Cortright and Szallasi 2004). Phosphorylation of TRPV1 by PKC results in reduction of its temperature threshold and potentiation of proton-evoked responses (Bhave et al. 2003; Studer and McNaughton 2010; Numazaki et al. 2002; Huang et al. 2006a, b). This PKC-mediated phosphorylation is also implicated in the potentiation of TRPV1 activation by NADA (Premkumar et al. 2004) and oleoylethanolamide (Ahern 2003) as well as in re-phosphorylation of TRPV1 after desensitization in the presence of Ca^{2+} (Mandadi et al. 2004).

2.3.3 Depolarisation

TRPV1 was initially considered to be a cation channel with no voltage sensitivity (Caterina et al. 1997) in accordance with its lack of positively charged residues in the fourth transmembrane domain. However, a pronounced outward rectification of capsaicin-induced membrane currents had previously been observed (Gunthorpe et al. 2000), suggesting the existence of a membrane depolarization-sensing domain in TRPV1. The C terminus of TRPV1 had recently been shown to influence both temperature and voltage-sensing (Vlachova et al. 2003). However, studies using chimeras between TRPV1 and another TRP channel, the cold receptor melastatin type 8 (TRPM8) channel, had demonstrated that the thermo-TRP-specific region is different from the voltage sensor region of these molecules (Brauchi et al. 2006).

2.4 Signal Integration

The fascinating polymodal nature of TRPV1 raises the question of how TRPV1 integrates the effects of its various activators. In recent years, two opposing views on this signal integration have developed. Bernd Nilius et al. have proposed a sequential model. In this model, various stimuli shift the voltage dependence of the channel from a physiologically uninteresting voltage range into a functionally relevant voltage (Nilius and Voets 2005). Hence, according to this model, all types of stimuli open the channel through modifying voltage-sensitivity. However, post-translational modifications as well as ligand binding also induces changes in temperature-sensitivity, which itself is connected to voltage dependence (Gunthorpe et al. 2000; Vlachova et al. 2003). Therefore, while a shift in the voltage-dependence may ultimately be responsible for opening the channel, ligand binding and post-translational modifications may act through modifying both temperature- and voltage-sensitivity.

An opposing view has been put forward by Latorre et al. who proposed an allosteric model. According to this model, while various sensors interact with each other, each sensor is linked directly to the gating apparatus. Hence, each stimulus is able to open the channel independently of each other (Latorre et al. 2007). The evidence that the C-terminus plays a role in temperature control while leaving voltage dependence unaffected (Brauchi et al. 2006) would support this view.

2.5 Mechanisms of TRPV1 Inactivation

Inactivation of TRPV1 can have potential therapeutic implication in a number of conditions, including pain (Roberts and Connor 2006; Jara-Oseguera et al. 2008), inflammation (Fernandes et al. 2012; Southall et al. 2003), chronic respiratory diseases (Preti et al. 2012) and conditions related to the cardiovascular system (Fernandes et al. 2012; Robbins et al. 2013). The action of TRPV1 may be negatively modulated by endogenous molecules, such as adenosine and cholesterol. Extracellular inactivation of TRPV1 may occur through antagonists (Roberts and Connor 2006) or through desensitisation (Touska et al. 2011) which may allow capsaicin and its analogues to be used as analgesics (Hoffmann et al. 2012; Maihofner and Heskamp 2013).

2.5.1 Endogenous Negative Modulators of TRPV1

Cholesterol, non-classic eicosanoids and adenosine have been proposed to negatively modulate TRPV1 (Morales-Lazaro et al. 2013). Picazo-Juarez et al. have demonstrated that cholesterol enrichment of excised patches from TRPV1-expressing HEK293 cells decreases capsaicin-induced TRPV1 currents as well as currents induced by temperature and voltage increase (Picazo-Juarez et al. 2011). The level of membrane cholesterol also appears essential for the expression of TRPV1. Earlier studies by Liu et al. (2006b) have demonstrated that depletion of cholesterol from membrane rafts reduces channel expression as well as capsaicin and proton-induced TRPV1 currents, probably through internalisation of TRPV1 channels on the membrane. The role of cholesterol might be multifaceted as depletion of cholesterol in trigeminal neurons was sufficient to diminish calcium uptake in response to capsaicin or resiniferatoxin (RTX). However, in rat TRPV1-transfected cells, cholesterol depletion was able to inhibit calcium influx in response to capsaicin and or N-oleoyl-dopamine, but not in response to anandamide, RTX or low pH (Szoke et al. 2010).

Other components of the lipid raft are likely to play additional, more complex roles in regulating the function and expression of TRPV1 channels. For example, treatment of sensory neurons with sphingomyelinase inhibited activation of TRPV1 by capsaicin and RTX, while inhibition of ganglioside synthesis reduced capsaicin- or RTX-evoked calcium influx (Szoke et al. 2010; Santha et al. 2010).

Resolvins are omega-3 fatty acids derivatives that have been shown to inhibit TRPV1-mediated currents in DRG neurons, with resolvin D2 being more potent that resolvin D1 or resolvin E1 (Park et al. 2011). The mechanism by which resolvins modulate TRPV1 activity is not clear, though it is likely to involve inhibition of the extracellular signal-regulated kinase (ERK) signalling pathway (Xu et al. 2010). In addition, inhibition of the Gi/o protein (Liu and Simon 1996; Caterina et al. 1997; Koplas et al. 1997) abolishes the inhibitory effects of resolvin D2 (Park et al. 2011; Morales-Lazaro et al. 2013). At a much higher concentration, resolvins are also inhibitors of TRPA1 and TRPV3 (Park et al. 2011; Bang et al. 2012). Intrathecal administration of resolvins at very low doses prevents spontaneous pain and mechanical hypersensitivity evoked by intrathecal capsaicin administration as well as formalin injection- and Complete Freund's Adjuvant injection-induced pain-related behaviour (Park et al. 2011; Xu et al. 2010).

Adenosine has also been suggested to negatively regulate the action of TRPV1, as its intrathecal injection has been shown to inhibit allodynia and mechanical hyperalgesia induced by intradermal injection of capsaicin in humans (Eisenach et al. 2002). In in vitro studies, adenosine analogues have been shown to inhibit capsaicin-induced TRPV1-mediated currents in TRPV1-expressing HEK293 cells and in DRG neurons in a competitive manner. Adenosine analogues compete for the ligand (resiniferatoxin and capsaicin)-binding site of TRPV1, indicating that the inhibitory effect is mediated via a direct interaction of these ligands with the ion channel (Puntambekar et al. 2004) rather than via the activation of adenosine receptors (Sawynok and Liu 2003). It is possible that adenosine mediates tonic suppression of TRPV1 activity in these conditions and thereby reduces the sensory inputs triggered by activation of this receptor (Puntambekar et al. 2004). TRPV1 activation has been suggested to promote adenosine release as its production depends on calcium availability, which is increased when TRPV1 is activated (Morales-Lazaro et al. 2013).

2.5.2 Desensitisation and Tachyphylaxis of TRPV1

Prolonged activation of TRPV1, for example by vanilloids or protons, induces acute desensitization of the receptor and insensitivity to subsequent stimuli (Liu and Simon 1996; Caterina et al. 1997; Koplas et al. 1997). Repeated applications of vanilloids also induce reduction in TRPV1-mediated responses, a phenomenon which is called tachyphylaxis (Liu and Simon 1996; Touska et al. 2011). It is not yet clear if tachyphylaxis is induced through the same mechanisms as desensitisation, but they are likely to share at least some molecular processes.

Desensitisation of TRPV1, which is largely a Ca^{2+}-depended process, is due to a rapid rise in intracellular calcium levels which occurs when TRPV1 is activated (Koplas et al. 1997; Mohapatra and Nau 2005; Cholewinski et al. 1993; Piper et al. 1999). In the absence of extracellular or intracellular Ca^{2+}, no desensitisation occurs (Koplas et al. 1997; Cholewinski et al. 1993). As mentioned, Ca^{2+} binds to CaM and activates the phosphatase calcineurin and CaMKII. This transient calmodulin binding is essential for TRPV1 desensitisation (Numazaki et al. 2003; Rosenbaum et al. 2004; Lishko et al. 2007). Rosenbaum et al. (2004) have demonstrated that overexpression of CaM in TRPV1-expressing cells potentiates the desensitising effects of Ca^{2+}, whereas co-expression of a mutant inactive form of CaM with TRPV1 results in a lack of Ca^{2+}-induced desensitisation. Dephosphorylation of the receptor by calcineurin, triggered by increased intracellular Ca^{2+} concentration, has been reported to enhance desensitisation (Docherty et al. 1996; Mohapatra and Nau 2005; Piper et al. 1999). Intracellular inhibition of calcineurin significantly decreases desensitization of TRPV1 by capsaicin or protons (Mohapatra and Nau 2005). On the other hand, PKA activity results in decreased desensitization and increased sensitivity to capsaicin, protons and anandamide (Mohapatra and Nau 2005; Di Marzo et al. 2002; Bhave et al. 2003). A balance between TRPV1 dephosphorylation by calcineurin and phosphorylation by different kinases, as mentioned earlier, is thought to regulate the Ca^{2+}-dependent desensitization of the channel (Jung et al. 2004; Cortright and Szallasi 2004; Docherty et al. 1996; Mohapatra and Nau 2005; Mandadi et al. 2004).

Upon desensitisation of TRPV1, a number of other molecular mechanisms contribute to further inhibition of the channel. Sanz-Salvador et al. (2012) have recently reported that TRPV1 agonists can downregulate the membrane expression of TRPV1 through endocytosis and lysosomal degradation, thus contributing further to agonist-insensitivity. This process is modulated by PKA-dependent phosphorylation (Sanz-Salvador et al. 2012). Capsaicin-desensitised TRPV1 also appears to have decreased affinity for capsaicin as, following the rapid onset of the first capsaicin evoked-response of TRPV1 in transfected HEK293T cells, the kinetics of subsequent responses become slower. In this case, desensitisation can be overcome with higher capsaicin concentrations (Vyklicky et al. 2008). However, the desensitisation is not due to the impairment of intrinsic gating mechanisms as the desensitised channel remains responsive to depolarisation (Yao and Qin 2009). Capsaicin-induced desensitisation of TRPV1 is also accompanied by a decrease in the responsiveness to heat (Vyklicky et al. 2008; Tominaga et al. 1998).

Other mechanisms, in addition to Ca^{2+}-dependent desensitisation are also involved in the receptor's desensitisation. As mentioned above, camphor activates TRPV1 independently of the vanilloid binding site and desensitises the channel in a Ca^{2+}-independent manner (Xu et al. 2005). Piperine has a propensity to cause greater desensitisation of TRPV1 than capsaicin, even in the absence of extracellular Ca^{2+} (McNamara et al. 2005).

Desensitisation of TRPV1 has been widely used to control pain for centuries and, in recent years, we have witnessed a revival of using capsaicin or its analogues in various concentrations. A formulation (WL-1002) from Winston Laboratories is in clinical trials for cluster headache, migraine and osteoarthritic pain, as is Compound 4975 from Anesina for neuropathic and musculoskeletal pain (Jara-Oseguera et al. 2008; Mandadi and Roufogalis 2008). At present, there are creams with a low concentration of capsaicin (0.075 %) available with no proof of desensitization (Szallasi and Sheta 2012) and a patch with an 8 % concentration of trans-capsaicin is available for the treatment of peripheral neuropathic and HIV-associated pain (Noto et al. 2009).

As application of capsaicin results in an unpleasant hot sensation and skin irritation, attempts have been made to develop TRPV1 agonists which produce less pungency, such as capsaite and olvanil (Brand et al. 1987; Iida et al. 2003). Such agonists have been shown to robustly activate TRPV1 and to present hyperalgesic effects in vivo (Wu et al. 2006; Appendino et al. 2005b; Phillips et al. 2004; Iida et al. 2003; Roberts and Connor 2006). However, the use of such synthetic agonists as analgesics has not been very successful in humans as they require direct contact with nerve endings before being broken down or sequestered (Cromer and McIntyre 2008).

In addition to desensitisation, other mechanisms have also been implicated in vanilloid-induce analgesia. Some studies reported degeneration of epidermal nerve fibers upon repeated or prolonged application of capsaicin (McMahon et al. 1991; Nolano et al. 1999; Simone et al. 1998; Knotkova et al. 2008) in parallel to reduction of pain responses. This capsaicin-induced degeneration of small nerve endings is a reversible process (Simone et al. 1998; McMahon et al. 1991) which may account for the long-lasting antinociceptive effects of capsaicin (Knotkova et al. 2008; Nagy et al. 2004; Jancsó et al. 2008; Tender et al. 2005). The vanilloid-induced degeneration is likely to occur through neurotoxicity due to excess Ca^{2+} influx (Olah et al. 2001; Szolcsányi 2004) or the production of intracellular reactive oxygen species (Hail 2003). In addition, a significant role for the vanilloid-induced inhibition of axonal transport (Santha and Jancso 2003) and decreased availability of nerve growth factor have also been suggested in the defunctionalisation of C-fibers (Jancsó et al. 2008). This may have additional effects on the availability of neuropeptides such as substance P and calcitonin gene-related peptide (CGRP), which have been implicated in nociceptive processes, thus further promoting anti-nociception (Jancsó et al. 2008).

2.5.3 Mechanisms of Action of TRPV1 Receptor Antagonists

The aim for the development of TRPV1 antagonists is to provide novel analgesic drugs which do not produce undesirable side effects (Gomtsyan et al. 2005; Roberts and Connor 2006). Non-competitive antagonists that interact with sites other than the agonist binding site prevent agonist-induced receptor opening or block the aqueous pore. This mode of action is thought to be more clinically relevant as, in a disease state, TRPV1 might already be activated. Competitive antagonists, on the other hand, bind to the agonist binding site and lock the channel in a closed, non-conductive state (Roberts and Connor 2006). TRPV1 is activated, through interactions with different binding sites by vanilloids, heat and protons (see below), which may all play a role in TRPV1 activation in pathological conditions. Therefore, antagonists should inhibit all binding sites. However, inhibition of the capsaicin binding site remains a critical requirement for TRPV1 antagonists and many have been developed by structurally altering capsaicin or other potent TRPV1 agonists such as RTX.

Capsazepine, an analogue of capsaicin, was the first synthetic competitive antagonist of TRPV1 (Bevan et al. 1992). Compared with other TRPV1 antagonists, capsazepine has a relatively low potency on TRPV1. Capsazepine has been shown to inhibit capsaicin-induced TRPV1 currents in sensory neurons and to compete with RTX for binding (Szallasi et al. 1993). Although capsazepine was shown to inhibit the behavioural nociceptive properties of capsaicin in vivo (Perkins and Campbell 1992), its effect on heat- and proton-induced TRPV1 activation appears to be species-dependant (Walker et al. 2003; Savidge et al. 2002). In humans, capsazepine has been reported to inhibit TRPV1 activation by heat and protons. However, due to low metabolic stability and poor pharmacokinetic properties, capsazepine did not reach clinical development (Gomtsyan et al. 2005). Capsazepine has also shown some effects on other channels, such as voltage-gated calcium channels, nicotinic receptors and TRPM8 (Roberts and Connor 2006). Although capsazepine has a low potency and exhibits unspecific binding, it has been used in many pharmacological studies and served as a pharmacological tool for comparing novel TRPV1 antagonists. In addition to capsazepine, other TRPV1 antagonists were also derived from TRPV1 agonists. Halogenation (i.e. iodine substitution) of vanillamide compounds, such as nonivamide and arvnil, produced potent TRPV1 antagonists (Appendino et al. 2003, 2005a, b; Roberts and Connor 2006; Wahl et al. 2001). Since then, a number of pharmaceutical companies have explored the development of novel TRPV1 antagonists such as fused pyridine, azabicyclic, heterocyclic and amide derivatives (Roberts and Connor 2006). Of them, fused pyridine derivatives have been shown to exhibit antinociceptive effects in rodent models of neuropathic pain at a low dose (0.1 mg kg^{-1}, (Roberts and Connor 2006). Other structural classes of TRPV1 antagonists include pyridyl piperazinyl ureas and cinnamides. Most of these compounds are potent TRPV1 antagonists that block capsaicin-, heat- and pH-evoked TRPV1 responses, with high efficacy in a number of pain models and good oral bioavailability (Swanson et al. 2005; Sun et al. 2003; El Kouhen et al. 2005; Honore et al. 2005; Tafesse et al. 2004; Gavva et al. 2005).

A number of novel TRPV1 antagonists produce long-lasting and dose-dependent hyperthermia (Roberts and Connor 2006; Swanson et al. 2005), which is thought to be due to the blocking of tonic TRPV1 activity which controls body temperature. In addition, the efficacy and potency of most novel TRPV1 antagonists has been assessed on peripherally produced analgesia. However, TRPV1 is also expressed in the central nervous system (Peters et al. 2011; Chavez et al. 2010; Matta and Ahern 2011; Kauer and Gibson 2009), as well as in various peripheral tissues where the role of TRPV1 is poorly defined. For example, TRPV1 is suggested to play a protective role against noxious stimuli in gastric mucosal epithelial cells (Kato et al. 2003; Holzer 2011; Faussone-Pellegrini et al. 2005), and a modulatory role in insulin secretion in the pancreas (Gram et al. 2007). Further, TRPV1 has been associated with a protective role against myocardial injury through the generation of chest pain in myocardial hypoxia (Robbins et al. 2013; Fernandes et al. 2012). Therefore, the blocking of TRPV1 activity by antagonists may have additional undesirable side-effects.

2.6 Stucture: Function Relationship in TRPV1

The TRPV1 protein consists of 838 or 839 amino acids in rats and humans respectively, and has an estimated relative molecular mass of 95,000 (Caterina et al. 1997). It can be divided into three structural components; the N- and C- termini, both of which are intracellular, and a transmembrane region consisting of six helices (S1-6) and a pore-forming loop between S5 and S6 (Fig. 2.1). The TRPV1 molecule possesses distinct protein moieties that enable it to complex with other molecules, or ‘subunits’, in order to form a tetrameric ion channel with fourfold symmetry and an aqueous pore. TRPV1 subunits typically self-associate, leading to TRPV1’s predominant expression as a homotetramer, though it may also contribute structurally to heteromers in the form of TRPV1 splice variants or functionally distinct complexes including other vanilloid type TRP channel subunits, such as TRPV2 and TRPV3 (Rutter et al. 2005; Smith et al. 2002). The resulting channel is integrated into a ‘transducisome’, a macromolecular complex including scaffolding proteins and downstream signalling molecules. The complex, derived from *Drosophila*

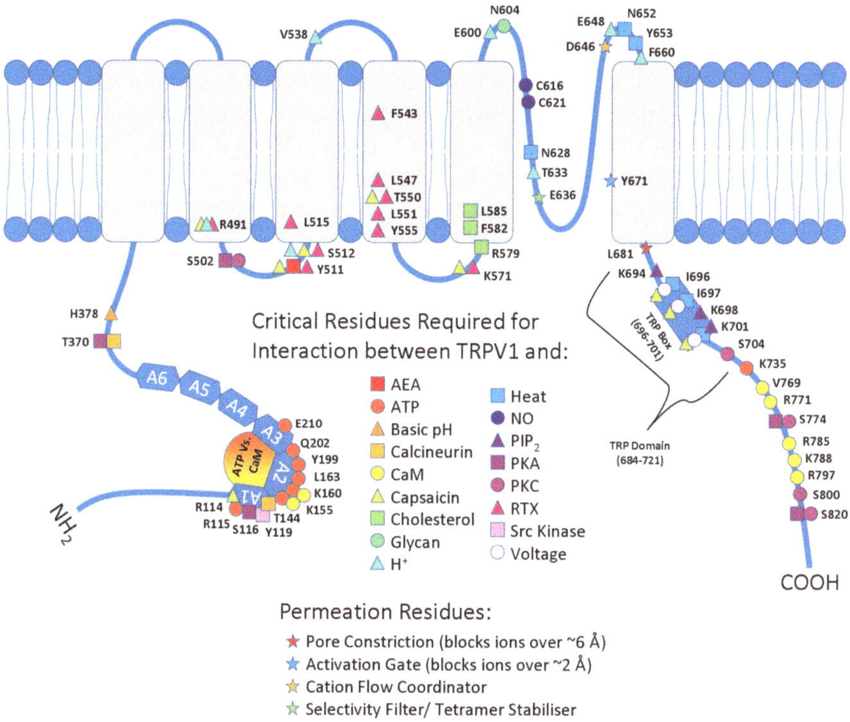

Fig. 2.1 Critical residues involved in TRPV1 function. TRPV1 topology highlighting residues implicated in the activation, sensitisation, desensitisation, gating properties or permeation of the channel

phototransduction machinery which includes the prototypical TRP channel (Vennekens et al. 2002), improves transduction efficiency by grouping components of the channel's intracellular signalling pathways, such as PKC, PLC (Vennekens et al. 2002), calmodulin (Docherty et al. 1996), phosphoinositide 3-kinase (Stein et al. 2006), SNAPIN and synaptotagmin IX (Morenilla-Palao et al. 2004). Within the channels at the centre of these signalling complexes, the structural divisions of each TRPV1 subunit also reflect functional distinctions determined by the localisation of activation sites where interactions with various endogenous and exogenous ligands, heat, protons and post-transcriptional modifications occur.

2.6.1 The N Terminus

Like other vanilloid type TRP proteins (Jin et al. 2006; McCleverty et al. 2006; Erler et al. 2004), TRPV1's cytosolic N-terminus hosts an ankyrin repeat domain (ARD) that contains six ankyrin repeats (Fig. 2.1). The 33-amino acid sequence of an ankyrin repeat can be found in many proteins with various responsibilities including cytoskeletal integrity, cell-cycle regulation, inflammation and transcription (Mosavi et al. 2004) and is required for channel function (Hellwig et al. 2005). Within the TRPV family, the ARD enables self-association between TRPV6 subunits (Erler et al. 2004) and the oligomerisation required for TRPV4 biogenesis (Arniges et al. 2006). Studies specifically investigating the TRPV1 ARD have identified a multi-ligand binding site for CaM and ATP which partly regulates the Ca^{2+}-dependent desensitisation discussed above (Koplas et al. 1997).

ATP binds to some transporters and receptors via nucleotide-binding sites known as ATP-binding cassettes (ABCs) containing the Walker A and B motifs and a signal sequence between their primary structures (Walker et al. 1982; Decottignies and Goffeau 1997; Hung et al. 1998). While TRPV1 does not possess the complete sequence, ATP was first proposed to interact with the N-terminus via a Walker B motif including D178. Mutation of D178 abolishes ATP-mediated potentiation of capsaicin-induced currents in TRPV1-expressing oocytes (Kwak et al. 2000), though Lishko's model shows that this residue lies within a helix of the second ARD rather than the typical Walker B β strand (Lishko et al. 2007).

As previously mentioned, extracellular acidity and intracellular alkalinity stimulate TRPV1 independently and the latter is mediated via the N-terminus. The alkaline deprotonation-underlying activation by an increase in cytosolic pH occurs at H378 (Fig. 2.1), a histidine residue located between the ARD and the first transmembrane segment (Dhaka et al. 2009). Point mutation studies have also shown that R114 within the N-terminus (Fig. 2.1) is a structural necessity for the channel's hydrophilic interaction with capsaicin and RTX (Jung et al. 2002).

In addition to binding sites, the N-terminus houses sites for post-transcriptional modifications. These sites include Y199 (or Y200 in humans; Fig. 2.1), the phosphorylation of which by Src kinase following nerve growth factor-induced activation of the tyrosine kinase A receptor promotes TRPV1 channel's insertion into the cell membrane (Zhang et al. 2005). The N-terminus is also suitably equipped for mediating the regulation of Ca^{2+}-dependent desensitisation; in addition to its above-mentioned CaM binding region it houses multiple consensus sites for PKA-mediated phosphorylation. Electrophysiological study of TRPV1 mutants has identified both S116 and T370 (Fig. 2.1) as major PKA phosphorylation sites required for reduction of TRPV1 desensitisation following capsaicin stimulation (Bhave et al. 2002; Mohapatra and Nau 2005). While phosphorylation at these sites reduces desensitisation, dephosphorylation at T144 and T370 (Fig. 2.1) by calcineurin promotes desensitisation (Jeske et al. 2006).

2.6.2 The C Terminus

TRPV1's C-terminus is composed of the distal 155 residues of the molecule (Fig. 2.1). Among its key structural features is the TRP domain (E684-R721; Fig. 2.1), a sequence located near the channel gate that is responsible for the tetramerisation of TRPV1 monomers (Garcia-Sanz et al. 2004) and modulating the channel's function. Functional TRPV chimaeras in which TRPV1's TRP domains are replaced with cognate domains from TRPV2-4 require capsaicin and/or heat to exhibit voltage-dependent gating. This, coupled with further biophysical analysis supporting the TRP domain's role in determining the activation energy of channel gating, supports the region's role in coupling stimulus reception with channel gating (Garcia-Sanz et al. 2007). Further study has localised key residues that determine activation energy to the TRP box, a region in the TRP domain that is highly conserved between the TRPV, the melastatin type (TRPM) and the canonical type (TRPC) TRP subfamilies. Alanine substitution of I696, W697 and R701 within this six-residue segment significantly impairs voltage-, heat- and capsaicin-induced channel activity in a manner consistent with modification of downstream signalling and TRP box-dependent channel subunit interaction (Valente et al. 2008). Consistent with the C-terminus' putative role in gating control, truncating the distal 31 or 72 amino acids of TRPV1 progressively reduces pH-, heat- and capsaicin-sensitivity, its thermal threshold and the onset, outward rectification and peak tail current amplitude of voltage-induced currents (Vlachova et al. 2003). Furthermore, TRP chimaeras coupling TRPV1 with the C-terminus of the cold-sensing TRPM8 molecule, or vice versa, exhibit the temperature sensitivity of the donor channel (Brauchi et al. 2006). This demonstrates that the C-terminus confers the channel's thermosensing phenotype. Subsequent investigation established that deletion of residues 741–752 abolishes TRPV1's heat-sensitivity and hence localised a major thermosensing region to the C-terminus (Brauchi et al. 2007). In experimenting with these chimaeric receptors, Brauchi noted the exchange of another important C-terminus feature; the modulation site of PIP2. PIP2 binding has been suggested to occur within residues 777–820 (Fig. 2.1) by Prescott and Julius (2003). However, homology modelling challenges the role of this region as a direct binding site and instead suggests that PIP2 makes contact with K694, K698 and K701 within the C-terminus (Fig. 2.1) (Brauchi et al. 2007). As discussed above, PIP_2's role in TRPV1 modulation remains unclear.

As with the proposed Walker B motif within the N-terminus, the C-terminus was proposed to contain the Walker A motif normally found within ABC transporters. Point mutation of a residue within this sequence at K735 prevents the sensitising effects of ATP in TRPV1-expressing oocytes (Kwak et al. 2000), suggesting the C-terminus possesses a nucleotide binding domain. Despite not possessing any previously defined CaM binding motifs, the C-terminus was also found to bind CaM within a 35-residue region (Numazaki et al. 2003). Point mutations within this region subsequently established the involvement of 5 residues in CaM binding (V769, R771, R785, K788 and R797). These findings were consistent with a model by which the C-terminus' binding motif docks into CaM as a basic amphiphilic α-helix (Grycova et al. 2008). Additionally, E761 was found to be of structural significance in vanilloid binding alongside R114 within the N-terminus (Jung et al. 2002).

There are further functional similarities between the structural components of the C- and N-termini. Point mutations of PKA consensus sites revealed that mimicking phosphorylation via S774D and S820D mutations significantly reduces capsaicin-induced desensitisation, demonstrating the presence of phosphorylation sites on the C-terminus. However, raising cAMP levels with forskolin pre-treatment in the presence of these mutants decreased tachyphylaxis further still. As this was not observed with S116D and T370D mutations, N-terminus-based phosphorylation sites appear to play the major roles in PKA-mediated TRPV1 modulation (Mohapatra and Nau 2003). Conversely, TRPV1 phosphorylation by PKC occurs at the C- rather than the N-terminus. Point mutation studies have identified that S800 is a major phosphorylation site underlying PKC's sensitising TRPV1 to capsaicin (Fig. 2.1) (Numazaki et al. 2002; Bhave et al. 2003), while S774 and S820 serve as minor PKC phosphorylation sites (Bhave et al. 2003). Furthermore, the ability of phorbol esters to activate TRPV1 in addition to stimulating PKC was identified and the potentiation of resulting currents by PKC was shown to be dependent on S704 (Fig. 2.1) (Bhave et al. 2003). The C-terminus hence hosts a variety of important structural features that regulate tetramerisation, gating properties, temperature sensitivity and channel sensitisation.

2.6.3 The Pore Domain

TRPV1's pore domain is formed by S5, S6 and the adjoining pore loop (P-loop) between them (Fig. 2.1). S6 constitutes the inner pore helix while the P-loop serves as the channel's selectivity filter. Subsequently, many key residues that determine the channel's gating and permeability properties have been identified here. Employing the substituted cysteine accessibility method to scan S6 of rat TRPV1 elucidated the presence of two intracellular constrictions that block the ion conduction pathway. One, located at L681, prevents the ingress of large (~6 Å) molecules. The other, at Y671, prevents the passage of small ions (~2 Å) and comprises TRPV1's activation gate in response to both capsaicin and heat (Fig. 2.1). Given the periodicity of an alpha helix, the accessibility of these residues was consistent with their positioning within the aqueous pore-facing side of a helical transmembrane domain (Salazar et al. 2009). This arrangement is consistent with the previous findings that T671 modulates Ca^{2+}-permeation properties and is implicated in Ca^{2+}-dependent desensitisation (Mohapatra et al. 2003). Beyond in addition to identifying pore constriction sites, point mutation studies have elucidated a range of residues with alternative functional relevance in the pore region. Following evidence that D646 neutralisation reduces divalent cation permeability, it has been suggested that this residue might form a ring of negative charges in order to construct a high affinity cation binding site near the channel's extracellular entrance. Such an arrangement could serve to coordinate cation movement and hence modulate channel permeation and blockade (Garcia-Martinez et al. 2000). Further, E636 mutation weakly modulated pore blockade consistently with this residue serving to stabilise the channel's selectivity filter or tetrameric structure. The suggested roles of these residues are consistent with TRPV1's proposed structural and operational similarity to the potassium crystallographically-sited activation channel KcsA (Garcia-Martinez et al. 2000).

While TRPV1's response to intracellular pH increase is mediated by the N-terminus, the effects of low pH, such as that occurring within damaged tissue due to local acidosis, are presumed to result from protonation of its extracellular acidic residues. Two such residues found near the channel's pore confer different means of proton-mediated gating (Fig. 2.1). E600 appears to determine the channel's response to other activators at low pH. Wild type TRPV1 exhibited dynamic heat-response potentiation when the extracellular pH decreased across a range reflecting tissue-damage associated local acidosis though, upon E600 mutation, the channel failed to exhibit such dynamic and robust response modulation (Jordt et al. 2000). E648 instead appears to confer the channel's direct activation by protons as its mutation selectively abrogates proton-induced channel activation while responses to capsaicin and heat remained unaffected (Jordt et al. 2000). The E648A mutation hence supports the co-existence of independent activation pathways for different stimuli within TRPV1. However, it is worth noting that an alternative mutation of this residue, E648Q, has conversely been reported to selectively potentiate responses to capsaicin and not protons. Furthermore, the study described this same effect as a result of mutating residues E636 and D646 (Welch et al. 2000), both discussed above. In addition to E600 and E648, a study demonstrating that both proton-induced activation and sensitisation of TRPV1 are mediated by shifting the voltage dependence of activation curves towards more physiological membrane potentials elucidated that both of these processes depend on F660 within the pore region (Aneiros et al. 2011). Further still, the hydrophobic interactions that appear to mediate the coupling of proton binding with channel gating appear to rely on additional residues, one of which is located in the pore region at T633 (Ryu et al. 2007).

The pore region has further function in addition to regulating TRPV1's permeability and mediating responses to acidic pH. S-nitrosylation of C616 and C621, which are located within the proximal pore domain, underlies NO-evoked responses of TRPV1 (Yoshida et al. 2006). Further, the lipid cholesterol, an essential structural component of cell membranes, has been shown to be an important regulator of TRPV1 and seems to bind to a cholesterol recognition amino acid consensus (CRAC) sequence within S5 (Liu et al. 2006b; Szoke et al. 2010; Jansson et al. 2013; Santha et al. 2010; Picazo-Juarez et al. 2011; Morales-Lazaro et al. 2013). The substitutions R579D and F582Q within this CRAC motif decrease the cholesterol response. However, depletion of cholesterol has also been shown to reduce TRPV1-mediated currents and, furthermore, decrease TRPV1 channel membrane expression (Liu et al. 2006b).

Along with the C-terminus (Brauchi et al. 2007), the pore domain appears to confer some of the channel's thermosensing capability as mutating residues 613–627, thereby giving TRPV1 an artificial pore turret sequence, prevents the channel from responding to heat. This region was then observed to undergo heat-induced conformational changes not observed with ligand- and voltage-dependent activation (Yang et al. 2010). In addition, triple (N628K, N652T and Y653T) and double (N652T and Y653T) point mutant channels exhibit a shorter open time specifically in response to heat, while responses to capsaicin and pH are unaffected (Grandl et al. 2010). Endogenous heat-induced TRPV1 gating incorporates multiple open states of varying durations; those of greater length are diminished in these mutants. As with other regions in the molecule, TRPV1's pore region appears to be functionally regulated by post-transcriptional modification. This was first established with the identification of an exclusive N-glycosylation site at N604 in cell lines (Jahnel et al. 2001). Western blotting of primary sensory nerve extracts later indicated the presence of both glycosylated and unglycosylated TRPV1. This variation in glycosylation state was observed in wild type TRPV1 (WT-TRPV1) but not the unglycosylated N604T mutant (N604T-TRPV1) upon expression in HEK293 cells. Variations in glycosylation state were reflected in the variability of capsaicin-induced currents and desensitisation observed across different WT-TRPV1-tranfected cells, while responses mediated by N604T-TRPV1 were uniform. Glycosylation ultimately appears to alter the maintenance of capsaicin-induced intracellular calcium level increases, acute desensitisation and pore dilation in a manner consistent with a substantial variability of endogenous TRPV1 glycosylation (Veldhuis et al. 2012).

2.6.4 The S1–S4 Module

The final TRPV1 component, the S1–S4 module (Fig. 2.1), confers many functional qualities also enabled by other regions of the molecule. However, by possessing the 'vanilloid pocket' between the first intracellular loop and S4, it is set apart by its predominant interaction with capsaicinoids and resiniferonoids. These compounds are highly lipophilic and it is presumed that they bind intracellularly having crossed the cell membrane. Mutational analysis supports an arrangement in which capsaicin interacts with the cytosolic aromatic residue Y511 via its vanillyl moiety and other polar residues such as S512 and R491 via hydrogen bonding (Jordt and Julius 2002). Alternatively, following the demonstration that I550T mutation in rabbit TRPV1 is sufficient to confer capsaicin sensitivity and that the reverse T550I mutation in rat and human TRPV1 prevents it, it has been suggested that capsaicin's vanillyl moiety interacts at T550 while hydrophobic interaction occurs at Y511 (Gavva et al. 2004). Similarly, an additional mutation, L547M, was sufficient to enable high affinity binding of the ultra-potent vanilloid RTX in rabbit TRPV1 and the reverse mutations at positions 550 and 547 caused a loss of RTX binding in human and rat TRPV1 (Gavva et al. 2004). It was also demonstrated that anandamide, an endocannabinoid and endovanilloid with significant structural similarity to capsaicin, failed to activate the Y511A mutant. It hence appears that there are shared structural determinants of sensitivity to capsaicin and endogenous ligands (Jordt and Julius 2002).

Consistent with these mutational analyses, a modelling study suggested that capsaicin's vanillyl moiety does indeed interact at Y511 via π–π and hydrophobic interactions and at S512 via hydrogen bonding, while its carbonyl group interacts via hydrogen bonds with both Y511 and K571 (Lee et al. 2011). The π–π and hydrophobic interactions at Y511 also appeared to occur with RTX binding while the residue's hydroxyl group formed a hydrogen bond with K571 in order to embrace RTX's phenyl ring. Additionally, RTX's longer tail region contributed to hydrophobic interaction with M547, its C_4-OH group hydrogen-bonded with T550 and its orthophenyl group exhibited hydrophobic interaction with L515. As the RTX molecule has phenyl rings at both ends, and there are hydrophobic residues at both ends of the binding region, the model also supported a secondary binding mode by which RTX's vanillyl moiety pointed towards M547, its orthophenyl group oriented towards Y511, its C_{20}-ester seemed to form hydrogen bonds with N551 and its C_{13}-propenyl group formed hydrophobic interaction with L515 (Lee et al. 2011). In addition, the importance of a second hydrophobic site at F543 (which had been implicated in a previous RTX model alongside Y555 (Chou et al. 2004)) in binding a simplified RTX analogue was established and has interesting implications for the design of novel ligands (Lee et al. 2011).

In addition to its major roles in vanilloid binding, the S1-4 module houses residues key to TRPV1's pH sensitivity. The mutational analyses that elucidated the above-described vanilloid binding site concomitantly established the involvement of S512 and R491 in mediating the channel's response to protons. R491G and S512F mutations dramatically reduced proton-induced currents, while alternative mutations of these residues would preserve the responses to a greater extent (Jordt and Julius 2002). Additionally, as with T633 within the pore region, V538 within the second extracellular loop is required for the hydrophobic interactions involved in coupling proton binding with channel gating (Ryu et al. 2007). The S1–S4 module enables further post-transcriptional modification via S502, a consensus phosphorylation site for both PKA and PKC located within the first intracellular loop. Upon comparison with other predicted phosphorylation site mutants including T370D, PKA-mediated potentiation of heat response currents were most prominently reduced with S502D (Rathee et al. 2002), supporting the particular functional significance of this PKA phosphorylation site. As with S800 within the C-terminus, mutation studies have demonstrated that phosphorylation of S502 by PKC potentiates capsaicin-induced currents (Numazaki et al. 2002). Although TRPV1's molecular determinants of voltage sensing have not yet been identified, such activation is generally associated with a series of positively charged amino acids within the channel's S4. This is supported by the effect of mutating such residues within various voltage-gated ion channels on gating charge (Stuhmer et al. 1989; Papazian et al. 1991). Employing this approach has since confirmed that S4 and the second intracellular loop do indeed constitute part of the voltage sensor in TRPM8, offering interesting insight into how TRPV1 might sense voltage (Voets et al. 2007).

References

Ahern GP (2003) Activation of TRPV1 by the satiety factor oleoylethanolamide. J Biol Chem 278:30429–30434
Ahern GP, Brooks IM, Miyares RL, Wang XB (2005a) Extracellular cations sensitize and gate capsaicin receptor TRPV1 modulating pain signaling. J Neurosci 25:5109–5116
Ahern GP, Brooks IM, Miyares RL, Wang XB (2005b) Extracellular cations sensitize and gate capsaicin receptor TRPV1 modulating pain signaling. J Neurosci: Official J Soc Neurosci 25:5109–5116
Almasi R, Szoke E, Bolcskei K, Varga A, Riedl Z, Sandor Z, Szolcsanyi J, Petho G (2008) Actions of 3-methyl-N-oleoyldopamine, 4-methyl-N-oleoyldopamine and N-oleoylethanolamide on the rat TRPV1 receptor in vitro and in vivo. Life Sci 82:644–651
Aneiros E, Cao L, Papakosta M, Stevens EB, Phillips S, Grimm C (2011) The biophysical and molecular basis of TRPV1 proton gating. EMBO J 30:994–1002
Appendino G, Daddario N, Minassi A, Moriello AS, de Petrocellis L, Di Marzo V (2005a) The taming of capsaicin. Reversal of the vanilloid activity of N-acylvanillamines by aromatic iodination. J Med Chem 48:4663–4669
Appendino G, de Petrocellis L, Trevisani M, Minassi A, Daddario N, Moriello AS, Gazzieri D, Ligresti A, Campi B, Fontana G, Pinna C, Geppetti P, Di Marzo V (2005b) Development of the first ultra-potent "capsaicinoid" agonist at transient receptor potential vanilloid type 1 (TRPV1) channels and its therapeutic potential. J Pharmacol Exp Ther 312:561–570
Appendino G, Harrison S, de Petrocellis L, Daddario N, Bianchi F, Schiano Moriello A, Trevisani M, Benvenuti F, Geppetti P, Di Marzo V (2003) Halogenation of a capsaicin analogue leads to novel vanilloid TRPV1 receptor antagonists. Br J Pharmacol 139: 1417–1424
Arniges M, Fernandez-Fernandez JM, Albrecht N, Schaefer M, Valverde MA (2006) Human TRPV4 channel splice variants revealed a key role of ankyrin domains in multimerization and trafficking. J Biol Chem 281:1580–1586
Bang S, Yoo S, Yang TJ, Cho H, Hwang SW (2012) 17(R)-resolvin D1 specifically inhibits transient receptor potential ion channel vanilloid 3 leading to peripheral antinociception. Br J Pharmacol 165:683–692
Baumann TK, Martenson ME (2000) Extracellular protons both increase the activity and reduce the conductance of capsaicin- gated channels. J Neurosci 20:RC80
Bevan S, Hothi S, Hughes G, James IF, Rang HP, Shah K, Walpole CS, Yeats JC (1992) Capsazepine: a competitive antagonist of the sensory neurone excitant capsaicin. Br J Pharmacol 107:544–552
Bhave G, Hu HJ, Glauner KS, Zhu W, Wang H, Brasier DJ, Oxford GS, Gereau RWT (2003) Protein kinase C phosphorylation sensitizes but does not activate the capsaicin receptor transient receptor potential vanilloid 1 (TRPV1). Proc Natl Acad Sci USA 100:12480–12485
Bhave G, Zhu W, Wang H, Brasier DJ, Oxford GS, Gereau RWT (2002) cAMP-dependent protein kinase regulates desensitization of the capsaicin receptor (VR1) by direct phosphorylation. Neuron 35:721–731
Blednov YA, Harris RA (2009) Deletion of vanilloid receptor (TRPV1) in mice alters behavioral effects of ethanol. Neuropharmacology 56:814–820
Bours MJ, Swennen EL, di Virgilio F, Cronstein BN, Dagnelie PC (2006) Adenosine 5'-triphosphate and adenosine as endogenous signaling molecules in immunity and inflammation. Pharmacol Ther 112:358–404
Brand L, Berman E, Schwen R, Loomans M, Janusz J, Bohne R, Maddin C, Gardner J, Lahann T, Farmer R et al (1987) NE-19550: a novel, orally active anti-inflammatory analgesic. Drugs Exp Clin Res 13:259–265
Brauchi S, Orta G, Mascayano C, Salazar M, Raddatz N, Urbina H, Rosenmann E, Gonzalez-Nilo F, Latorre R (2007) Dissection of the components for PIP2 activation and thermosensation in TRP channels. Proc Natl Acad Sci USA 104:10246–10251

Brauchi S, Orta G, Salazar M, Rosenmann E, Latorre R (2006) A hot-sensing cold receptor: C-terminal domain determines thermosensation in transient receptor potential channels. J Neurosci 26:4835–4840
Burnstock G (2008) Purinergic signalling and disorders of the central nervous system. Nat Rev Drug Discov 7:575–590
Burnstock G (2009) Purinergic receptors and pain. Curr Pharm Des 15:1717–1735
Burnstock G, Kennedy C (2011) P2X receptors in health and disease. Adv Pharmacol 61:333–372
Carrier EJ, Kearn CS, Barkmeier AJ, Breese NM, Yang W, Nithipatikom K, Pfister SL, Campbell WB, Hillard CJ (2004) Cultured rat microglial cells synthesize the endocannabinoid 2-arachidonylglycerol, which increases proliferation via a CB2 receptor-dependent mechanism. Mol Pharmacol 65:999–1007
Caterina MJ, Schumacher MA, Tominaga M, Rosen TA, Levine JD, Julius D (1997) The capsaicin receptor: a heat-activated ion channel in the pain pathway. Nature 389:816–824
Cavanaugh DJ, Chesler AT, Braz JM, Shah NM, Julius D, Basbaum AI (2011) Restriction of transient receptor potential vanilloid-1 to the peptidergic subset of primary afferent neurons follows its developmental downregulation in nonpeptidergic neurons. J Neurosci 31:10119–10127
Cesare P, Dekker LV, Sardini A, Parker PJ, McNaughton PA (1999) Specific involvement of PKC-epsilon in sensitization of the neuronal response to painful heat. Neuron 23:617–624
Cesare P, McNaughton P (1996) A novel heat-activated current in nociceptive neurons and its sensitization by bradykinin. Proc Natl Acad Sci U S A 93:15435–15439
Chavez AE, Chiu CQ, Castillo PE (2010) TRPV1 activation by endogenous anandamide triggers postsynaptic long-term depression in dentate gyrus. Nat Neurosci 13:1511–1518
Cho W, Stahelin RV (2005) Membrane-protein interactions in cell signaling and membrane trafficking. Annu Rev Biophys Biomol Struct 34:119–151
Cholewinski A, Burgess GM, Bevan S (1993) The role of calcium in capsaicin-induced desensitization in rat cultured dorsal root ganglion neurons. Neuroscience 55:1015–1023
Chou MZ, Mtui T, Gao YD, Kohler M, Middleton RE (2004) Resiniferatoxin binds to the capsaicin receptor (TRPV1) near the extracellular side of the S4 transmembrane domain. Biochemistry 43:2501–2511
Chuang HH, Prescott ED, Kong H, Shields S, Jordt SE, Basbaum AI, Chao MV, Julius D (2001) Bradykinin and nerve growth factor release the capsaicin receptor from PtdIns(4,5) P2-mediated inhibition. Nature 411:957–962
Cortright DN, Szallasi A (2004) Biochemical pharmacology of the vanilloid receptor TRPV1. An update. Europ J Biochem/FEBS 271:1814–1819
Cromer BA, McIntyre P (2008) Painful toxins acting at TRPV1. Toxicon 51:163–173
Culotta E, Koshland DE Jr (1992) No news is good news. Science 258:1862–1865
Decottignies A, Goffeau A (1997) Complete inventory of the yeast ABC proteins. Nat Genet 15:137–145
Devane WA, Hanus L, Breuer A, Pertwee RG, Stevenson LA, Griffin G, Gibson D, Mandelbaum A, Etinger A, Mechoulam R (1992) Isolation and structure of a brain constituent that binds to the cannabinoid receptor. Science 258:1946–1949
Dhaka A, Uzzell V, Dubin AE, Mathur J, Petrus M, Bandell M, Patapoutian A (2009) TRPV1 is activated by both acidic and basic pH. J Neurosci 29:153–158
Di Marzo V, Blumberg PM, Szallasi A (2002) Endovanilloid signaling in pain. Curr Opin Neurobiol 12:372–379
Di Marzo V, de Petrocellis L, Sepe N, Buono A (1996) Biosynthesis of anandamide and related acylethanolamides in mouse J774 macrophages and N18 neuroblastoma cells. Biochem J 316(Pt 3):977–984
Di Marzo V, Fontana A, Cadas H, Schinelli S, Cimino G, Schwartz JC, Piomelli D (1994) Formation and inactivation of endogenous cannabinoid anandamide in central neurons. Nature 372:686–691

Dietrich A, Kalwa H, Rost BR, Gudermann T (2005) The diacylgylcerol-sensitive TRPC3/6/7 subfamily of cation channels: functional characterization and physiological relevance. Pflugers Arch 451:72–80

Dinitto JP, Cronin TC, Lambright DG (2003) Membrane recognition and targeting by lipid-binding domains. Sci STKE: Sig Transduct Knowl Environ 213:re16

Docherty RJ, Yeats JC, Bevan S, Boddeke HW (1996) Inhibition of calcineurin inhibits the desensitization of capsaicin-evoked currents in cultured dorsal root ganglion neurones from adult rats. Pflugers Arch 431:828–837

Dray A (1992) Neuropharmacological mechanisms of capsaicin and related substances. Biochem Pharmacol 44:611–615

Eisenach JC, Hood DD, Curry R (2002) Preliminary efficacy assessment of intrathecal injection of an American formulation of adenosine in humans. Anesthesiology 96:29–34

el Kouhen R, Surowy CS, Bianchi BR, Neelands TR, McDonald HA, Niforatos W, Gomtsyan A, Lee CH, Honore P, Sullivan JP, Jarvis MF, Faltynek CR (2005) A-425619 [1-isoquinolin-5-yl-3-(4-trifluoromethyl-benzyl)-urea], a novel and selective transient receptor potential type V1 receptor antagonist, blocks channel activation by vanilloids, heat, and acid. J Pharmacol Exp Ther 314:400–409

Erler I, Hirnet D, Wissenbach U, Flockerzi V, Niemeyer BA (2004) Ca^{2+}-selective transient receptor potential V channel architecture and function require a specific ankyrin repeat. J Biol Chem 279:34456–34463

Everaerts W, Gees M, Alpizar YA, Farre R, Leten C, Apetrei A, Dewachter I, van Leuven F, Vennekens R, de Ridder D, Nilius B, Voets T, Talavera K (2011) The capsaicin receptor TRPV1 is a crucial mediator of the noxious effects of mustard oil. Curr Biol 21:316–321

Fajardo O, Meseguer V, Belmonte C, Viana F (2008) TRPA1 channels mediate cold temperature sensing in mammalian vagal sensory neurons: pharmacological and genetic evidence. J Neurosci 28:7863–7875

Faussone-Pellegrini MS, Taddei A, Bizzoco E, Lazzeri M, Vannucchi MG, Bechi P (2005) Distribution of the vanilloid (capsaicin) receptor type 1 in the human stomach. Histochem Cell Biol 124:61–68

Fernandes ES, Fernandes MA, Keeble JE (2012) The functions of TRPA1 and TRPV1: moving away from sensory nerves. Br J Pharmacol 166:510–521

Fischer MJ, Btesh J, McNaughton PA (2013) Disrupting sensitization of transient receptor potential vanilloid subtype 1 inhibits inflammatory hyperalgesia. J Neurosci 33:7407–7414

Fu J, Gaetani S, Oveisi F, Lo Verme J, Serrano A, Rodriguez de Fonseca F, Rosengarth A, Luecke H, di Giacomo B, Tarzia G, Piomelli D (2003) Oleylethanolamide regulates feeding and body weight through activation of the nuclear receptor PPAR-alpha. Nature 425:90–93

Fujiwake H, Suzuki T, Oka S, Iwai K (1980) Enzymatic formation of capsaicinoid from vanillylamine and iso-type fatty acids by cell-free extracts of Capsicum annuum var. annuum cv. Karayatsubus. Agric Biol Chem 44:2907–2912

Garcia-Martinez C, Morenilla-Palao C, Planells-Cases R, Merino JM, Ferrer-Montiel A (2000) Identification of an aspartic residue in the P-loop of the vanilloid receptor that modulates pore properties. J Biol Chem 275:32552–32558

Garcia-Sanz N, Fernandez-Carvajal A, Morenilla-Palao C, Planells-Cases R, Fajardo-Sanchez E, Fernandez-Ballester G, Ferrer-Montiel A (2004) Identification of a tetramerization domain in the C terminus of the vanilloid receptor. J Neurosci 24:5307–5314

Garcia-Sanz N, Valente P, Gomis A, Fernandez-Carvajal A, Fernandez-Ballester G, Viana F, Belmonte C, Ferrer-Montiel A (2007) A role of the transient receptor potential domain of vanilloid receptor I in channel gating. J Neurosci 27:11641–11650

Gau P, Poon J, Ufret-Vincenty C, Snelson CD, Gordon SE, Raible DW, Dhaka A (2013) The zebrafish ortholog of TRPV1 is required for heat-induced locomotion. J Neurosci 33:5249–5260

Gavva NR, Bannon AW, Surapaneni S, Hovland DN Jr, Lehto SG, Gore A, Juan T, Deng H, Han B, Klionsky L, Kuang R, Le A, Tamir R, Wang J, Youngblood B, Zhu D, Norman MH, Magal E, Treanor JJ, Louis JC (2007) The vanilloid receptor TRPV1 is tonically activated in vivo and involved in body temperature regulation. J Neurosci 27:3366–3374

Gavva NR, Klionsky L, Qu Y, Shi L, Tamir R, Edenson S, Zhang TJ, Viswanadhan VN, Toth A, Pearce LV, Vanderah TW, Porreca F, Blumberg PM, Lile J, Sun Y, Wild K, Louis JC, Treanor JJ (2004) Molecular determinants of vanilloid sensitivity in TRPV1. J Biol Chem 279:20283–20295

Gavva NR, Tamir R, Qu Y, Klionsky L, Zhang TJ, Immke D, Wang J, Zhu D, Vanderah TW, Porreca F, Doherty EM, Norman MH, Wild KD, Bannon AW, Louis JC, Treanor JJ (2005) AMG 9810 [(E)-3-(4-t-butylphenyl)-N-(2,3-dihydrobenzo[b][1,4] dioxin-6-yl)acrylamide], a novel vanilloid receptor 1 (TRPV1) antagonist with antihyperalgesic properties. J Pharmacol Exp Ther 313:474–484

Gees M, Alpizar YA, Boonen B, Sanchez A, Everaerts W, Segal A, Xue F, Janssens A, Owsianik G, Nilius B, Voets T, Talavera K (2013) Mechanisms of TRPV1 activation and sensitization by Allyl Isothiocyanate. Mol Pharmacol 84:325–334

Glendinning JI, Simons YM, Youngentob L, Youngentob SL (2012) Fetal ethanol exposure attenuates aversive oral effects of TrpV1, but not TrpA1 agonists in rats. Exp Biol Med (Maywood) 237:236–240

Gomtsyan A, Bayburt EK, Schmidt RG, Zheng GZ, Perner RJ, Didomenico S, Koenig JR, Turner S, Jinkerson T, Drizin I, Hannick SM, Macri BS, McDonald HA, Honore P, Wismer CT, Marsh KC, Wetter J, Stewart KD, Oie T, Jarvis MF, Surowy CS, Faltynek CR, Lee CH (2005) Novel transient receptor potential vanilloid 1 receptor antagonists for the treatment of pain: structure-activity relationships for ureas with quinoline, isoquinoline, quinazoline, phthalazine, quinoxaline, and cinnoline moieties. J Med Chem 48:744–752

Goodfellow CE, Glass M (2009) Anandamide receptor signal transduction. Vitam Horm 81:79–110

Goswami C, Dreger M, Jahnel R, Bogen O, Gillen C, Hucho F (2004) Identification and characterization of a Ca^{2+} -sensitive interaction of the vanilloid receptor TRPV1 with tubulin. J Neurochem 91:1092–1103

Gram DX, Ahren B, Nagy I, Olsen UB, Brand CL, Sundler F, Tabanera R, Svendsen O, Carr RD, Santha P, Wierup N, Hansen AJ (2007) Capsaicin-sensitive sensory fibers in the islets of Langerhans contribute to defective insulin secretion in Zucker diabetic rat, an animal model for some aspects of human type 2 diabetes. Eur J Neurosci 25:213–223

Grandl J, Kim SE, Uzzell V, Bursulaya B, Petrus M, Bandell M, Patapoutian A (2010) Temperature-induced opening of TRPV1 ion channel is stabilized by the pore domain. Nat Neurosci 13:708–714

Green BG, Hayes JE (2003) Capsaicin as a probe of the relationship between bitter taste and chemesthesis. Physiol Behav 79:811–821

Grycova L, Lansky Z, Friedlova E, Obsilova V, Janouskova H, Obsil T, Teisinger J (2008) Ionic interactions are essential for TRPV1 C-terminus binding to calmodulin. Biochem Biophys Res Commun 375:680–683

Gunthorpe MJ, Harries MH, Prinjha RK, Davis JB, Randall A (2000) Voltage- and time-dependent properties of the recombinant rat vanilloid receptor (rVR1). J Physiol 525(Pt 3):747–759

Hail N Jr (2003) Mechanisms of vanilloid-induced apoptosis. Apoptosis: Int J Program Cell Death 8:251–262

Helgren FJ, Lynch MJ, Kirchmeyer FJ (1955) A taste panel study of the saccharin off-taste. J Am Pharm Assoc Am Pharm Assoc (Baltim) 44:353–355

Hellwig N, Albrecht N, Harteneck C, Schultz G, Schaefer M (2005) Homo- and heteromeric assembly of TRPV channel subunits. J Cell Sci 118:917–928

Hoffmann J, Supronsinchai W, Andreou AP, Summ O, Akerman S, Goadsby PJ (2012) Olvanil acts on transient receptor potential vanilloid channel 1 and cannabinoid receptors to modulate neuronal transmission in the trigeminovascular system. Pain 153:2226–2232

Hőgyes E (1878a) Adatok a paprika (Capsicum annuum) élettani hatásához. Orvosi Hetilap 10/V

Hőgyes E (1878b) Beitrage zur physiologischen Wirkung der Bestandtheile des Capiscum annuum (Spanischer Pfeffer). Archiv für Experimentelle Pathologie und Pharmakologie 9:117–130

Holzer P (2008) The pharmacological challenge to tame the transient receptor potential vanilloid-1 (TRPV1) nocisensor. Br J Pharmacol 155:1145–1162

Holzer P (2011) Acid sensing by visceral afferent neurones. Acta Physiol (Oxf) 201:63–75

Honore P, Wismer CT, Mikusa J, Zhu CZ, Zhong C, Gauvin DM, Gomtsyan A, el Kouhen R, Lee CH, Marsh K, Sullivan JP, Faltynek CR, Jarvis MF (2005) A-425619 [1-isoquinolin-5-yl-3-(4-trifluoromethyl-benzyl)-urea], a novel transient receptor potential type V1 receptor antagonist, relieves pathophysiological pain associated with inflammation and tissue injury in rats. J Pharmacol Exp Ther 314:410–421

Huang J, Zhang X, McNaughton PA (2006a) Inflammatory pain: the cellular basis of heat hyperalgesia. Curr Neuropharmacol 4:197–206

Huang J, Zhang X, McNaughton PA (2006b) Modulation of temperature-sensitive TRP channels. Semin Cell Dev Biol 17:638–645

Huang RF, Huang SM, Lin BS, Hung CY, Lu HT (2002a) N-Acetylcysteine, vitamin C and vitamin E diminish homocysteine thiolactone-induced apoptosis in human promyeloid HL-60 cells. J Nutr 132:2151–2156

Huang SM, Bisogno T, Trevisani M, Al-Hayani A, De Petrocellis L, Fezza F, Tognetto M, Petros TJ, Krey JF, Chu CJ, Miller JD, Davies SN, Geppetti P, Walker JM, Di Marzo V (2002b) An endogenous capsaicin-like substance with high potency at recombinant and native vanilloid VR1 receptors. Proc Natl Acad Sci USA 99:8400–8405

Hung LW, Wang IX, Nikaido K, Liu PQ, Ames GF, Kim SH (1998) Crystal structure of the ATP-binding subunit of an ABC transporter. Nature 396:703–707

Hwang SW, Cho H, Kwak J, Lee SY, Kang CJ, Jung J, Cho S, Min KH, Suh YG, Kim D, Oh U (2000) Direct activation of capsaicin receptors by products of lipoxygenases: endogenous capsaicin-like substances. Proc Natl Acad Sci USA 97:6155–6160

Iida T, Moriyama T, Kobata K, Morita A, Murayama N, Hashizume S, Fushiki T, Yazawa S, Watanabe T, Tominaga M (2003) TRPV1 activation and induction of nociceptive response by a non-pungent capsaicin-like compound, capsiate. Neuropharmacology 44:958–967

Izzo AA, Capasso R, Pinto L, di Carlo G, Mascolo N, Capasso F (2001) Effect of vanilloid drugs on gastrointestinal transit in mice. Br J Pharmacol 132:1411–1416

Jahnel R, Dreger M, Gillen C, Bender O, Kurreck J, Hucho F (2001) Biochemical characterization of the vanilloid receptor 1 expressed in a dorsal root ganglia derived cell line. Eur J Biochem 268:5489–5496

Jancsó-Gábor A, Szolcsányi J, Jancsó N (1970) Irreversible impairment of thermoregulation induced by capsaicin and similar pungent substances in rats and guinea-pigs. J Physiol 206:495–507

Jancsó G, Dux M, Oszlacs O, Santha P (2008) Activation of the transient receptor potential vanilloid-1 (TRPV1) channel opens the gate for pain relief. Br J Pharmacol 155:1139–1141

Jancsó G, Király E, Jancsó-Gábor A (1977) Pharmacologically induced selective degeneration of chemosensitive primary sensory neurones. Nature 270:741–743

Jancsó M, Jancsóné M (1949) Érzőidegvégződések desensibilizálása Kísérletes. Orvostudomány 2:15

Jancsó N, Jancsó-Gábor A, Szolcsányi J (1967) Direct evidence for neurogenic inflammation and its prevention by denervation and by pretreatment with capsaicin. Br J Pharmacol Chemother 31:138–151

Jansson ET, Trkulja CL, Ahemaiti A, Millingen M, Jeffries GD, Jardemark K, Orwar O (2013) Effect of cholesterol depletion on the pore dilation of TRPV1. Mol Pain 9:1

Jara-Oseguera A, Simon SA, Rosenbaum T (2008) TRPV1: on the road to pain relief. Curr Mol Pharmacol 1:255–269

Jeske NA, Patwardhan AM, Gamper N, Price TJ, Akopian AN, Hargreaves KM (2006) Cannabinoid WIN 55,212-2 regulates TRPV1 phosphorylation in sensory neurons. J Biol Chem 281:32879–32890

Jeske NA, Patwardhan AM, Ruparel NB, Akopian AN, Shapiro MS, Henry MA (2009) A-kinase anchoring protein 150 controls protein kinase C-mediated phosphorylation and sensitization of TRPV1. Pain 146:301–307

Jin X, Touhey J, Gaudet R (2006) Structure of the N-terminal ankyrin repeat domain of the TRPV2 ion channel. J Biol Chem 281:25006–25010

Jordt SE, Julius D (2002) Molecular basis for species-specific sensitivity to "hot" chili peppers. Cell 108:421–430

Jordt SE, Tominaga M, Julius D (2000) Acid potentiation of the capsaicin receptor determined by a key extracellular site. Proc Natl Acad Sci USA 97:8134–8139

Jung J, Lee SY, Hwang SW, Cho H, Shin J, Kang YS, Kim S, Oh U (2002) Agonist recognition sites in the cytosolic tails of vanilloid receptor 1. J Biol Chem 277:44448–44454

Jung J, Shin JS, Lee SY, Hwang SW, Koo J, Cho H, Oh U (2004) Phosphorylation of vanilloid receptor 1 by Ca^{2+}/calmodulin-dependent kinase II regulates its vanilloid binding. J Biol Chem 279:7048–7054

Kass GE, Orrenius S (1999) Calcium signaling and cytotoxicity. Environ Health Perspect 107(Suppl 1):25–35

Kato S, Aihara E, Nakamura A, Xin H, Matsui H, Kohama K, Takeuchi K (2003) Expression of vanilloid receptors in rat gastric epithelial cells: role in cellular protection. Biochem Pharmacol 66:1115–1121

Kauer JA, Gibson HE (2009) Hot flash: TRPV channels in the brain. Trends Neurosci 32:215–224

Kim AY, Tang Z, Liu Q, Patel KN, Maag D, Geng Y, Dong X (2008) Pirt, a phosphoinositide-binding protein, functions as a regulatory subunit of TRPV1. Cell 133:475–485

Knotkova H, Pappagallo M, Szallasi A (2008) Capsaicin (TRPV1 Agonist) therapy for pain relief: farewell or revival? Clin J Pain 24:142–154

Koplas PA, Rosenberg RL, Oxford GS (1997) The role of calcium in the desensitization of capsaicin responses in rat dorsal root ganglion neurons. J Neurosci: Official J Soc Neurosci 17:3525–3537

Kwak J, Wang MH, Hwang SW, Kim TY, Lee SY, Oh U (2000) Intracellular ATP increases capsaicin-activated channel activity by interacting with nucleotide-binding domains. J Neurosci 20:8298–8304

Lainez S, Valente P, Ontoria-Oviedo I, Estevez-Herrera J, Camprubi-Robles M, Ferrer-Montiel A, Planells-Cases R (2010) GABAA receptor associated protein (GABARAP) modulates TRPV1 expression and channel function and desensitization. FASEB J: Official Publ Fed Am Soc Exp Biol 24:1958–1970

Latorre R, Brauchi S, Orta G, Zaelzer C, Vargas G (2007) ThermoTRP channels as modular proteins with allosteric gating. Cell Calcium 42:427–438

Lau SY, Procko E, Gaudet R (2012) Distinct properties of Ca^{2+}-calmodulin binding to N- and C-terminal regulatory regions of the TRPV1 channel. J Gen Physiol 140:541–555

Lee JH, Lee Y, Ryu H, Kang DW, Lee J, Lazar J, Pearce LV, Pavlyukovets VA, Blumberg PM, Choi S (2011) Structural insights into transient receptor potential vanilloid type 1 (TRPV1) from homology modeling, flexible docking, and mutational studies. J Comput Aided Mol Des 25:317–327

Lemmon MA (2003) Phosphoinositide recognition domains. Traffic 4:201–213

Levine JD, Lam D, Taiwo YO, Donatoni P, Goetzl EJ (1986) Hyperalgesic properties of 15-lipoxygenase products of arachidonic acid. Proc Natl Acad Sci USA 83:5331–5334

Levine JD, Taiwo YO (1990) Hyperalgesic pain: a review. Anesth prog 37:133–135

Lim J, Green BG (2007) The psychophysical relationship between bitter taste and burning sensation: evidence of qualitative similarity. Chem Senses 32:31–39

Lishko PV, Procko E, Jin X, Phelps CB, Gaudet R (2007) The ankyrin repeats of TRPV1 bind multiple ligands and modulate channel sensitivity. Neuron 54:905–918

Liu L, Simon SA (1996) Capsaicin-induced currents with distinct desensitization and Ca^{2+} dependence in rat trigeminal ganglion cells. J Neurophysiol 75:1503–1514

Liu B, Hui K, Qin F (2003) Thermodynamics of heat activation of single capsaicin ion channels VR1. Biophys J 85:2988–3006

Liu B, Zhang C, Qin F (2005) Functional recovery from desensitization of vanilloid receptor TRPV1 requires resynthesis of phosphatidylinositol 4,5-bisphosphate. J Neurosci: Official J Soc Neurosci 25:4835–4843

Liu J, Wang L, Harvey-White J, Huang BX, Kim HY, Luquet S, Palmiter RD, Krystal G, Rai R, Mahadevan A, Razdan RK, Kunos G (2008) Multiple pathways involved in the biosynthesis of anandamide. Neuropharmacology 54:1–7

Liu J, Wang L, Harvey-White J, Osei-Hyiaman D, Razdan R, Gong Q, Chan AC, Zhou Z, Huang BX, Kim HY, Kunos G (2006a) A biosynthetic pathway for anandamide. Proc Natl Acad Sci U S A 103:13345–13350

Liu M, Huang W, Wu D, Priestley JV (2006b) TRPV1, but not P2X, requires cholesterol for its function and membrane expression in rat nociceptors. Europ J Neurosci 24:1–6

Lopshire JC, Nicol GD (1998) The cAMP transduction cascade mediates the prostaglandin E2 enhancement of the capsaicin-elicited current in rat sensory neurons: whole-cell and single-channel studies. J Neurosci 18:6081–6092

Lukacs V, Thyagarajan B, Varnai P, Balla A, Balla T, Rohacs T (2007) Dual regulation of TRPV1 by phosphoinositides. J Neurosci: Official J Soc Neurosci 27:7070–7080

Macpherson LJ, Geierstanger BH, Viswanath V, Bandell M, Eid SR, Hwang S, Patapoutian A (2005) The pungency of garlic: activation of TRPA1 and TRPV1 in response to allicin. Curr Biol 15:929–934

Mahmud A, Santha P, Paule CC, Nagy I (2009) Cannabinoid 1 receptor activation inhibits transient receptor potential vanilloid type 1 receptor-mediated cationic influx into rat cultured primary sensory neurons. Neuroscience 162:1202–1211

Maihofner C, Heskamp ML (2013) Prospective, non-interventional study on the tolerability and analgesic effectiveness over 12 weeks after a single application of capsaicin 8 % cutaneous patch in 1044 patients with peripheral neuropathic pain: first results of the QUEPP study. Curr Med Res Opin 29:673–683

Mandadi S, Numazaki M, Tominaga M, Bhat MB, Armati PJ, Roufogalis BD (2004) Activation of protein kinase C reverses capsaicin-induced calcium-dependent desensitization of TRPV1 ion channels. Cell Calcium 35:471–478

Mandadi S, Roufogalis BD (2008) ThermoTRP channels in nociceptors: taking a lead from capsaicin receptor TRPV1. Curr Neuropharmacol 6:21–38

Matsuda LA, Lolait SJ, Brownstein MJ, Young AC, Bonner TI (1990) Structure of a cannabinoid receptor and functional expression of the cloned cDNA. Nature 346:561–564

Matta JA, Ahern GP (2011) TRPV1 and synaptic transmission. Curr Pharm Biotechnol 12:95–101

McCleverty CJ, Koesema E, Patapoutian A, Lesley SA, Kreusch A (2006) Crystal structure of the human TRPV2 channel ankyrin repeat domain. Protein Sci 15:2201–2206

McLatchie LM, Bevan S (2001) The effects of pH on the interaction between capsaicin and the vanilloid receptor in rat dorsal root ganglia neurons. Br J Pharmacol 132:899–908

McMahon SB, Lewin G, Bloom SR (1991) The consequences of long-term topical capsaicin application in the rat. Pain 44:301–310

McNamara FN, Randall A, Gunthorpe MJ (2005) Effects of piperine, the pungent component of black pepper, at the human vanilloid receptor (TRPV1). Br J Pharmacol 144:781–790

Mercado J, Gordon-Shaag A, Zagotta WN, Gordon SE (2010) Ca^{2+}-dependent desensitization of TRPV2 channels is mediated by hydrolysis of phosphatidylinositol 4,5-bisphosphate. J Neurosci: Official J Soc Neurosci 30:13338–13347

Mohapatra DP, Nau C (2003) Desensitization of capsaicin-activated currents in the vanilloid receptor TRPV1 is decreased by the cyclic AMP-dependent protein kinase pathway. J Biol Chem 278:50080–50090

Mohapatra DP, Nau C (2005) Regulation of Ca^{2+}-dependent desensitization in the vanilloid receptor TRPV1 by calcineurin and cAMP-dependent protein kinase. J Biol Chem 280:13424–13432

Mohapatra DP, Wang SY, Wang GK, Nau C (2003) A tyrosine residue in TM6 of the Vanilloid Receptor TRPV1 involved in desensitization and calcium permeability of capsaicin-activated currents. Mol Cell Neurosci 23:314–324

Morales-Lazaro SL, Simon SA, Rosenbaum T (2013) The role of endogenous molecules in modulating pain through transient receptor potential vanilloid 1 (TRPV1). J Physiol 591:3109–3121

Morenilla-Palao C, Planells-Cases R, Garcia-Sanz N, Ferrer-Montiel A (2004) Regulated exocytosis contributes to protein kinase C potentiation of vanilloid receptor activity. J Biol Chem 279:25665–25672

Moriyama T, Higashi T, Togashi K, Iida T, Segi E, Sugimoto Y, Tominaga T, Narumiya S, Tominaga M (2005a) Sensitization of TRPV1 by EP1 and IP reveals peripheral nociceptive mechanism of prostaglandins. Mol Pain 1:3

Moriyama T, Higashi T, Togashi K, Iida T, Segi E, Sugimoto Y, Tominaga T, Narumiya S, Tominaga M (2005b) Sensitization of TRPV1 by EP1 and IP reveals peripheral nociceptive mechanism of prostaglandins. Mol Pain 1:3

Moriyama T, Iida T, Kobayashi K, Higashi T, Fukuoka T, Tsumura H, Leon C, Suzuki N, Inoue K, Gachet C, Noguchi K, Tominaga M (2003) Possible involvement of P2Y2 metabotropic receptors in ATP-induced transient receptor potential vanilloid receptor 1-mediated thermal hypersensitivity. J Neurosci: Official J Soc Neurosci 23:6058–6062

Mosavi LK, Cammett TJ, Desrosiers DC, Peng ZY (2004) The ankyrin repeat as molecular architecture for protein recognition. Protein Sci 13:1435–1448

Movahed P, Jonsson BA, Birnir B, Wingstrand JA, Jorgensen TD, Ermund A, Sterner O, Zygmunt PM, Hogestatt ED (2005) Endogenous unsaturated C18 N-acylethanolamines are vanilloid receptor (TRPV1) agonists. J Biol Chem 280:38496–38504

Nagy B, Fedonidis C, Photiou A, Wahba J, Paule CC, Ma D, Buluwela L, Nagy I (2009) Capsaicin-sensitive primary sensory neurons in the mouse express N-Acyl phosphatidylethanolamine phospholipase D. Neuroscience 161:572–577

Nagy I (2004) Sensory processing: primary afferent neurons/DRG. In: Maze EA (ed) Anesthetic pharmacology: physiologic principles and clinical practice. Churchill Livingstone, Philadelphia

Nagy I, Santha P, Jancso G, Urban L (2004) The role of the vanilloid (capsaicin) receptor (TRPV1) in physiology and pathology. Eur J Pharmacol 500:351–369

Nieto-Posadas A, Picazo-Juarez G, Llorente I, Jara-Oseguera A, Morales-Lazaro S, Escalante-Alcalde D, Islas LD, Rosenbaum T (2012) Lysophosphatidic acid directly activates TRPV1 through a C-terminal binding site. Nat Chem Biol 8:78–85

Nilius B, Appendino G (2011) Tasty and healthy TR(i)Ps. The human quest for culinary pungency. EMBO Rep 12:1094–1101

Nilius B, Voets T (2005) TRP channels: a TR(I)P through a world of multifunctional cation channels. Pflugers Arch 451:1–10

Noguchi K, Herr D, Mutoh T, Chun J (2009) Lysophosphatidic acid (LPA) and its receptors. Curr Opin Pharmacol 9:15–23

Nolano M, Simone DA, Wendelschafer-Crabb G, Johnson T, Hazen E, Kennedy WR (1999) Topical capsaicin in humans: parallel loss of epidermal nerve fibers and pain sensation. Pain 81:135–145

Noto C, Pappagallo M, Szallasi A (2009) NGX-4010, a high-concentration capsaicin dermal patch for lasting relief of peripheral neuropathic pain. Curr Opin Investig Drugs 10:702–710

Numazaki M, Tominaga T, Takeuchi K, Murayama N, Toyooka H, Tominaga M (2003) Structural determinant of TRPV1 desensitization interacts with calmodulin. Proc Natl Acad Sci USA 100:8002–8006

Numazaki M, Tominaga T, Toyooka H, Tominaga M (2002) Direct phosphorylation of capsaicin receptor VR1 by protein kinase Cepsilon and identification of two target serine residues. J Biol Chem 277:13375–13378

Oh U, Hwang SW, Kim D (1996) Capsaicin activates a nonselective cation channel in cultured neonatal rat dorsal root ganglion neurons. J Neurosci 16:1659–1667

Ohta T, Imagawa T, Ito S (2007) Novel agonistic action of mustard oil on recombinant and endogenous porcine transient receptor potential V1 (pTRPV1) channels. Biochem Pharmacol 73:1646–1656

Okamoto Y, Morishita J, Tsuboi K, Tonai T, Ueda N (2004) Molecular characterization of a phospholipase D generating anandamide and its congeners. J Biol Chem 279:5298–5305

Olah Z, Szabo T, Karai L, Hough C, Fields RD, Caudle RM, Blumberg PM, Iadarola MJ (2001) Ligand-induced dynamic membrane changes and cell deletion conferred by vanilloid receptor 1. J Biol Chem 276:11021–11030

Papazian DM, Timpe LC, Jan YN, Jan LY (1991) Alteration of voltage-dependence of Shaker potassium channel by mutations in the S4 sequence. Nature 349:305–310

Park CK, Xu ZZ, Liu T, Lu N, Serhan CN, Ji RR (2011) Resolvin D2 is a potent endogenous inhibitor for transient receptor potential subtype V1/A1, inflammatory pain, and spinal cord synaptic plasticity in mice: distinct roles of resolvin D1, D2, and E1. J Neurosci 31:18433–18438

Perkins MN, Campbell EA (1992) Capsazepine reversal of the antinociceptive action of capsaicin in vivo. Br J Pharmacol 107:329–333

Peters JH, McDougall SJ, Fawley JA, Andresen MC (2011) TRPV1 marks synaptic segregation of multiple convergent afferents at the rat medial solitary tract nucleus. PLoS ONE 6:e25015

Phelps CB, Wang RR, Choo SS, Gaudet R (2010) Differential regulation of TRPV1, TRPV3, and TRPV4 sensitivity through a conserved binding site on the ankyrin repeat domain. J Biol Chem 285:731–740

Phillips E, Reeve A, Bevan S, McIntyre P (2004) Identification of species-specific determinants of the action of the antagonist capsazepine and the agonist PPAHV on TRPV1. J Biol Chem 279:17165–17172

Picazo-Juarez G, Romero-Suarez S, Nieto-Posadas A, Llorente I, Jara-Oseguera A, Briggs M, McIntosh TJ, Simon SA, Ladron-De-guevara E, Islas LD, Rosenbaum T (2011) Identification of a binding motif in the S5 helix that confers cholesterol sensitivity to the TRPV1 ion channel. J Biol Chem 286:24966–24976

Piper AS, Yeats JC, Bevan S, Docherty RJ (1999) A study of the voltage dependence of capsaicin-activated membrane currents in rat sensory neurones before and after acute desensitization. J Physiol 518(Pt 3):721–733

Por ED, Bierbower SM, Berg KA, Gomez R, Akopian AN, Wetsel WC, Jeske NA (2012) beta-Arrestin-2 desensitizes the transient receptor potential vanilloid 1 (TRPV1) channel. J Biol Chem 287:37552–37563

Pórszász J, Jancsó N (1959) Studies on the action potentials of sensory nerves in animals desensitized with capsaicine. Acta Physiol Acad Sci Hung 16:299–306

Premkumar LS, Ahern GP (2000) Induction of vanilloid receptor channel activity by protein kinase C. Nature 408:985–990

Premkumar LS, Qi ZH, van Buren J, Raisinghani M (2004) Enhancement of potency and efficacy of NADA by PKC-mediated phosphorylation of vanilloid receptor. J Neurophysiol 91:1442–1449

Prescott ED, Julius D (2003) A modular PIP2 binding site as a determinant of capsaicin receptor sensitivity. Science 300:1284–1288

Preti D, Szallasi A, Patacchini R (2012) TRP channels as therapeutic targets in airway disorders: a patent review. Expert Opin Ther Pat 22:663–695

Puntambekar P, van Buren J, Raisinghani M, Premkumar LS, Ramkumar V (2004) Direct interaction of adenosine with the TRPV1 channel protein. J Neurosci: Official J Soc Neurosci 24:3663–3671

Raisinghani M, Pabbidi RM, Premkumar LS (2005) Activation of transient receptor potential vanilloid 1 (TRPV1) by resiniferatoxin. J Physiol 567:771–786

Rathee PK, Distler C, Obreja O, Neuhuber W, Wang GK, Wang SY, Nau C, Kress M (2002) PKA/AKAP/VR-1 module: a common link of Gs-mediated signaling to thermal hyperalgesia. J Neurosci: Official J Soc Neurosci 22:4740–4745

Riera CE, Vogel H, Simon SA, le Coutre J (2007) Artificial sweeteners and salts producing a metallic taste sensation activate TRPV1 receptors. Am J Physiol Regul Integr Comp Physiol 293:R626–R634

Robbins N, Koch SE, Rubinstein J (2013) Targeting TRPV1 and TRPV2 for potential therapeutic interventions in cardiovascular disease. Transl Res: J Lab Clin Med 161:469–476

Roberts LA, Connor M (2006) TRPV1 antagonists as a potential treatment for hyperalgesia. Recent Pat CNS Drug Discov 1:65–76

Rosenbaum T, Gordon-Shaag A, Munari M, Gordon SE (2004) Ca^{2+}/calmodulin modulates TRPV1 activation by capsaicin. J Gen Physiol 123:53–62
Rutter AR, Ma QP, Leveridge M, Bonnert TP (2005) Heteromerization and colocalization of TrpV1 and TrpV2 in mammalian cell lines and rat dorsal root ganglia. NeuroReport 16:1735–1739
Ryu S, Liu B, Yao J, Fu Q, Qin F (2007) Uncoupling proton activation of vanilloid receptor TRPV1. J Neurosci 27:12797–12807
Saito S, Shingai R (2006) Evolution of thermoTRP ion channel homologs in vertebrates. Physiol Genomics 27:219–230
Salazar H, Jara-Oseguera A, Hernandez-Garcia E, Llorente I, Arias O II, Soriano-Garcia M, Islas LD, Rosenbaum T (2009) Structural determinants of gating in the TRPV1 channel. Nat Struct Mol Biol 16:704–710
Salazar H, Llorente I, Jara-Oseguera A, Garcia-Villegas R, Munari M, Gordon SE, Islas LD, Rosenbaum T (2008) A single N-terminal cysteine in TRPV1 determines activation by pungent compounds from onion and garlic. Nat Neurosci 11:255–261
Samuelsson B (1983) Leukotrienes: mediators of immediate hypersensitivity reactions and inflammation. Science 220:568–575
Santha P, Jancso G (2003) Transganglionic transport of choleragenoid by capsaicin-sensitive C-fibre afferents to the substantia gelatinosa of the spinal dorsal horn after peripheral nerve section. Neuroscience 116:621–627
Santha P, Oszlacs O, Dux M, Dobos I, Jancso G (2010) Inhibition of glucosylceramide synthase reversibly decreases the capsaicin-induced activation and TRPV1 expression of cultured dorsal root ganglion neurons. Pain 150:103–112
Sanz-Salvador L, Andres-Borderia A, Ferrer-Montiel A, Planells-Cases R (2012) Agonist- and Ca^{2+}-dependent desensitization of TRPV1 channel targets the receptor to lysosomes for degradation. J Biol Chem 287:19462–19471
Savidge J, Davis C, Shah K, Colley S, Phillips E, Ranasinghe S, Winter J, Kotsonis P, Rang H, McIntyre P (2002) Cloning and functional characterization of the guinea pig vanilloid receptor 1. Neuropharmacology 43:450–456
Sawynok J, Liu XJ (2003) Adenosine in the spinal cord and periphery: release and regulation of pain. Prog Neurobiol 69:313–340
Schiffman SS, Suggs MS, Abou Donia MB, Erickson RP, Nagle HT (1995) Environmental pollutants alter taste responses in the gerbil. Pharmacol Biochem Behav 52:189–194
Shin HJ, Gye MH, Chung KH, Yoo BS (2002) Activity of protein kinase C modulates the apoptosis induced by polychlorinated biphenyls in human leukemic HL-60 cells. Toxicol Lett 135:25–31
Siemens J, Zhou S, Piskorowski R, Nikai T, Lumpkin EA, Basbaum AI, King D, Julius D (2006) Spider toxins activate the capsaicin receptor to produce inflammatory pain. Nature 444:208–212
Simon GM, Cravatt BF (2008) Anandamide biosynthesis catalyzed by the phosphodiesterase GDE1 and detection of glycerophospho-N-acyl ethanolamine precursors in mouse brain. J Biol Chem 283:9341–9349
Simone DA, Baumann TK, Lamotte RH (1989) Dose-dependent pain and mechanical hyperalgesia in humans after intradermal injection of capsaicin. Pain 38:99–107
Simone DA, Nolano M, Johnson T, Wendelschafer-Crabb G, Kennedy WR (1998) Intradermal injection of capsaicin in humans produces degeneration and subsequent reinnervation of epidermal nerve fibers: correlation with sensory function. J Neurosci: Official J Soc Neurosci 18:8947–8959
Smith GD, Gunthorpe MJ, Kelsell RE, Hayes PD, Reilly P, Facer P, Wright JE, Jerman JC, Walhin JP, Ooi L, Egerton J, Charles KJ, Smart D, Randall AD, Anand P, Davis JB (2002) TRPV3 is a temperature-sensitive vanilloid receptor-like protein. Nature 418:186–190
Southall MD, Li T, Gharibova LS, Pei Y, Nicol GD, Travers JB (2003) Activation of epidermal vanilloid receptor-1 induces release of proinflammatory mediators in human keratinocytes. J Pharmacol Exp ther 304:217–222

Stein AT, Ufret-Vincenty CA, Hua L, Santana LF, Gordon SE (2006) Phosphoinositide 3-kinase binds to TRPV1 and mediates NGF-stimulated TRPV1 trafficking to the plasma membrane. J Gen Physiol 128:509–522

Storti B, Bizzarri R, Cardarelli F, Beltram F (2012) Intact microtubules preserve transient receptor potential vanilloid 1 (TRPV1) functionality through receptor binding. J Biol Chem 287:7803–7811

Studer M, McNaughton PA (2010) Modulation of single-channel properties of TRPV1 by phosphorylation. J Physiol 588:3743–3756

Stuhmer W, Conti F, Suzuki H, Wang XD, Noda M, Yahagi N, Kubo H, Numa S (1989) Structural parts involved in activation and inactivation of the sodium channel. Nature 339:597–603

Sun Q, Tafesse L, Islam K, Zhou X, Victory SF, Zhang C, Hachicha M, Schmid LA, Patel A, Rotshteyn Y, Valenzano KJ, Kyle DJ (2003) 4-(2-pyridyl)piperazine-1-carboxamides: potent vanilloid receptor 1 antagonists. Bioorg Med Chem Lett 13:3611–3616

Sun YX, Tsuboi K, Okamoto Y, Tonai T, Murakami M, Kudo I, Ueda N (2004) Biosynthesis of anandamide and N-palmitoylethanolamine by sequential actions of phospholipase A2 and lysophospholipase D. Biochem J 380:749–756

Swanson DM, Dubin AE, Shah C, Nasser N, Chang L, Dax SL, Jetter M, Breitenbucher JG, Liu C, Mazur C, Lord B, Gonzales L, Hoey K, Rizzolio M, Bogenstaetter M, Codd EE, Lee DH, Zhang SP, Chaplan SR, Carruthers NI (2005) Identification and biological evaluation of 4-(3-trifluoromethylpyridin-2-yl)piperazine-1-carboxylic acid (5-trifluoromethylpyridin-2-yl) amide, a high affinity TRPV1 (VR1) vanilloid receptor antagonist. J Med Chem 48:1857–1872

Szallasi A, Blumberg PM (1990) Specific binding of resiniferatoxin, an ultrapotent capsaicin analog, by dorsal root ganglion membranes. Brain Res 524:106–111

Szallasi A, Goso C, Blumberg PM, Manzini S (1993) Competitive inhibition by capsazepine of [3H]resiniferatoxin binding to central (spinal cord and dorsal root ganglia) and peripheral (urinary bladder and airways) vanilloid (capsaicin) receptors in the rat. J Pharmacol Exp Ther 267:728–733

Szallasi A, Sheta M (2012) Targeting TRPV1 for pain relief: limits, losers and laurels. Expert Opin Investig Drugs 21:1351–1369

Szoke E, Borzsei R, Toth DM, Lengl O, Helyes Z, Sandor Z, Szolcsanyi J (2010) Effect of lipid raft disruption on TRPV1 receptor activation of trigeminal sensory neurons and transfected cell line. Eur J Pharmacol 628:67–74

Szolcsányi J (2004) Forty years in capsaicin research for sensory pharmacology and physiology. Neuropeptides 38:377–384

Tafesse L, Sun Q, Schmid L, Valenzano KJ, Rotshteyn Y, Su X, Kyle DJ (2004) Synthesis and evaluation of pyridazinylpiperazines as vanilloid receptor 1 antagonists. Bioorg Med Chem Lett 14:5513–5519

Taiwo YO, Bjerknes LK, Goetzl EJ, Levine JD (1989) Mediation of primary afferent peripheral hyperalgesia by the cAMP second messenger system. Neuroscience 32:577–580

Taiwo YO, Levine JD (1990) Effects of cyclooxygenase products of arachidonic acid metabolism on cutaneous nociceptive threshold in the rat. Brain Res 537:372–374

Tender GC, Walbridge S, Olah Z, Karai L, Iadarola M, Oldfield EH, Lonser RR (2005) Selective ablation of nociceptive neurons for elimination of hyperalgesia and neurogenic inflammation. J Neurosurg 102:522–525

Thresh JC (1876a) Capsaicin, the active principle in Capsicum fruits. The Analyst 1:148–149

Thresh JC (1876b) Isolation of capsaicin. Pharm J Trans 3:941–947

Tominaga M, Caterina MJ, Malmberg AB, Rosen TA, Gilbert H, Skinner K, Raumann BE, Basbaum AI, Julius D (1998) The cloned capsaicin receptor integrates multiple pain-producing stimuli. Neuron 21:531–543

Tominaga M, Wada M, Masu M (2001) Potentiation of capsaicin receptor activity by metabotropic ATP receptors as a possible mechanism for ATP-evoked pain and hyperalgesia. Proc Natl Acad Sci USA 98:6951–6956

Touska F, Marsakova L, Teisinger J, Vlachova V (2011) A "cute" desensitization of TRPV1. Curr Pharm Biotechnol 12:122–129

Trevisani M, Smart D, Gunthorpe MJ, Tognetto M, Barbieri M, Campi B, Amadesi S, Gray J, Jerman JC, Brough SJ, Owen D, Smith GD, Randall AD, Harrison S, Bianchi A, Davis JB, Geppetti P (2002) Ethanol elicits and potentiates nociceptor responses via the vanilloid receptor-1. Nat Neurosci 5:546–551

Ueda H, Matsunaga H, Olaposi OI, Nagai J (2013a) Lysophosphatidic acid: chemical signature of neuropathic pain. Biochim Biophys Acta 1831:61–73

Ueda N, Tsuboi K, Uyama T (2013b) Metabolism of endocannabinoids and related N-acylethanolamines: canonical and alternative pathways. FEBS J 280:1874–1894

Valente P, Garcia-Sanz N, Gomis A, Fernandez-Carvajal A, Fernandez-Ballester G, Viana F, Belmonte C, Ferrer-Montiel A (2008) Identification of molecular determinants of channel gating in the transient receptor potential box of vanilloid receptor I. FASEB J 22:3298–3309

van der Stelt M, Di Marzo V (2005) Anandamide as an intracellular messenger regulating ion channel activity. Prostaglandins Other Lipid Mediat 77:111–122

van der Stelt M, Trevisani M, Vellani V, de Petrocellis L, Schiano Moriello A, Campi B, Mcnaughton P, Geppetti P, Di Marzo V (2005) Anandamide acts as an intracellular messenger amplifying Ca^{2+} influx via TRPV1 channels. EMBO J 24:3026–3037

Varga A, Jenes A, Marczylo TH, Sousa-Valente J, Chen J, Austin J, Selvarajah S, Piscitelli F, Andreou AP, Taylor AH, Kyle F, Yaqoob M, Brain S, White JP, Csernoch L, Di Marzo V, Buluwela L, Nagy I (2013) Anandamide produced by Ca^{2+}-insensitive enzymes induces excitation in primary sensory neurons. Pflugers Archiv: Europ J Physiol In Press. PMID: 24114173

Veldhuis NA, Lew MJ, Abogadie FC, Poole DP, Jennings EA, Ivanusic JJ, Eilers H, Bunnett NW, McIntyre P (2012) N-glycosylation determines ionic permeability and desensitization of the TRPV1 capsaicin receptor. J Biol Chem 287:21765–21772

Vellani V, Mapplebeck S, Moriondo A, Davis JB, McNaughton PA (2001) Protein kinase C activation potentiates gating of the vanilloid receptor VR1 by capsaicin, protons, heat and anandamide. J Physiol 534:813–825

Vellani V, Petrosino S, de Petrocellis L, Valenti M, Prandini M, Magherini PC, McNaughton PA, Di Marzo V (2008) Functional lipidomics. Calcium-independent activation of endocannabinoid/endovanilloid lipid signalling in sensory neurons by protein kinases C and A and thrombin. Neuropharmacology 55:1274–1279

Vennekens R, Voets T, Bindels RJ, Droogmans G, Nilius B (2002) Current understanding of mammalian TRP homologues. Cell Calcium 31:253–264

Vetter SW, Leclerc E (2003) Novel aspects of calmodulin target recognition and activation. Europ J Biochem/FEBS 270:404–414

Vincent HC, Lynch MJ, Pohley FM, Helgren FJ, Kirchmeyer FJ (1955) A taste panel study of cyclamate-saccharin mixture and of its components. J Am Pharm Assoc Am Pharm Assoc (Baltim) 44:442–446

Vlachova V, Teisinger J, Susankova K, Lyfenko A, Ettrich R, Vyklicky L (2003) Functional role of C-terminal cytoplasmic tail of rat vanilloid receptor 1. J Neurosci 23:1340–1350

Voets T, Owsianik G, Janssens A, Talavera K, Nilius B (2007) TRPM8 voltage sensor mutants reveal a mechanism for integrating thermal and chemical stimuli. Nat Chem Biol 3:174–182

Volff JN (2005) Genome evolution and biodiversity in teleost fish. Heredity (Edinb) 94:280–294

Vyklicky L, Novakova-Tousova K, Benedikt J, Samad A, Touska F, Vlachova V (2008) Calcium-dependent desensitization of vanilloid receptor TRPV1: a mechanism possibly involved in analgesia induced by topical application of capsaicin. Physiol Res/Academia Scientiarum Bohemoslovaca 57(Suppl 3):S59–S68

Wahl P, Foged C, Tullin S, Thomsen C (2001) Iodo-resiniferatoxin, a new potent vanilloid receptor antagonist. Mol Pharmacol 59:9–15

Walker JE, Saraste M, Runswick MJ, Gay NJ (1982) Distantly related sequences in the alpha- and beta-subunits of ATP synthase, myosin, kinases and other ATP-requiring enzymes and a common nucleotide binding fold. EMBO J 1:945–951

Walker KM, Urban L, Medhurst SJ, Patel S, Panesar M, Fox AJ, McIntyre P (2003) The VR1 antagonist capsazepine reverses mechanical hyperalgesia in models of inflammatory and neuropathic pain. J Pharmacol Exp Ther 304:56–62

Wang X, Miyares RL, Ahern GP (2005) Oleoylethanolamide excites vagal sensory neurones, induces visceral pain and reduces short-term food intake in mice via capsaicin receptor TRPV1. J Physiol 564:541–547

Webster LR, Peppin JF, Murphy FT, Lu B, Tobias JK, Vanhove GF (2011) Efficacy, safety, and tolerability of NGX-4010, capsaicin 8 % patch, in an open-label study of patients with peripheral neuropathic pain. Diab Res Clin Pract 93:187–197

Welch JM, Simon SA, Reinhart PH (2000) The activation mechanism of rat vanilloid receptor 1 by capsaicin involves the pore domain and differs from the activation by either acid or heat. Proc Natl Acad Sci U S A 97:13889–13894

White JP, Urban L, Nagy I (2011) TRPV1 function in health and disease. Curr Pharm Biotechnol 12:130–144

Woo DH, Jung SJ, Zhu MH, Park CK, Kim YH, Oh SB, Lee CJ (2008a) Direct activation of transient receptor potential vanilloid 1(TRPV1) by diacylglycerol (DAG). Mol pain 4:42

Woo DH, Jung SJ, Zhu MH, Park CK, Kim YH, Oh SB, Lee CJ (2008b) Direct activation of transient receptor potential vanilloid 1(TRPV1) by diacylglycerol (DAG). Mol Pain 4:42

Wood JN, Winter J, James IF, Rang HP, Yeats J, Bevan S (1988) Capsaicin-induced ion fluxes in dorsal root ganglion cells in culture. J Neurosci 8:3208–3220

Wu ZZ, Chen SR, Pan HL (2006) Signaling mechanisms of down-regulation of voltage-activated Ca^{2+} channels by transient receptor potential vanilloid type 1 stimulation with olvanil in primary sensory neurons. Neuroscience 141:407–419

Xu H, Blair NT, Clapham DE (2005) Camphor activates and strongly desensitizes the transient receptor potential vanilloid subtype 1 channel in a vanilloid-independent mechanism. J Neurosci 25:8924–8937

Xu ZZ, Zhang L, Liu T, Park JY, Berta T, Yang R, Serhan CN, Ji RR (2010) Resolvins RvE1 and RvD1 attenuate inflammatory pain via central and peripheral actions. Nat Med 16:592–597. 1p following 597

Yang F, Cui Y, Wang K, Zheng J (2010) Thermosensitive TRP channel pore turret is part of the temperature activation pathway. Proc Natl Acad Sci U S A 107:7083–7088

Yao J, Qin F (2009) Interaction with phosphoinositides confers adaptation onto the TRPV1 pain receptor. PLoS Biol 7:e46

Yoshida T, Inoue R, Morii T, Takahashi N, Yamamoto S, Hara Y, Tominaga M, Shimizu S, Sato Y, Mori Y (2006) Nitric oxide activates TRP channels by cysteine S-nitrosylation. Nat Chem Biol 2:596–607

Zhang X, Huang J, McNaughton PA (2005) NGF rapidly increases membrane expression of TRPV1 heat-gated ion channels. EMBO J 24:4211–4223

Zhang X, Li L, McNaughton PA (2008) Proinflammatory mediators modulate the heat-activated ion channel TRPV1 via the scaffolding protein AKAP79/150. Neuron 59:450–461

Zygmunt PM, Petersson J, Andersson DA, Chuang H, Sorgard M, Di Marzo V, Julius D, Hogestatt ED (1999) Vanilloid receptors on sensory nerves mediate the vasodilator action of anandamide. Nature 400:452–457

Chapter 3
TRPV1 in the Central Nervous System: Synaptic Plasticity, Function, and Pharmacological Implications

Jeffrey G. Edwards

Abstract The function of TRPV1 in the peripheral nervous system is increasingly being investigated for its anti-inflammatory and antinociceptive properties in an effort to find a novel target to fight pain that is nonaddictive. However, in recent years, it was discovered that TRPV1 is also associated with a wide array of functions and behaviors in the central nervous system, such as fear, anxiety, stress, thermoregulation, pain, and, more recently, synaptic plasticity, the cellular mechanism that allows the brain to adapt to its environment. This suggests a new role for brain TRPV1 in areas such as learning and memory, reward and addiction, and development. This wide array of functional aspects of TRPV1 in the central nervous system (CNS) is in part due to its multimodal form of activation and highlights the potential pharmacological implications of TRPV1 in the brain. As humans also express a TRPV1 homologue, it is likely that animal research will be translational to humans and therefore worthy of exploration. This review outlines the basic expression patterns of TRPV1 in the CNS along with what is known regarding its signaling mechanisms and its role in the aforementioned brain functions. As TRPV1 involvement in synaptic plasticity has never been fully reviewed elsewhere, it will be a focus of this review. The chapter concludes with some of the potential pharmaceutical implications of further TRPV1 research.

3.1 Introduction

TRPV1 is a nonselective calcium-permeable cation channel involved in nociceptive circuits in the peripheral nervous system (PNS) and various functions including synaptic plasticity in the central nervous system (CNS). TRPV1 is highly

---

J. G. Edwards (✉)
Physiology and Developmental Biology, Brigham Young University, Neuroscience Center
575 WIDB, Provo, UT 84602, USA
e-mail: Jeffrey_edwards@byu.edu

O. M. E. Abdel-Salam (ed.), *Capsaicin as a Therapeutic Molecule*, Progress in Drug Research 68, DOI: 10.1007/978-3-0348-0828-6_3, © Springer Basel 2014

expressed in the PNS, including in dorsal root ganglia, trigeminal ganglia, and primary sensory neurons (Szallasi and Blumberg 1991; Helliwell et al. 1998), where it is being examined for its anti-inflammatory and antinociceptive properties (Caterina et al. 2000; Nagy et al. 2004; Palazzo et al. 2008). This is important considering its multimodal activation properties that could integrate many types of painful stimuli (Tominaga et al. 1998) as it is activated by low pH, various ligands, and physical stimuli such as temperature. In addition, TRPV1 is also present, albeit at lower levels, in the brain (Mezey et al. 2000), including hippocampus, amygdala, and hypothalamus, where it was identified using various techniques, including immunocytochemistry, quantitative RT-PCR, and in situ hybridization (Mezey et al. 2000; Cristino et al. 2006; Toth et al. 2005; Roberts et al. 2004; Merrill et al. 2012).

It should be noted, however, that TRPV1 expression in the CNS has been debated for two main reasons. First, in contrast to previous studies, one report using TRPV1 reporter mice identified very restricted TRPV1 expression in the brain, with the highest levels primarily in the hypothalamus (Cavanaugh et al. 2011). Second, considering the important role TRPV1 plays as a sensory receptor in the PNS, some have questioned the necessity of a function for TRPV1 in the CNS as TRPV1 is thermal sensitive and thus activated by moderate thermal stimuli at a temperature >42–43 °C. It is also activated exogenously by capsaicin (Tominaga and Tominaga 2005; Caterina et al. 1997; Caterina 2007), the component in chili peppers that mediates the "hot" or pain sensation of spicy foods. Therefore, the question is could TRPV1, which is highly expressed in the PNS and involved in sensation, be involved in brain function where it has ~20–25-fold lower expression in rodents (Sanchez et al. 2001; Han et al. 2013), and are these lower expression levels even physiologically or behaviorally relevant? One part of this question could be answered by the fact that TRPV1 is both multimodal and is activated by many different ligands, suggesting that activation of TRPV1 may be variable depending on the specific region in which it is expressed.

Recently, several studies attempted to answer the question regarding the physiological and behavioral relevance of TRPV1 in the CNS. First, endogenous ligands (in addition to exogenous capsaicin) for TRPV1 and enzymes that produce these ligands are expressed in the brain. These include endocannabinoids/eicosanoids/endovanilloids, such as N-arachidonoyl-ethanolamine (anandamide), N-arachidonoyl-dopamine (NADA) (Huang et al. 2002), oleoylethanolamide (Ahern 2003), and N-oleoyldopamine (Chu et al. 2003), arachidonic acid derivatives, such as 12-hydroperoxyeicosa-tetraenoic acid (12-HPETE) (Gibson et al. 2008), and finally N-acylethanolamines (Movahed et al. 2005), among others. This extremely large number of endogenous ligands for one receptor has been the topic of a recent review (Di Marzo and De Petrocellis 2012) and suggests a role for this TRPV1 characteristic in potential function. Second, many studies now illustrate that TRPV1 is physiologically relevant in the CNS where reported functions include behavioral anxiolytic effects following TRPV1 antagonism (Santos et al. 2008; Kasckow et al. 2004; Micale et al. 2008), contextual fear learning and plasticity using TRPV1 knockout (TRPV1$^{-/-}$) mice (Marsch et al. 2007), visual development in the superior colliculus (Maione et al. 2009), and improved spatial memory retrieval under stressful conditions in response to TRPV1 activation (Li et al. 2008). In addition, presynaptic TRPV1 in the hippocampus is involved in inhibitory interneuron synaptic plasticity (Gibson et al. 2008). This was the first demonstration of TRPV1 involvement in synaptic plasticity, the critical cellular mechanism used by the brain to allow animals to adapt and respond to changes in their environment, a function known as experience-dependent or use-dependent plasticity. Following this initial description of TRPV1 involvement in hippocampal plasticity, other researchers identified TRPV1-dependent plasticity in other brain regions, suggesting it could be an important mechanism used throughout the brain. Therefore, just like many other proteins that can be present and necessary in both the PNS and CNS, such as the Na^+/K^+ ATP-ase transporter, which is expressed in both the brain and kidney, TRPV1 appears to play important yet distinct roles in both the PNS and the CNS.

In summary, while there has been some debate regarding TRPV1 expression in the brain, there is now a substantial accumulation of data demonstrating TRPV1 function in the CNS. One of the focuses of this chapter will be the role TRPV1 plays in CNS synaptic plasticity and signaling pathways, with a focus particularly on the hippocampus, the declarative memory center of the brain. This chapter also presents other major functions of TRPV1 in the CNS, such as its association with anxiety, analgesia, behavior, thermoregulation, etc., as well as its potential pharmaceutical applications. In order to provide a framework for the following chapter review of TRPV1 function in the CNS, I will first outline CNS TRPV1 expression and function.

3.2 Brain TRPV1 Expression and Function

Using radiolabeled TRPV1 ligand, RNA expression and PCR, western blot, and immunoprecipitation, TRPV1 has been identified in the CNS of humans, rats, and mice. In rodents, TRPV1 expression is located in major brain areas, including the forebrain, the limbic system, the diencephalon, and midbrain. Regional expression of these major areas include cerebellum, cortex, hippocampus, dentate gyrus, amygdala, habenula, hypothalamus, suprachiasmatic nucleus, inferior olive, substantia nigra, among others (Mezey et al. 2000; Sanchez et al. 2001; Roberts et al. 2004; Szabo et al. 2002; Acs et al. 1996; Cortright et al. 2001; Han et al. 2013; Hayes et al. 2000). It is important to highlight that a TRPV1 homologue with 92 % similarity to rats is present in humans (Hayes et al. 2000). Human TRPV1 is located on the chromosome site 17p13, and similar to rodents is activated by capsaicin, low pH, and temperature. Also similar to rodent TRPV1, human TRPV1 is expressed in the cerebellum, the hippocampus, and the frontal cortex as well as in the dorsal root ganglia. Interestingly, while rat TRPV1 is expressed ~25 times higher in dorsal root ganglia than in the CNS, human TRPV1 is expressed only 6–7 times higher in the dorsal root ganglia than in the CNS, suggesting an even greater potential for TRPV1 functionality in the human CNS. Human TRPV1 expression is an important consideration as it suggests that studies of rodent TRPV1 are likely translational in nature to humans. Therefore, information gleaned from research with rodents, where most TRPV1 data originates, will likely apply to humans, which is the focus of this chapter.

In outlining TRPV1 expression, this chapter will begin with the hippocampus, a major emphasis of this review. In the hippocampus, cellular localization of TRPV1 was identified within hippocampal pyramidal cells and astrocytes but is absent from most, but not all, interneurons. Expression was noted using varied techniques, including examination through either (1) protein expression via standard immunocytochemistry, electron microscopy, or western blot; (2) mRNA expression via RT-PCR; or (3) whole cell recordings (Cristino et al. 2006; Toth et al. 2005; Gibson et al. 2008; Bennion et al. 2011; Merrill et al. 2012; Cristino et al. 2008). Specifically, TRPV1 is present in CA1 and CA3 pyramidal cell somas; the dentate gyrus, including the molecular layer; and punctate of hippocampal layers within the stratum oriens and stratum radiatum. This punctate was located in postsynaptic dendrites along with some expression in presynaptic terminals in CA1. Using immunocytochemistry, TRPV1 expression in CA3 and CA1 pyramidal cells was determined to be homogeneous within most cells and within just some interneurons of the oriens (Cristino et al. 2008). Using RT-PCR, TRPV1 was identified within 50 % of CA3 cells (Merrill et al. 2012), while CA1 cells were not examined. Rare interneurons of the stratum radiatum are positive for TRPV1 using RT-PCR (unpublished observation of the author).

The location of expression of physiologically relevant TRPV1 includes both presynaptic and postsynaptic domains. When expressed presynaptically, TRPV1 usually enhances the release of the excitatory neurotransmitter glutamate, for example, in the substantia nigra (Marinelli et al. 2003; Starowicz et al. 2007), hypothalamus (Sasamura et al. 1998), and other regions (Jennings et al. 2003). However, there are some important exceptions in which presynaptic TRPV1 depressed glutamate release in synaptic plasticity (Gibson et al. 2008; Maione et al. 2009). Postsynaptically TRPV1often activates calcium-sensitive signaling pathways and in several cases mediates synaptic plasticity as well (Chavez et al. 2010).

In the hippocampus TRPV1 is physiologically present and modulates synaptic activity (Gibson et al. 2008; Marsch et al. 2007; Santos et al. 2008; Al-Hayani et al. 2001; Li et al. 2008; Chavez et al. 2010; Bennion et al. 2011). Al-Hayani et al. (2001) reported that TRPV1 agonists selectively increase paired-pulse depression in a dose-dependent fashion, which was blocked by the TRPV1 antagonist capsazepine; this is the first demonstration of TRPV1 functioning in the hippocampus at the synaptic level. Subsequently, other studies demonstrated TRPV1 involvement in the plasticity of synapses causing long-term changes, beginning with the finding that TRPV1 was required for a novel form of plasticity known as long-term depression (Gibson et al. 2008). As the study of the TRPV1 involvement in plasticity is fairly new and has been only briefly reviewed previously (Cachope 2012; Di Marzo and De Petrocellis 2012), it will be a primary focus of this chapter.

3.3 Synaptic Plasticity

Synaptic plasticity is a critical phenomenon used by the brain for adapting or learning from experiences in our environment, also known as experience-dependent plasticity. The study of synaptic plasticity involves determining how mammalian brains can alter their synapses, a cellular mechanism involved in functions ranging from learning and memory, to reward and addiction, to brain development. Many types of plasticity are dependent on the N-methyl-D-aspartate (NMDA) glutamate receptors, which function as a coincidence detector of simultaneous presynaptic and postsynaptic activity. If a receptor or signaling molecule is required for a certain type of plasticity, such as the NMDA receptor, it is a mediator. If a receptor alters the properties of the plasticity but is not required for it, it is a modulator.

For NMDA-dependent plasticity, calcium entry via NMDA receptors activates signaling pathways that either enhance or inhibit synaptic neurotransmission. Enhanced neurotransmission is known as long-term potentiation (LTP) and is usually due to increased presynaptic neurotransmitter release or increased postsynaptic receptors, such as insertion of α-amino-3-hydroxy-5-methyl-4-isoxazolepropionic acid (AMPA) glutamate receptors into the postsynaptic membrane. Depressed neurotransmission is long-term depression (LTD) and results from decreased presynaptic neurotransmitter release or decreased postsynaptic receptor numbers that are removed from the synapse. Both LTP and LTD occur in the hippocampus, the critical brain region required for declarative and spatial memories. Both can be induced in vitro using various stimulation protocols. High-frequency stimulation (50–100 Hz) usually induces LTP and low-frequency stimulation (1–5 Hz) induces LTD. The hippocampus is made up of a trisynaptic pathway with information coming from the entorhinal cortex into the dentate gyrus subfield and from there to the Cornu Ammonis 3 (CA3) and CA1 subfields. CA1 LTP is one of the most heavily studied types of plasticity in the brain. As TRPV1 is highly calcium-permeable, similar to NMDA, it is also a great candidate for triggering calcium-induced cell signaling, such as occurs to initiate plasticity.

3.3.1 Hippocampal Long-Term Potentiation

Regarding studies of TRPV1 involvement in NMDA receptor-dependent hippocampal CA1 LTP, TRPV1 *modulation* of plasticity was first demonstrated when CA1 LTP in TRPV1$^{-/-}$ mice was reduced compared to wild-type control mice (Marsch et al. 2007). This illustrated for the first time that TRPV1 could modulate this highly studied type of plasticity. A study published the following year supported this finding as TRPV1 agonists facilitated NMDA receptor-dependent CA1 LTP, albeit in rats, which was blocked by TRPV1 antagonists, capsazepine, and SB366791 (Li et al. 2008). Collectively, the genetic elimination of TRPV1 reduced LTP, while TRPV1 activation by agonists enhanced LTP, suggesting a real role for TRPV1 in modulating CA1 LTP.

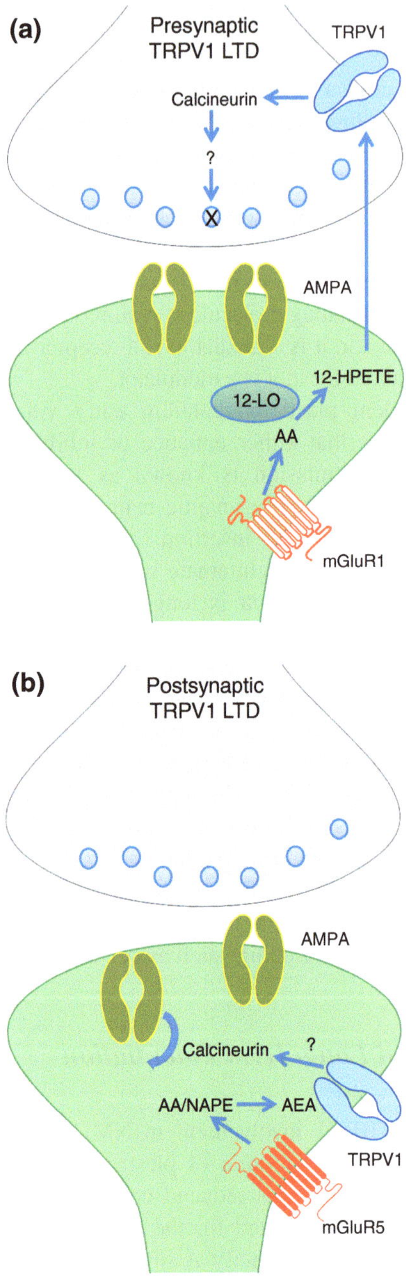
(a)
Presynaptic
TRPV1 LTD
TRPV1
Calcineurin
?
X
AMPA
12-HPETE
12-LO
AA
mGluR1
(b)
Postsynaptic
TRPV1 LTD
AMPA
Calcineurin
?
AA/NAPE
AEA
TRPV1
mGluR5

◀ **Fig. 3.1** Schematic Representation of TRPV1 LTD. **a** Presynaptic TRPV1 LTD, while mediated at the presynaptic terminal depressing glutamate neurotransmitter release, requires formation of postsynaptic 12-HPETE in order to activate TRPV1. 12-HPETE is formed by the enzyme 12-lipoxygenase (12-LO) using arachidonic acid (AA) as a metabolic precursor, which is liberated subsequent to mGluR1 activation. Once TRPV1 is activated presynaptically, it results in activation of the protein phosphatase calcineurin, which through an unknown mechanism (?) inhibits neurotransmission (as illustrated with an 'x'). **b** Postsynaptic LTD results from endocytosis of AMPA glutamate receptors. Postsynaptic mGluR5 and TRPV1 activation along with anandamide (AEA) formation are required for this LTD. While the exact pathway of AEA formation and its effect is not completely known, AEA usually is formed from the conversion of metabolic precursor N-arachidonoyl phosphatidylethanolamine (NAPE) phospholipase D, and once formed AEA likely targets TRPV1. TRPV1 then potentially results in the activation of calcineurin (?), which through clathrin-dependent mechanisms induces endocytosis of AMPA receptors. It should be noted that the exact location of TRPV1 in both cases is not specifically known as TRPV1 could be expressed by the plasma membrane or by intracellular membranes regulating internal calcium release

While these data illustrate TRPV1 involvement in hippocampal plasticity, the mechanism by which TRPV1 modulates hippocampal CA1 LTP was not determined. This mechanism was later identified which will be described below, but only after the discovery of a novel form of hippocampal plasticity that was directly *mediated* by TRPV1. In this case, TRPV1 directly induced plasticity of inhibitory hippocampal GABAergic interneurons (Gibson et al. 2008). Hippocampal inhibitory feedforward interneurons in the stratum radiatum underwent high-frequency stimulus-induced LTD. This LTD was dependent on postsynaptic activation of metabotropic glutamate receptor 1 (mGluR1) followed by presynaptic TRPV1 stimulation. In this pathway, mGluR1 induced increases in intracellular calcium, resulting in the formation of 12-(S)-Hydroperoxyeicosa-5Z, 8Z, 10E, 14Z-tetraenoic acid (12-HPETE) from arachidonic acid cleavage via the enzyme 12-lipoxygenase. 12-HPETE was then retrogradely diffused or transported across the synapse and activated presynaptic TRPV1 receptors on glutamate inputs, depressing transmitter release (Fig. 3.1a). The identification of this plasticity suggested a possible mechanism for TRPV1 enhancement of CA1 NMDA-dependent LTP. When inhibitory feedforward interneurons, which innervate pyramidal cells in the CA1, are depressed by LTD, CA1 pyramidal cells could be disinhibited, allowing them to exhibit larger LTP. This was confirmed by the fact that the $GABA_A$ antagonist picrotoxin blocked CA1 LTP enhancement by TRPV1 agonists resiniferatoxin and capsaicin (Fig. 3.2a, b). In essence picrotoxin eliminates fast inhibition mediated by interneurons from the circuit (Bennion et al. 2011) (see Fig. 3.2c). Therefore, TRPV1 activation reduced GABA inhibition onto CA1 pyramidal cells, allowing for enhanced LTP. This was later supported by a genetic study in which the reduction in CA1 LTP in $TRPV1^{-/-}$ mice could be rescued back to wild-type levels by picrotoxin (Brown et al. 2013). Therefore, TRPV1 modulates LTP of hippocampal output CA1 pyramidal cells via synaptic plasticity of feedforward interneurons.

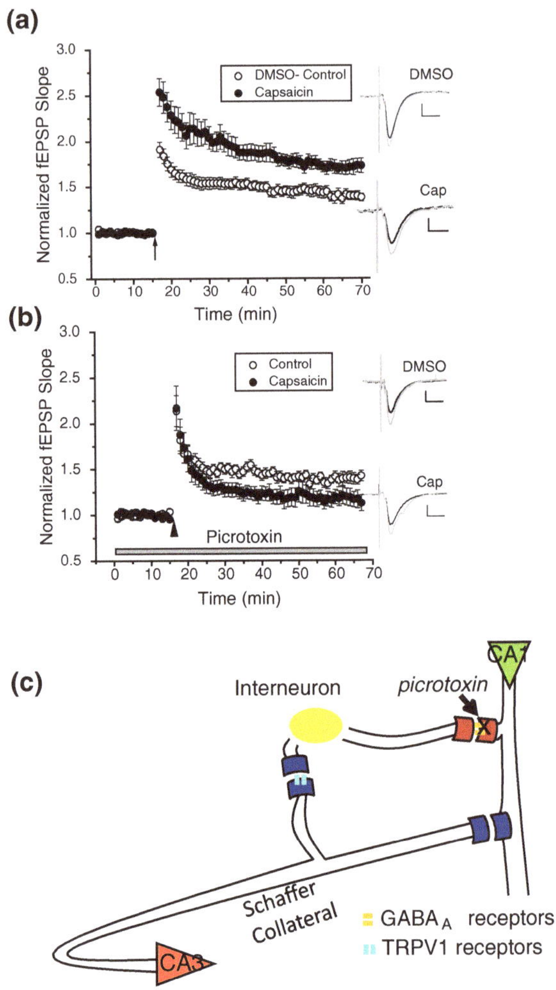

One interesting conundrum concerning the TRPV1-mediated LTD is that while normally presynaptic TRPV1 enhances glutamate neurotransmission, as TRPV1 is calcium-permeable and thus enhances presynaptic calcium and transmitter release levels, in this case TRPV1 depressed transmitter release. It turns out that TRPV-mediated LTD requires activation of the phosphatase calcineurin by TRPV1, in order to induce LTD. This data will be more fully addressed later on.

Collectively, these data suggest that TRPV1 is normally involved in NMDA receptor-dependent LTP. Since TRPV1 plays a role in plasticity, TRPV1 could be used as a neuromodulator target in the effort to potentially enhance plasticity and therefore theoretically enhance memory formation.

◀ **Fig. 3.2** TRPV1-induced enhancement of CA1 pyramidal cell long-term potentiation (LTP) is blocked by $GABA_A$ antagonist picrotoxin. **a** The TRPV1 agonist capsaicin (1 μM), significantly increased ($p < 0.05$; $n = 14$) theta burst (*arrow*)-induced LTP as compared to dimethyl sulfoxide (DMSO) vehicle control (0.1 % DMSO; $n = 20$), as measured using field excitatory postsynaptic potentials (fEPSPs). **b** Picrotoxin (100 μM) significantly blocked the capsaicin-induced enhancement of LTP ($p < 0.05$; $n = 8$) compared to control ($n = 17$). Insets: an average of 15 traces either just before (*black*) or 28–30 min after (*gray*) conditioning stimulus. Scale Bars: 0.25 mV, 10 ms. Figure 3.2 parts a and b were reprinted with permission from Bennion et al. (2011). **c** A schematic model representing the effect of picrotoxin in the hippocampal circuit. CA3 pyramidal cell axons form the Schaffer Collateral pathway innervate the CA1 subfield and synapse onto both CA1 pyramidal cells and CA1 inhibitory interneurons. Interneurons use GABA as an inhibitory neurotransmitter that binds to postsynaptic $GABA_A$ receptors, which mediate fast inhibition onto pyramidal cells. TRPV1 located presynaptically at the Schaffer Collateral synapse onto the interneurons induce LTD when activated (see Fig. 3.1a) and thus reduce inhibition from the interneurons to the CA1 pyramidal cells, known as disinhibition. In the presence of capsaicin to induce TRPV1 LTD, LTP of CA1 pyramidal cells is enhanced (see **a** this figure). In the presence of picrotoxin, which eliminates the effect of the interneurons from the hippocampal circuit, this capsaicin-induced enhancement of CA1 LTP is blocked (see **b** this figure); indicating TRPV1 acting through the interneuron pathway is required for enhanced CA1 pyramidal cell LTP

3.3.2 Hippocampal Long-Term Depression

Recent studies examined TRPV1 modulation of various forms of hippocampal LTD following the demonstration of TRPV1 modulation of NMDA receptor-dependent LTP in CA1 pyramidal cells. Hippocampal LTD is a mechanism thought to depotentiate synapses that have undergone LTP and could be used to eliminate harmful memories or allow for new memory formation, among other potential options. These studies identified that TRPV1 is indeed likely involved in several types of hippocampal LTD, including (1) in the dentate gyrus, (2) mGluR-dependent CA1 LTD, and (3) NMDA-dependent CA1 LTD, which will be discussed in turn.

A novel postsynaptic LTD mediated by TRPV1 was identified in the dentate gyrus (Chavez et al. 2010). Dentate gyrus granule cells innervated by the medial perforant pathway underwent postsynaptic LTD via clathrin-dependent internalization of AMPA receptors in response to capsaicin application or a 1 Hz pairing protocol that was TRPV1-dependent. TRPV1-induced LTD in the dentate gyrus was confirmed using $TRPV1^{-/-}$ mice, supporting the study's pharmacological data (see model in Fig. 3.1b). Interestingly, in contrast to CA1, where presynaptic TRPV1 activation required postsynaptic mGluR1 and 12-HPETE formation; in the dentate gyrus, postsynaptic TRPV1 activation required postsynaptic mGluR5 and anandamide production. Therefore, TRPV1-dependent LTD in the hippocampus can differ fairly dramatically depending on the hippocampal subfield. However, similar to CA1, dentate gyrus LTD was also calcineurin-dependent, suggesting calcineurin may play a key role in TRPV1 signaling in the hippocampus.

Another major type of hippocampal synaptic plasticity is mGluR-dependent LTD, in contrast to NMDA-dependent LTD. Regarding CA1 mGluR-dependent

LTD, previous studies proposed that the initial acute depression of it was mediated by a cannabinoid receptor 1 (CB1)–independent endocannabinoid pathway (Rouach and Nicoll 2003), though what this endocannabinoid pathway could be, was not known. One report suggests this CB1-independent acute depression could be TRPV1 induced. In this case, initiating mGluR-dependent LTD using the type I mGluR agonist DHPG while examining the acute depression phase, the TRPV1 antagonist capsazepine actually caused an increase in the depression (Bennion et al. 2011). This implied a role for TRPV1, though capsaicin application caused no further change in the depression. Taken together, however, the fact that capsazepine caused an increase in depression suggests that when activated normally, TRPV1 mitigates some of the acute depression of mGluR-dependent LTD, and since capsaicin had no effect, TRPV1 is already probably close to being fully activated in response to DHPG application. Type I mGluRs activated by DHPG thus likely result in the production of a TRPV1 agonist, such as anandamide or 12-HPETE, to activate TRPV1. Thus when TRPV1 is blocked, the acute depression is even greater by eliminating the mitigating effect of TRPV1 on depressed glutamate neurotransmission. The TRPV1 involved in acute DHPG-induced depression is most likely present on CA1 pyramidal cells rather than the TRPV1 modulating interneuron activity, as the acute depression in the presence of capsazepine is not altered by the $GABA_A$ antagonist picrotoxin. While TRPV1 altered acute short-term depression, it was not involved in true LTD or long-lasting depression of duration greater than 15 min.

Regarding CA1 NMDA-dependent LTD, in one report, TRPV1 agonist capsaicin (1 mM) caused a reduction of LTD induced by 3 Hz stimulation, an effect that was eliminated by capsazepine (Li et al. 2008), suggesting that TRPV1 can modulate CA1 NMDA-dependent LTD. However, while this study enticingly suggests that TRPV1 is involved in CA1 LTD, the concentration of capsaicin used can have off-target effects, including increasing intracellular calcium in a TRPV1-indendent manner. A subsequent study using a lower, more TRPV1-specific concentration of capsaicin (1–10 μM) and 5 Hz stimulation noted no change in LTD (Bennion et al. 2011). While several variables differed between these two reports and could be the reason for the discrepancy, no conclusive evidence can be reached at this time regarding TRPV1 involvement in CA1 NMDA-dependent LTD.

Collectively, while TRPV1 involvement in CA1 NMDA-dependent LTD is debatable, TRPV1 is likely involved in short-term acute depression of mGluR-dependent LTD, and strong evidence supports it mediating a novel form of LTD in the CA1 and dentate gyrus.

3.3.3 Plasticity in Other CNS Regions

After TRPV1-dependent synaptic plasticity was reported in the hippocampus, TRPV1-dependent types of plasticity were identified in other brain regions as well. One such example is in the superior colliculus, which is a classic model used to examine the synaptic refinement or pruning that occurs in the developing visual system via mechanisms such as LTD, which can cause a weakening or loss of synapses. High-frequency stimulus-induced LTD of the superior colliculus, as measured using field excitatory postsynaptic potentials, was blocked with TRPV1 antagonists and mimicked using TRPV1 agonists (Maione et al. 2009). The developmental timing of the ability to induce LTD also coincided with temporal TRPV1 expression as measured using TRPV1 antibodies. TRPV1 receptor expression and TRPV1-dependent LTD were both present in young animals but absent in adults. Juvenile TRPV1 expression occurs in GABAergic cells of the superior colliculus and on glutamatergic retinal inputs to the superior colliculus where TRPV1 is likely presynaptically expressed in the latter, similar to glutamatergic input to CA1 stratum radiatum interneurons. It appears that this plasticity modulates the GABA pathway to induce LTD as GABA receptor blockers eliminated this LTD. In summary, TRPV1 could be developmentally involved in the CNS by regulating synaptic pruning, the elimination of incorrect and unnecessary synapses.

In addition to the superior colliculus, the amygdala, which is part of the limbic system along with the hippocampus, has also altered plasticity in the presence of capsaicin (Zschenderlein et al. 2011). Interestingly, TRPV1-induced alteration of amygdalar LTP was dependent on the type of anesthetic used on the animal, with ether producing decreased LTP and isoflurane producing increased LTP. These results were confirmed using TRPV1$^{-/-}$ mice. In addition, in the presence of ether, the TRPV1 agonist N-oleoyldopamine also depressed amygdala lateral nucleus LTP (Kulisch and Albrecht 2013). In this case stress was also examined, and research demonstrated that TRPV1 activation by N-oleoyldopamine inhibited stress-induced depression of LTP by forced swim test. The exact mechanism of this TRPV1 pathway and how TRPV1 altered amygdala LTP was not completely determined, though nitric oxide synthase was required. Along with modulation of amygdala LTP, TRPV1 was also required for a type of amygdala LTD. In the extended amygdala, neurons from the bed nucleus of the stria terminalis exhibit TRPV1-dependent LTD (Puente et al. 2011). This postsynaptic form of plasticity required the activation of postsynaptic TRPV1 via anandamide, which was formed as a result of postsynaptic mGluR5 stimulation, very similar to TRPV1-dependent LTD in the dentate gyrus (Chavez et al. 2010).

The midbrain also demonstrates plasticity via TRPV1 in both the nucleus accumbens and the substantia nigra. The nucleus accumbens is especially important for reward and reward-dependent learning, which can be modulated by the drugs of abuse that alter normal plasticity, leading to addictive states. Addiction results in behaviors and actions that are carried out inspite of the negative consequences. In medium spiny neurons of the nucleus accumbens, mGluR5-induced endocannabinoid production is required for postsynaptic TRPV1-mediated LTD initiated by either low-frequency stimulus or the type I mGluR agonist DHPG (Grueter et al. 2010). This LTD required activation of both mGluR5 and TRPV1 receptors as demonstrated using various antagonists and TRPV1$^{-/-}$ mice. TRPV1 induced postsynaptic AMPA receptor endocytosis, again similar to TRPV1-LTD in the hippocampus and amygdala. Interestingly, the injection of cocaine 24 h prior to the physiological experiments altered this plasticity by blocking it. This suggests that TRPV1 plays a role synaptically and behaviorally in the reward pathways of the brain and could be involved in addiction at the nucleus accumbens level. In this study TRPV1$^{-/-}$ mice also demonstrated enhanced locomotion in response to cocaine injection, supporting a role for TRPV1 in motor pathways. Finally, dopamine release in the nucleus accumbens can also be enhanced by TRPV1 activation of dopamine neurons in the ventral tegmental area via glutamate, which activates the nucleus accumbens following noxious stimulation (Marinelli et al. 2005). This further supports a role for TRPV1 in the midbrain reward pathways.

As a note, it is worth mentioning that a form of TRPV-like mediated LTD is exhibited in leeches, an invertebrate. This LTD occurs at nociceptive synapses and is dependent on presynaptic TRPV-like receptors activated by postsynaptically produced endocannabinoids and is also calcineurin-dependent (Yuan and Burrell 2010, 2012). This type of plasticity is extremely similar to presynaptic TRPV1-mediated LTD in hippocampal interneurons (Gibson et al. 2008) and is also dependent on presynaptic protein synthesis and postsynaptic synthesis of mRNA and protein (Yuan and Burrell 2013). While the requirement of transcription and translation in mammalian CNS TRPV1 plasticity has yet to be investigated, it is likely similar to leeches as many forms of plasticity are dependent on protein synthesis.

In summary, there is now substantial data supporting the role of TRPV1 in synaptic plasticity in divergent brain regions, including acting as a mediator of LTD and a modulator of LTP. Therefore, TRPV1 has the potential to be a widespread regulator of adaptive brain function via synaptic alterations in brain areas required for learning and memory, visual development, and the reward pathways, including drug-induced alterations in reward plasticity. The involvement of TRPV1 in synaptic plasticity is summarized in Table 3.1.

3.4 Endogenous TRPV1 Activity

3.4.1 Endogenous CNS TRPV1 Ligands

As changes in pH and temperature are relatively small and likely insufficient to activate TRPV1 in the CNS, lipid-based ligands are the most likely endogenous activators. Various fatty acid derivatives that activate TRPV1 are endogenously produced in the CNS. These ligands are thought not to be released by standard vesicle chemical neurotransmission mechanisms but are locally acting signal molecules, functioning in paracrine/autocrine or intracellular messenger fashion. Endogenously produced TRPV1 CNS ligands include several

Table 3.1 TRPV1 involvement in the modulation and mediation of mammalian CNS synaptic plasticity

	Plasticity type	Location	TRPV1- pre or post	Effect	mGluR	eCB	Induction	Signal molecule	Reference
Modulate	LTP	Hippocampal CA1 pyramidal cells		Enhanced LTP			HFS (100 Hz)	ND	Li et al. (2008)
		Hippocampal CA1 pyramidal cells	Postsynaptic likely	Enhanced LTP mediated by disinhibition via interneurons			Theta burst, HFS	ND	Bennion et al. (2011)
		Hippocampal CA1 pyramidal cells		Reduced LTP in $TRPV1^{-/-}$			HFS (100 Hz)	ND	Marsch et al. (2007)
		Hippocampal CA1 pyramidal cells		Reduced LTP in $TRPV1^{-/-}$ rescued to WT with GABA antagonist			HFS (100 Hz)	ND	Brown et al. (2013)
		Amygdala, lateral nucleus	Pre and Postsynaptic, alters glutamate	Depressed LTP in ether, enhanced LTP in isoflurane		Anandamide likely	HFS (100 Hz), capsaicin	Nitric Oxide Synthase	Zschenderlein et al. (2011)
		Amygdala, lateral nucleus	Pre and Postsynaptic, alters glutamate	Depressed LTP (ether), blocked stress-induced impairment of LTP		N-oleoyldopamine	HFS (100 Hz), w/w out N-oleoyldopamine		Kulisch and Albrecht (2013)
	LTD	Hippocampal CA1 pyramidal cells		Reduction in LTD			LFS (3 Hz)	ND	Li et al. (2008)

(continued)

Table 3.1 (continued)

	Plasticity type	Location	TRPV1- pre or post	Effect	mGluR	eCB	Induction	Signal molecule	Reference
		Hippocampal CA1 pyramidal cells	Postsynaptic likely	No change in LTD			LFS (5 Hz)	ND	Bennion et. al. (2011)
	mGluR-LTD	Hippocampal CA1 pyramidal cells	Postsynaptic likely	Mitigate acute depression, no effect on LTD	Type I mGluRs		DHPG	ND	Bennion et al. (2011)
Mediate	LTD	Hippocampal CA1 interneurons	Presynaptic	Depressed glutamate release	mGluR1	12-HPETE	HFS, TRPV1 agonists	Calcineurin, Ca^{2+}	Gibson et al. (2008); Jensen and Edwards (2012)
		Superior colliculus	Presynaptic likely	Induce LTD, GABA system involved	ND	Anandamide or 12-HPETE possibly	HFS (50 Hz), TRPV1 agonist	ND	Maione et al. (2009)
		Hippocampal dentate gyrus	Postsynaptic	AMPA receptor endocytosis	mGluR5	Anandamide	LFS, TRPV1 agonists	Calcineurin, Ca^{2+}	Chavez et al. (2010)
		Nucleus accumbens-MSNs	Postsynaptic	AMPA receptor endocytosis	mGluR5	ND	LFS (3 Hz); Capsaicin	Ca^{2+}	Grueter et al. (2010)
		Amygdala, stria terminalis	Postsynaptic	ND	mGluR5	Anandamide	LFS (10 Hz)	Ca^{2+}	Puente et al. (2011)

Abbreviations: ND, not determined; HFS, high frequency stimulus; LFS, low frequency stimulus

C18 N-acylethanolamines, such as endovanilloid N-oleoylethanolamine (Movahed et al. 2005), N-arachidonoyl-dopamine, 12-HPETE, and anandamide (Tóth et al. 2009). These all bind TRPV1 in the hippocampus (Ahern 2003; Al-Hayani et al. 2001; Gibson et al. 2008; Huang et al. 2002). 12-HPETE is also produced in the hippocampus by stimulation protocols used for synaptic plasticity (Feinmark et al. 2003). Therefore, theoretically these all could be involved in the induction of TRPV1 plasticity or TRPV1-induced behavior in vivo. For example, as activation of endogenous anandamide (Al-Hayani et al. 2001) or N-arachidonoyl-dopamine (NADA) (Huang et al. 2002) in the hippocampus both increase paired-pulse depression of population spikes, and 12-HPETE mediates CA1 stratum radiatum interneuron LTD (Gibson et al. 2008), hippocampal TRPV1 could likely influence synaptic plasticity in vivo/in vitro. Enzymes that form anandamide and 12-HPETE are respectively N-acyl-phosphatidylethanolamine-specific phospholipase D (NAPE-PLD) (Di Marzo et al. 1994) and 12-lipoxygenase (Hwang et al. 2000). mRNA for these enzymes are expressed by both hippocampal pyramidal cells and inhibitory interneurons as demonstrated using RT-PCR (Merrill et al. 2012), suggesting that both cells express enzymes to produce TRPV1 ligands and thus modulate hippocampal TRPV1 activity. That interneurons can produce endocannabinoids in addition to pyramidal cells was also recently demonstrated electrophysiologically (Péterfi et al. 2012). Immunocytochemical localization of TRPV1 alongside biosynthesis or biodegradation enzymes of TRPV1 endogenous ligands in the hippocampus and cerebellum support an endogenous role of TRPV1 in the brain (Cristino et al. 2008). Involvement of TRPV1 in normal, in vivo/in vitro hippocampal function is also supported by the fact that TRPV1$^{-/-}$ mice show reduced CA1 LTP as compared to littermate controls (Marsch et al. 2007). In addition to the hippocampus, in the superior colliculus, TRPV1 expression was co-localized in young animals (P14-28) to NAPE-PLD and 12-lipoxygenase (Maione et al. 2009). The demonstration of TRPV1 expression near the enzymes that produce TRPV1 endovanilloid ligands illustrates that all the components necessary for TRPV1 to be endogenously active in vivo present in specific regions. It also strongly suggests that TRPV1 could be used as a target of pharmaceutical agents that alter TRPV1 activity in order to achieve a particular benefit.

3.4.2 *Tonic Activation*

Similar to the PNS, where tonic activation of TRPV1 seems to be especially important for pain and inflammatory conditions (Premkumar and Abooj 2013), endogenously produced ligands also appear to tonically activate CNS TRPV1, where it alters basal neurotransmission. For example, in the hippocampus, where the previously described TRPV1-mediated interneuron LTD occurs in response to mGluR1 activation followed by 12-HPETE formation, there is actually an increase in glutamate neurotransmission in response to mGluR1

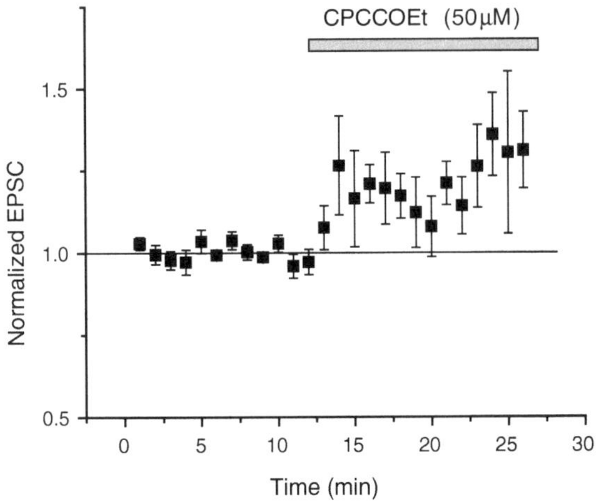

Fig. 3.3 TRPV1 is likely tonically activated in CA1 causing basal depression of neurotransmitter release onto hippocampal stratum radiatum interneurons. The metabotropic glutamate receptor 1 (mGluR1) antagonist CPCCOEt significantly increases ($p < 0.05$; $n = 7$) excitatory postsynaptic currents (EPSCs). EPSCs increased by 27.6 ± 3.8 % (STE) at 10–15 min after drug application. As mGluR1 is required to synthesize 12-HPETE to induce LTD via TRPV1 (Gibson et al. 2008), this suggests there is tonic activation of mGluR1 and thus TRPV1 stimulation under basal conditions in vitro, which is uncovered by blocking mGluR1

antagonists, suggesting that the interneurons were tonically inhibited by TRPV1 via mGluR1 (see Fig. 3.3). In other brain regions TRPV1 is also tonically activated, such as in the substantia nigra, in response to tonic anandamide release (Marinelli et al. 2003), and in the brain stem, where TRPV1 antagonists altered increased activity in the rostral ventromedial medulla (Starowicz et al. 2007). While the significance of tonic action of CNS TRPV1 is currently unknown, the cannabinoid receptor CB1 is also often tonically activated (Cachope 2012) and it could be a shared property of cannabinoid/endovanilloid receptors.

3.5 TRPV1 Signaling in CNS

TRPV1 can be expressed both presynaptically and postsynaptically, and depending on the specific synapse, it can either increase or decrease neurotransmission. Therefore, TRPV1 may have various signaling roles and mechanisms that are unique in different brain regions. As stated previously, presynaptic TRPV1 normally enhances glutamate neurotransmission by increasing presynaptic calcium (Musella et al. 2009; Marinelli et al. 2003; Marinelli et al. 2007; Doyle et al. 2002). However, presynaptic TRPV1 can also depress neurotransmission, as in hippocampal LTD (Gibson et al. 2008). While initially contradictory, it is possible that in this case calcium entry via TRPV1 could be activating a calcium-sensitive pathway to depress transmitter release. Supportive of this was evidence that blockade of the protein phosphatase calcineurin, also known as protein phosphatase 3/protein phosphatase 2B, eliminated both high-frequency stimulus-induced and TRPV1 agonist-induced LTD in interneurons (Jensen and Edwards 2012). Thus TRPV1 mediated this LTD or depression of neurotransmission via activation of a calcineurin-dependent pathway (see Fig. 3.1a). Supportive of this are the many studies that have linked calcineurin activity to synaptic plasticity, including presynaptic plasticity (Heifets et al. 2008; Zeng et al. 2001). In addition, a link between TRPV1 and calcineurin in depressing neurotransmission was identified in dorsal root ganglion cells where TRPV1-mediated Ca^{2+} currents activated calcineurin, causing reduced neurotransmitter release (Wu et al. 2005). In this study dephosphorylation via calcineurin had the dual effect of both decreasing activity of voltage-gated calcium channels in the presynaptic terminal and endocytosing them. It is possible that a similar mechanism mediates depression of neurotransmission via calcineurin in the hippocampus as well. These data also suggest that TRPV1 is closely coupled with calcineurin in the presynaptic terminal. While the exact location of TRPV1 is not known, as it could be expressed in the plasma membrane or on intracellular membranes, TRPV1 activates calcineurin that likely depresses voltage-gated calcium channels and reduces neurotransmission overall at the synapse. Another possibility is that TRPV1 mediates activation of a kinase such as PKA, which alters the vesicle release machinery of the cell through RIM1α, as has been reported for CB1 plasticity (Marinelli et al. 2007). This seems less likely based on our unpublished data using the PKA/kinase antagonist staurosporine that did not block LTD. In regions such as the superior colliculus, presynaptic TRPV1 may be functioning in a similar fashion, though to date the presynaptic TRPV1 signaling pathway is not known in other brain regions.

Interestingly, postsynaptic TRPV1 also mediates a signal cascade triggered by calcineurin in the dentate gyrus (Chavez et al. 2010) (see Fig. 3.1b). Therefore, calcineurin is a potential common downstream target of TRPV1 and is likely closely associated with TRPV1 by a protein binding domain such as AKAP (Schnizler et al. 2008) in a type of supramolecular signaling complex. This would allow calcineurin activation by calcium, which is specifically entering the synapse terminal via TRPV1, similar to sensory neurons (Schnizler et al. 2008). Finally, calcineurin desensitizes TRPV1 (Mohapatra and Nau 2005), suggesting this could serve as a kind of negative feedback system as well; however, this has yet to be investigated specifically in the CNS. While much is known about TRPV1 in the PNS (or through expression systems, e.g., HEK cells), including its reversible phosphorylation via PKA/PKC and calcineurin, along with factors involved in sensitization, desensitization, and TRPV1 activation (Cortright and Szallasi 2004; Mohapatra and Nau 2005; Zhang et al. 2007; Mandadi et al. 2004; Woo et al. 2008), much less is known regarding signaling in the CNS, which remains to be fully explored.

3.6 TRPV1 in CNS Behavior

3.6.1 Stress and Anxiety

In the CNS, TRPV1 seems especially relevant in stress- and anxiety-related behaviors. TRPV1 has recently been reviewed as an important stress-response protein in the CNS (Ho et al. 2012). TRPV1$^{-/-}$ mice exhibit several behavioral changes, including reduced anxiety, fear conditioning (amygdala-dependent), and stress sensitization (Marsch et al. 2007; Santos et al. 2008), while wild-type mice infused with capsaicin exhibit anxiety-like behaviors (Hakimizadeh et al. 2012). TRPV1$^{-/-}$ mice had less anxiety in elevated maze, and light-dark tests and less freezing response following fear conditioning in tone and stress sensitization compared to wild-type littermates (Marsch et al. 2007). Similarly, following the infusion of TRPV1 antagonists in the ventral hippocampus or by intraperitoneal injection, rats and mice exhibit reduced anxiety in the elevated plus-maze test (Santos et al. 2008; Kasckow et al. 2004; Micale et al. 2008). Microinjection of the CB1/TRPV1 agonist anandamide into the prefrontal cortex suggests that TRPV1 plays a role in anxiety, with CB1 activation being more anxiolytic and TRPV1 activation being more anxiogenic (Rubino et al. 2008). In this study, higher dose injections of the nonhydrolysable anandamide analog methananandamide produced an anxiogenic effect, which was blocked by TRPV1 antagonist capsazepine. URB597, the selective inhibitor of fatty acid amide hydrolase, the anandamide degrading enzyme, which induces increased endogenous anandamide, was somewhat anxiogenic as well. These data indicate a role for TRPV1 in anxiety in various brain regions.

Regarding stressful events, TRPV1 activation proved to enhance spatial memory retrieval in response to stress (Li et al. 2008). While TRPV1 agonist capsaicin application by itself, either via intrahippocampal or intragastric infusion, did not enhance memory as measured using a Morris water maze behavioral assay, capsaicin did eliminate the deficits in spatial memory associated with stress from forced swim. This suggests that TRPV1 may play a protective role on short-term memory following stress. Similar findings were also demonstrated in the lateral nucleus of the amygdala where TRPV1 agonists eliminate stress-induced decreases in LTP (Kulisch and Albrecht 2013). Therefore, TRPV1 appears to play a significant role in anxiety and stress in the CNS.

3.6.2 Alcohol Consumption

As TRPV1 is also activated by ethanol, it has the potential to induce CNS ethanol-mediated behaviors. Indeed, TRPV1$^{-/-}$ mice had a higher preference for and consumption of ethanol (Blednov and Harris 2009) than wild-type mice. In addition, TRPV1$^{-/-}$ mice had a faster recovery from ethanol-induced motor incoordination and loss of righting reflex than wild-type mice. Injection of TRPV1 antagonist into wild-type mice resulted in the same phenotype as the TRPV1$^{-/-}$ mice. Decreased ethanol avoidance, associated with no change in consumption of sweet and bitter, was also noted by others (Ellingson et al. 2009), supporting this general find. It should be highlighted that while ethanol consumption in TRPV1$^{-/-}$ mice could still be mediated by lack of TRPV1 in the PNS trigeminal nerve in the oral cavity, effects on motor coordination are likely mediated by TRPV1 in the midbrain.

3.7 Thermoregulation/Analgesia

3.7.1 Thermoregulation/Hypothalamus

As TRPV1 is thermosensitive and has been noted to be present in the hypothalamus by almost every study examining its CNS expression, it is now being studied in the CNS for its role in thermoregulation, as well as other hypothalamic functions. As early as 1970, a study examined the effect of capsaicin injection into the hypothalamus and demonstrated a dose-dependent decrease in temperature (Jancsó-Gábor et al. 1970), though no TRPV1 antagonist was known at the time to confirm the specificity of capsaicin action. More recent data also suggests that TRPV1 plays a role in thermoregulation, including in humans, where TRPV1-specific blockade induces hyperthermia (Gavva et al. 2008). However, the case for TRPV1 or other TRP channels in thermoregulation is currently debated. I will not go into further discussion of TRPV1-mediated thermoregulation here as this has been reviewed by others (Caterina 2007; Romanovsky et al. 2009).

Hypothalamic TRPV1 function is also involved in osmoregulation, as sweat production and water-regulating mechanisms in the kidney are linked to thermoregulation. TRPV1 is connected to the regulation of the vasopressin/antidiuretic hormone that contributes to thermal control in vivo (Naeini et al. 2006; Sharif-Naeini et al. 2008). For review see Sudbury et al. (2010).

3.7.2 Pain/Analgesia

Of great importance was the initial identification that TRPV1$^{-/-}$ mice have decreased pain response (Caterina et al. 2000). Currently, TRPV1 (along with other TRPs) is considered a critical target for second-generation analgesics (Premkumar and Abooj 2013), which have been reviewed by many others particularly in the PNS (Gavva et al. 2008; Cortright and Szallasi 2009; Brederson et al. 2013; Schumacher 2010). Antagonism of brain TRPV1 is thought to play a role in broad-spectrum analgesia via central desensitization (Cui et al. 2006). However, a major issue with TRPV1 antagonists is that they induce hyperthermia (Gavva et al. 2008), likely caused by hypothalamic TRPV1. Interestingly, TRPV1 also plays a role in pain transmission in the CNS. For example, in descending antinociceptive pain pathways in the brain stem, TRPV1 agonists suppress nociception (Maione et al. 2006). For review see Palazzo et al. (2008). The mechanism is enhanced glutamate release in the rostral ventromedial medulla activating antinociceptive neurons subsequent to TRPV1 stimulation (Starowicz et al. 2007). TRPV1 involvement in pain analgesia in the CNS was also evidenced using N-arachidonoyl-serotonin, a combination fatty acid amine hydrolase (FAAH)/TRPV1 antagonist (de Novellis et al. 2011). This antagonist blocked a significant amount of neuropathic pain induced by spared nerve injury as monitored in the prelimbic cortex subsequent to basolateral amygdala stimulation. In this study, the spared nerve injury model resulted in increased local glutamate, and enhanced TRPV1 and FAAH protein expression. This pain processing mediated by TRPV1 appears to be dependent on glial caspases (Giordano et al. 2012). The aforementioned FAAH/TRPV1 antagonist was also examined for analgesic effects in this and other brain regions (de Novellis et al. 2008). TRPV1 involvement in pain also extends to the spinal cord (Morisset et al. 2001). Collectively, the data suggest that not only could TRPV1 play a role in anti-inflammatory/antinociception pathways in the PNS but could also have an analgesic effect in the CNS, including in the brain and spinal cord.

3.8 Potential Pharmacological Implications

TRPV1 is the most highly studied of all the TRP channels and has been shown to have therapeutic value (Di Marzo et al. 2002; Cortright and Szallasi 2004; Starowicz et al. 2008). Based on this review, it is evident that TRPV1 could have potential pharmacological implications in the CNS for anxiety; learning and memory; protection from stress-induced memory loss; motor control, especially during ethanol intoxication; analgesia; thermoregulation; and more. Because of the multimodal characteristics of TRPV1 and its widespread distribution in the CNS (Di Marzo and De Petrocellis 2012), several therapeutic approaches in the CNS could be illuminated for the benefit of humans. This includes drugs or agents that not only block or activate TRPV1 directly, but that also alter TRPV1 ligand biosynthesis or degradation, which could be especially important given that TRPV1 seems to be under tonic regulation. The side effects of such drugs, however, should be taken into account since they could adversely impact the control of body temperature, memory, etc.

Regarding learning and memory, TRPV1 in CA1 hippocampus could be a target to facilitate LTP or alter interneuron activity. Facilitation of LTP is important as many studies have correlated depressed LTP to poorer performance on memory tests, such as the Morris water maze, while increased LTP corresponds to better performance. As TRPV1 activation enhances hippocampal LTP (Li et al. 2008; Bennion et al. 2011), and genetic deletion of TRPV1 depresses LTP (Marsch et al. 2007), it is tempting to postulate that TRPV1 activity in the hippocampus could be a potential target for enhancing memory in those with memory deficits such as Alzheimer's disease. In addition, as stress is one factor that impairs LTP and performance on memory tests (Li et al. 2008) and TRPV1 appears to be protective of LTP during stress, TRPV1 could be targeted to mitigate stress-mediated memory loss. Understanding how TRPV1 controls interneuron activity could also be critical, as interneurons play a crucial role in the function and rhythm of pyramidal cells, the output cells of the hippocampus. A single interneuron innervates hundreds of pyramidal cells (Freund and Buzsaki 1996). Interneurons synchronize the firing and oscillatory behavior of CA1 pyramidal cells (Cobb et al. 1995) as well as create the gamma rhythm (30–80 Hz) and theta rhythm (5–12 Hz) (Whittington and Traub 2003; McBain and Fisahn 2001), the latter of which is critical for normal memory formation. Importantly, interneurons also quiet the excitatory circuit in the hippocampus that forms a loop with the entorhinal cortex, thus preventing epileptic activity due to over-excitation. Those with temporal lobe seizures are thought to have reduced interneuron numbers or function, which is often associated with stroke or other neurological damage. Therefore, as TRPV1 appears to be under basal activation, partially inhibiting CA1 hippocampal interneurons, TRPV1 antagonism could increase interneuron activity, thereby reducing seizure activity. Modulating TRPV1 activity could also have an effect on hippocampal synchronization and oscillation. Collectively, while none of these potential outcomes of hippocampal TRPV1 have been fully investigated, they are enticing avenues of future research in the areas of learning and memory, stress effects on learning and memory, and epilepsy.

Understanding the role of CNS expressed TRPV1 in analgesia is also an exciting avenue of research as we struggle to find a nonaddictive treatment to alleviate pain. While opiates are the current major class of drug to block pain, typically blocking pain at the level of the spinal cord, they are also the number one reason drug addicts enroll in drug rehabilitation clinics. Thus, the need for alternative analgesics that are nonaddictive is great.

Two additional topics not yet highlighted are TRPV1 involvement in locomotion and neuroprotection. Neuroprotection subsequent to cerebral ischemia by TRPV1 antagonism was observed via increased cell survival of hippocampal CA1 pyramidal cells and, interestingly, prevented ischemia-induced hyperlocomotion (Pegorini et al. 2006). Direct TRPV1 activation can also induce hypolocomotion (Di Marzo et al. 2001). This suggests a direct correlation between Parkinson's disease and TRPV1 function, as TRPV1 suppresses locomotion in normal animals and alters behaviors induced by L-DOPA (Lee et al. 2006). This study builds upon others and suggests a role for TRPV1 in voluntary movement.

While there is great deal of potential, many of the therapeutic pharmacological applications of TRPV1 research in the CNS are currently unexplored. Hopefully, in the coming years those researching TRPV1 in the CNS will investigate the many potential applications and uncover some of the benefits that the examination of TRPV1 will provide. These applications include Parkinson's disease (locomotion/dopamine cells), cognition and learning disorders such as Alzheimer's disease (hippocampus/limbic system), reward (dopaminergic cells), pain (spinal cord and brain), temperature regulation (hypothalamus), etc.

3.9 Conclusion

The data on TRPV1 in the CNS illustrate its important role as it is involved in an impressive array of behaviors and functions, indicating the need for further exploration. As TRPV1 is expressed in humans, knowledge gained regarding its function in rodents could be translational in nature. For example, drugs targeting TRPV1 and other TRP channels are being investigated for pain treatment in humans and in animals (Salat et al. 2013), and enhanced TRPV1 expression has been illustrated in the human cortex in association with epilepsy (Shu et al. 2013). The development of second-generation TRPV1 antagonists for analgesia has been encouraged (Szolcsányi and Pintér 2013). These, among many other evidences of TRPV1 in humans, suggest that TRPV1 research in animals and humans has therapeutic value. The potential therapeutic applications of brain TRPV1 have been reviewed by others (Starowicz et al. 2008; Morelli et al. 2013), including the role of TRPV1 in anxiety, locomotion, body temperature, pain, etc. However, TRPV1 is also involved in other brain functions, such as synaptic plasticity and development, as reviewed here. It appears very likely that the study of TRPV1 will provide additional insight into the understanding of the brain and open up new applications in pharmacological research using TRPV1 as the target molecule.

References

Acs G, Palkovits M, Blumberg PM (1996) Specific binding of [3H] resiniferatoxin by human and rat preoptic area, locus ceruleus, medial hypothalamus, reticular formation and ventral thalamus membrane preparations. Life Sci 59(22):1899–1908. http://dx.doi.org/10.1016/S0024-3205(96)00537-1

Ahern GP (2003) Activation of TRPV1 by the satiety factor Oleoylethanolamide. J Biol Chem 278(33):30429–30434. doi:10.1074/jbc.M305051200

Al-Hayani A, Wease KN, Ross RA, Pertwee RG, Davies SN (2001) The endogenous cannabinoid anandamide activates vanilloid receptors in the rat hippocampal slice. Neuropharmacology 41(8):1000–1005

Bennion D, Jensen T, Walther C, Hamblin J, Wallmann A, Couch J, Blickenstaff J, Castle M, Dean L, Beckstead S, Merrill C, Muir C, St Pierre T, Williams B, Daniel S, Edwards JG (2011) Transient receptor potential vanilloid 1 agonists modulate hippocampal CA1 LTP via the GABAergic system. Neuropharmacology. doi: 10.1016/j.neuropharm.2011.05.018 [pii] S0028-3908(11)00208-5

Blednov YA, Harris RA (2009) Deletion of vanilloid receptor (TRPV1) in mice alters behavioral effects of ethanol. Neuropharmacology 56(4):814–820. http://dx.doi.org/10.1016/j.neuropharm.2009.01.007

Brederson J-D, Kym PR, Szallasi A (2013) Targeting TRP channels for pain relief. Eur J Pharmacol (Epub ahead of print). http://dx.doi.org/10.1016/j.ejphar.2013.03.003

Brown TE, Chirila AM, Schrank BR, Kauer JA (2013) Loss of interneuron LTD and attenuated pyramidal cell LTP in Trpv1 and Trpv3 KO mice. Hippocampus (Epub ahead of print). 10.1002/hipo.22125

Cachope R (2012) Functional diversity on synaptic plasticity mediated by endocannabinoids. Philos Trans R Soc B Biol Sci 367(1607):3242–3253. doi:10.1098/rstb2011.0386

Caterina MJ (2007) Transient receptor potential ion channels as participants in thermosensation and thermoregulation. Am J Physiol Regul Integr Comp Physiol 292(1):R64–R76. doi:10.1152/ajpregu.00446.2006

Caterina MJ, Leffler A, Malmberg AB, Martin WJ, Trafton J, Petersen-Zeitz KR, Koltzenburg M, Basbaum AI, Julius D (2000) Impaired Nociception and pain sensation in Mice Lacking the Capsaicin receptor. Science 288(5464):306–313. doi:10.1126/science.288.5464.306

Caterina MJ, Schumacher MA, Tominaga M, Rosen TA, Levine JD, Julius D (1997) The capsaicin receptor: a heat-activated ion channel in the pain pathway. Nature 389(6653):816–824

Cavanaugh DJ, Chesler AT, Jackson AC, Sigal YM, Yamanaka H, Grant R, O'Donnell D, Nicoll RA, Shah NM, Julius D, Basbaum AI (2011) Trpv1 reporter mice reveal highly restricted brain distribution and functional expression in arteriolar smooth muscle cells. J Neurosci 31(13):5067–5077 31/13/5067 [pii] 10.1523/JNEUROSCI.6451-10.2011

Chavez AE, Chiu CQ, Castillo PE (2010) TRPV1 activation by endogenous anandamide triggers postsynaptic long-term depression in dentate gyrus. Nat Neurosci 13(12):1511–1518. http://www.nature.com/neuro/journal/v13/n12/abs/nn.2684.html#supplementary-information

Chu CJ, Huang SM, De Petrocellis L, Bisogno T, Ewing SA, Miller JD, Zipkin RE, Daddario N, Appendino G, Di Marzo V, Walker JM (2003) N-Oleoyldopamine, a novel endogenous Capsaicin-like lipid that produces Hyperalgesia. J Biol Chem 278(16):13633–13639. doi:10.1074/jbc.M211231200

Cobb SR, Buhl EH, Halasy K, Paulsen O, Somogyi P (1995) Synchronization of neuronal activity in hippocampus by individual GABAergic interneurons. Nature 378(6552):75–78

Cortright DN, Crandall M, Sanchez JF, Zou T, Krause JE, White G (2001) The Tissue Distribution and Functional Characterization of Human VR1. Biochem Biophys Res Commun 281(5):1183–1189. http://dx.doi.org/10.1006/bbrc.2001.4482

Cortright DN, Szallasi A (2004) Biochemical pharmacology of the vanilloid receptor TRPV1. An update. Eur J Biochem 271(10):1814–1819. doi:10.1111/j.1432-1033.2004.04082.x

Cortright DN, Szallasi A (2009) TRP Channels and Pain. Curr Pharm Des 15(15). 10.2174/138161209788186308

Cristino L, de Petrocellis L, Pryce G, Baker D, Guglielmotti V, Di Marzo V (2006) Immunohistochemical localization of cannabinoid type 1 and vanilloid transient receptor potential vanilloid type 1 receptors in the mouse brain. Neuroscience 139(4):1405–1415

Cristino L, Starowicz K, De Petrocellis L, Morishita J, Ueda N, Guglielmotti V, Di Marzo V (2008) Immunohistochemical localization of anabolic and catabolic enzymes for anandamide and other putative endovanilloids in the hippocampus and cerebellar cortex of the mouse brain. Neuroscience 151(4):955–968

Cui M, Honore P, Zhong C, Gauvin D, Mikusa J, Hernandez G, Chandran P, Gomtsyan A, Brown B, Bayburt EK, Marsh K, Bianchi B, McDonald H, Niforatos W, Neelands TR, Moreland RB, Decker MW, Lee C-H, Sullivan JP, Faltynek CR (2006) TRPV1 Receptors in the CNS play a key role in Broad-Spectrum Analgesia of TRPV1 antagonists. J Neurosci 26(37):9385–9393. doi:10.1523/jneurosci.1246-06.2006

de Novellis V, Palazzo E, Rossi F, De Petrocellis L, Petrosino S, Guida F, Luongo L, Migliozzi A, Cristino L, Marabese I, Starowicz K, Di Marzo V, Maione S (2008) The analgesic effect of N-arachidonoyl-serotonin, a FAAH inhibitor and TRPV1 receptor antagonist, associated with changes in rostral ventromedial medulla and locus coeruleus cell activity in rats. Neuropharmacology 55(7):1105–1113. http://dx.doi.org/10.1016/j.neuropharm.2008.06.023

de Novellis V, Vita D, Gatta L, Luongo L, Bellini G, De Chiaro M, Marabese I, Siniscalco D, Boccella S, Piscitelli F, Di Marzo V, Palazzo E, Rossi F, Maione S (2011) The blockade of the transient receptor potential vanilloid type 1 and fatty acid amide hydrolase decreases symptoms and central sequelae in the medial prefrontal cortex of neuropathic rats. Mol Pain 7(1):7

Di Marzo V, Blumberg PM, Szallasi A (2002) Endovanilloid signaling in pain. Curr Opin Neurobiol 12(4):372–379. http://dx.doi.org/10.1016/S0959-4388(02)00340-9

Di Marzo V, De Petrocellis L (2012) Why do cannabinoid receptors have more than one endogenous ligand? Philos Trans R Soc B Biol Sci 367(1607):3216–3228. doi:10.1098/rstb2011.0382

Di Marzo V, Fontana A, Cadas H, Schinelli S, Cimino G, Schwartz J-C, Piomelli D (1994) Formation and inactivation of endogenous cannabinoid anandamide in central neurons. Nature 372(6507):686–691

Di Marzo V, Lastres-Becker I, Bisogno T, De Petrocellis L, Milone A, Davis JB, Fernandez-Ruiz JJ (2001) Hypolocomotor effects in rats of capsaicin and two long chain capsaicin homologues. Eur J Pharmacol 420(2–3):123–131. http://dx.doi.org/10.1016/S0014-2999(01)01012-3

Doyle MW, Bailey TW, Jin Y-H, Andresen MC (2002) Vanilloid receptors presynaptically modulate cranial visceral Afferent synaptic transmission in nucleus tractus solitarius. J Neurosci 22(18):8222–8229

Ellingson J, Silbaugh B, Brasser S (2009) Reduced oral ethanol avoidance in mice lacking transient receptor potential channel vanilloid receptor 1. Behav Genet 39(1):62–72. doi:10.1007/s10519-008-9232-1

Feinmark SJ, Begum R, Tsvetkov E, Goussakov I, Funk CD, Siegelbaum SA, Bolshakov VY (2003) 12-lipoxygenase metabolites of arachidonic acid mediate metabotropic glutamate receptor-dependent long-term depression at hippocampal CA3-CA1 synapses. J Neurosci 23(36):11427–11435

Freund TF, Buzsaki G (1996) Interneurons of the hippocampus. Hippocampus 6(4):347–470

Gavva NR, Treanor JJS, Garami A, Fang L, Surapaneni S, Akrami A, Alvarez F, Bak A, Darling M, Gore A, Jang GR, Kesslak JP, Ni L, Norman MH, Palluconi G, Rose MJ, Salfi M, Tan E, Romanovsky AA, Banfield C, Davar G (2008) Pharmacological blockade of the vanilloid receptor TRPV1 elicits marked hyperthermia in humans. Pain 136(1–2):202–210

Gibson HE, Edwards JG, Page RS, Van Hook MJ, Kauer JA (2008) TRPV1 channels mediate long-term depression at synapses on hippocampal interneurons. Neuron 57(5):746–759

Giordano C, Cristino L, Luongo L, Siniscalco D, Petrosino S, Piscitelli F, Marabese I, Gatta L, Rossi F, Imperatore R, Palazzo E, de Novellis V, Di Marzo V, Maione S (2012) TRPV1-dependent and -independent alterations in the limbic cortex of neuropathic mice: Impact on glial caspases and pain perception. Cereb Cortex 22(11):2495–2518. doi:10.1093/cercor/bhr328

Grueter BA, Brasnjo G, Malenka RC (2010) Postsynaptic TRPV1 triggers cell type-specific long-term depression in the nucleus accumbens. Nat Neurosci 13(12):1519–1525. http://www.nature.com/neuro/journal/v13/n12/abs/nn.2685.html#supplementary-information

Hakimizadeh E, Oryan S, Hajizadeh moghaddam A, Roohbakhsh A (2012) Endocannabinoid system and TRPV1 receptors in the dorsal hippocampus of the rats modulate anxiety-like behaviors. Iran J Basic Med Sci 15(3):795–802

Han P, Korepanova A, Vos M, Moreland R, Chiu M, Faltynek C (2013) Quantification of TRPV1 protein levels in rat tissues to understand its physiological roles. J Mol Neurosci 50(1):23–32. doi:10.1007/s12031-012-9849-7

Hayes P, Meadows HJ, Gunthorpe MJ, Harries MH, Duckworth DM, Cairns W, Harrison DC, Clarke CE, Ellington K, Prinjha RK, Barton AJL, Medhurst AD, Smith GD, Topp S, Murdock P, Sanger GJ, Terrett J, Jenkins O, Benham CD, Randall AD, Gloger IS, Davis JB (2000) Cloning and functional expression of a human orthologue of rat vanilloid receptor-1. Pain 88(2):205–215. http://dx.doi.org/10.1016/S0304-3959(00)00353-5

Heifets BD, Chevaleyre V, Castillo PE (2008) Interneuron activity controls endocannabinoid-mediated presynaptic plasticity through calcineurin. Proc Natl Acad Sci 105(29):10250–10255. doi:10.1073/pnas.0711880105

Helliwell RJA, McLatchie LM, Clarke M, Winter J, Bevan S, McIntyre P (1998) Capsaicin sensitivity is associated with the expression of the vanilloid (capsaicin) receptor (VR1) mRNA in adult rat sensory ganglia. Neurosci Lett 250(3):177–180. http://dx.doi.org/10.1016/S0304-3940(98)00475-3

Ho KW, Ward NJ, Calkins DJ (2012) TRPV1: a stress response protein in the central nervous system. Am J Neurodegener Dis 1(1):1–14
Huang SM, Bisogno T, Trevisani M, Al-Hayani A, De Petrocellis L, Fezza F, Tognetto M, Petros TJ, Krey JF, Chu CJ, Miller JD, Davies SN, Geppetti P, Walker JM, Di Marzo V (2002) An endogenous capsaicin-like substance with high potency at recombinant and native vanilloid VR1 receptors. Proc Natl Acad Sci USA 99(12):8400–8405
Hwang SW, Cho H, Kwak J, Lee S-Y, Kang C-J, Jung J, Cho S, Min KH, Suh Y-G, Kim D, Oh U (2000) Direct activation of capsaicin receptors by products of lipoxygenases: endogenous capsaicin-like substances. PNAS 97(11):6155–6160. doi:10.1073/pnas.97.11.6155
Jancsó-Gábor A, Szolcsányi J, Jancsó N (1970) Stimulation and desensitization of the hypothalamic heat-sensitive structures by capsaicin in rats. J Physiol 208(2):449–459
Jennings EA, Vaughan CW, Roberts LA, Christie MJ (2003) The actions of anandamide on rat superficial medullary dorsal horn neurons in vitro. J Physiol 548(1):121–129. doi:10.1113/jphysiol.2002.035063
Jensen T, Edwards JG (2012) Calcineurin is required for TRPV1-induced long-term depression of hippocampal interneurons. Neurosci Lett 510(2):82–87. http://dx.doi.org/10.1016/j.neulet.2012.01.006
Kasckow JW, Mulchahey JJ, Geracioti TD Jr (2004) Effects of the vanilloid agonist olvanil and antagonist capsazepine on rat behaviors. Prog Neuropsychopharmacol Biol Psychiatry 28(2):291–295
Kulisch C, Albrecht D (2013) Effects of single swim stress on changes in TRPV1-mediated plasticity in the amygdala. Behav Brain Res 236(0):344–349. http://dx.doi.org/10.1016/j.bbr.2012.09.003
Lee J, Di Marzo V, Brotchie JM (2006) A role for vanilloid receptor 1 (TRPV1) and endocannabinnoid signalling in the regulation of spontaneous and L-DOPA induced locomotion in normal and reserpine-treated rats. Neuropharmacology 51(3):557–565. http://dx.doi.org/10.1016/j.neuropharm.2006.04.016
Li H-B, Mao R-R, Zhang J-C, Yang Y, Cao J, Xu L (2008) Antistress effect of TRPV1 channel on synaptic plasticity and spatial memory. Biol Psychiatry 64(4):286–292. doi:10.1016/j.biopsych.2008.02.020
Maione S, Bisogno T, de Novellis V, Palazzo E, Cristino L, Valenti M, Petrosino S, Guglielmotti V, Rossi F, Marzo VD (2006) Elevation of endocannabinoid levels in the ventrolateral periaqueductal grey through inhibition of fatty acid amide hydrolase affects descending nociceptive pathways via both cannabinoid receptor type 1 and transient receptor potential vanilloid Type-1 receptors. J Pharmacol Exp Ther 316(3):969–982. doi:10.1124/jpet.105.093286
Maione S, Cristino L, Migliozzi AL, Georgiou AL, Starowicz K, Salt TE, Di Marzo V (2009) TRPV1 channels control synaptic plasticity in the developing superior colliculus. J Physiol 587(11):2521–2535. doi:10.1113/jphysiol.2009.171900
Mandadi S, Numazaki M, Tominaga M, Bhat MB, Armati PJ, Roufogalis BD (2004) Activation of protein kinase C reverses capsaicin-induced calcium-dependent desensitization of TRPV1 ion channels. Cell Calcium 35(5):471–478
Marinelli S, Di Marzo V, Berretta N, Matias I, Maccarrone M, Bernardi G, Mercuri NB (2003) Presynaptic facilitation of glutamatergic synapses to dopaminergic neurons of the rat substantia nigra by endogenous stimulation of vanilloid receptors. J Neurosci 23(8):3136–3144
Marinelli S, Di Marzo V, Florenzano F, Fezza F, Viscomi MT, van der Stelt M, Bernardi G, Molinari M, Maccarrone M, Mercuri NB (2007) N-arachidonoyl-dopamine tunes synaptic transmission onto dopaminergic neurons by activating both cannabinoid and vanilloid receptors. Neuropsychopharmacology 32(2):298–308. doi: 10.1038/sj.npp.1301118 (1301118 [pii])
Marinelli S, Pascucci T, Bernardi G, Puglisi-Allegra S, Mercuri NB (2005) Activation of TRPV1 in the VTA excites dopaminergic neurons and increases chemical-and noxious-induced dopamine release in the nucleus accumbens. Neuropsychopharmacology 30(5):864–870. doi: 10.1038/sj.npp.1300615

Marsch R, Foeller E, Rammes G, Bunck M, Kossl M, Holsboer F, Zieglgansberger W, Landgraf R, Lutz B, Wotjak CT (2007) Reduced anxiety, conditioned fear, and hippocampal long-term potentiation in transient receptor potential vanilloid type 1 receptor-deficient mice. J Neurosci 27(4):832–839. doi:10.1523/jneurosci.3303-06.2007

McBain CJ, Fisahn A (2001) Interneurons unbound. Nat Rev Neurosci 2(1):11–23

Merrill CB, McNeil M, Williamson RC, Poole BR, Nelson B, Sudweeks S, Edwards JG (2012) Identification of mRNA for endocannabinoid biosynthetic enzymes within hippocampal pyramidal cells and CA1 stratum radiatum interneuron subtypes using quantitative real-time polymerase chain reaction. Neuroscience 218:89–99. http://dx.doi.org/10.1016/j.neuroscience.2012.05.012

Mezey E, Toth ZE, Cortright DN, Arzubi MK, Krause JE, Elde R, Guo A, Blumberg PM, Szallasi A (2000) Distribution of mRNA for vanilloid receptor subtype 1 (VR1), and VR1-like immunoreactivity, in the central nervous system of the rat and human. PNAS 97(7):3655–3660. doi:10.1073/pnas.060496197

Micale V, Cristino L, Tamburella A, Petrosino S, Leggio GM, Drago F, Di Marzo V (2008) Anxiolytic effects in mice of a dual blocker of fatty acid amide hydrolase and transient receptor potential vanilloid type-1 channels. Neuropsychopharmacology 34(3):593–606

Mohapatra DP, Nau C (2005) Regulation of Ca2+-dependent Desensitization in the Vanilloid Receptor TRPV1 by Calcineurin and cAMP-dependent Protein Kinase. J Biol Chem vol 280. doi:10.1074/jbc.M410917200

Morelli MB, Amantini C, Liberati S, Santoni M, Nabissi M (2013) TRP channels: new potential therapeutic approaches in CNS neuropathies. CNS Neurol Disord Drug Targets 12(2):274–293

Morisset V, Ahluwalia J, Nagy I, Urban L (2001) Possible mechanisms of cannabinoid-induced antinociception in the spinal cord. Eur J Pharmacol 429(1–3):93–100

Movahed P, Jönsson BAG, Birnir B, Wingstrand JA, Jørgensen TD, Ermund A, Sterner O, Zygmunt PM, Högestätt ED (2005) Endogenous unsaturated C18 N-acylethanolamines are vanilloid receptor (TRPV1) agonists. J Biol Chem 280(46):38496–38504. doi:10.1074/jbc.M507429200

Musella A, De Chiara V, Rossi S, Prosperetti C, Bernardi G, Maccarrone M, Centonze D (2009) TRPV1 channels facilitate glutamate transmission in the striatum. Mol Cell Neurosci 40(1):89–97

Naeini RS, Witty M-F, Seguela P, Bourque CW (2006) An N-terminal variant of Trpv1 channel is required for osmosensory transduction. Nat Neurosci 9(1):93–98

Nagy I, Sántha P, Jancsó G, Urbán L (2004) The role of the vanilloid (capsaicin) receptor (TRPV1) in physiology and pathology. Eur J Pharmacol 500(1–3):351–369. doi:10.1016/j.ejphar.2004.07.037

Palazzo E, Rossi F, Maione S (2008) Role of TRPV1 receptors in descending modulation of pain. Mol Cell Endocrinol 286(1–2, Supplement 1):S79–S83

Pegorini S, Zani A, Braida D, Guerini-Rocco C, Sala M (2006) Vanilloid VR1 receptor is involved in rimonabant-induced neuroprotection. Br J Pharmacol 147(5):552–559. doi:10.1038/sj.bjp.0706656

Péterfi Z, Urbán GM, Papp OI, Németh B, Monyer H, Szabó G, Erdélyi F, Mackie K, Freund TF, Hájos N, Katona I (2012) Endocannabinoid-Mediated Long-Term Depression of Afferent Excitatory Synapses in Hippocampal Pyramidal Cells and GABAergic Interneurons. J Neurosci 32(41):14448–14463. doi:10.1523/jneurosci.1676-12.2012

Premkumar LS, Abooj M (2013) TRP channels and analgesia. Life Sci 92(8–9):415–424. http://dx.doi.org/10.1016/j.lfs.2012.08.010

Puente N, Cui Y, Lassalle O, Lafourcade M, Georges F, Venance L, Grandes P, Manzoni OJ (2011) Polymodal activation of the endocannabinoid system in the extended amygdala. Nat Neurosci 14(12):1542–1547. http://www.nature.com/neuro/journal/v14/n12/abs/nn.2974.html#supplementary-information

Roberts JC, Davis JB, Benham CD (2004) [3H] Resiniferatoxin autoradiography in the CNS of wild-type and TRPV1 null mice defines TRPV1 (VR-1) protein distribution. Brain Res 995(2):176–183

Romanovsky AA, Almeida MC, Garami A, Steiner AA, Norman MH, Morrison SF, Nakamura K, Burmeister JJ, Nucci TB (2009) The transient receptor potential Vanilloid-1 channel in thermoregulation: A thermosensor it is not. Pharmacol Rev 61(3):228–261. doi:10.1124/pr.109.001263

Rouach N, Nicoll RA (2003) Endocannabinoids contribute to short-term but not long-term mGluR-induced depression in the hippocampus. Eur J Neurosci 18(4):1017–1020. doi:10.1046/j.1460-9568.2003.02823.x

Rubino T, Realini N, Castiglioni C, Guidali C, Viganó D, Marras E, Petrosino S, Perletti G, Maccarrone M, Di Marzo V, Parolaro D (2008) Role in anxiety behavior of the endocannabinoid system in the prefrontal cortex. Cereb Cortex 18(6):1292–1301. doi:10.1093/cercor/bhm161

Salat K, Moniczewski A, Librowski T (2013) Transient receptor potential channels—emerging novel drug targets for the treatment of pain. Curr Med Chem 20(11):1409–1436

Sanchez JF, Krause JE, Cortright DN (2001) The distribution and regulation of vanilloid receptor VR1 and VR1 5' splice variant RNA expression in rat. Neuroscience 107(3):373–381

Santos CJPA, Stern CAJ, Bertoglio LJ (2008) Attenuation of anxiety-related behaviour after the antagonism of transient receptor potential vanilloid type 1 channels in the rat ventral hippocampus. Behav Pharmacol 19(4):357–360

Sasamura T, Sasaki M, Tohda C, Kuraishi Y (1998) Existence of capsaicin-sensitive glutamatergic terminals in rat hypothalamus. NeuroReport 9(9):2045–2048

Schnizler K, Shutov LP, Van Kanegan MJ, Merrill MA, Nichols B, McKnight GS, Strack S, Hell JW, Usachev YM (2008) Protein kinase A anchoring via AKAP150 is essential for TRPV1 modulation by forskolin and prostaglandin E2 in mouse sensory neurons. J Neurosci 28(19):4904–4917. doi:10.1523/jneurosci.0233-08.2008

Schumacher MA (2010) Transient receptor potential channels in pain and inflammation: therapeutic opportunities. Pain Pract 10(3):185–200. doi:10.1111/j.1533-2500.2010.00358.x

Sharif-Naeini R, Ciura S, Bourque CW (2008) TRPV1 gene required for thermosensory transduction and anticipatory secretion from vasopressin neurons during hyperthermia. Neuron 58(2):179–185

Shu HF, Yu SX, Zhang CQ, Liu SY, Wu KF, Zang ZL, Yang H, Zhou SW, Yin Q (2013) Expression of TRPV1 in cortical lesions from patients with tuberous sclerosis complex and focal cortical dysplasia type IIb. Brain Dev 35(3):252–260. doi:10.1016/j.braindev.2012.04.007

Starowicz K, Cristino L, Di Marzo V (2008) TRPV1 receptors in the central nervous system: potential for previously unforeseen therapeutic applications. Curr Pharm Des 14(1):42–54

Starowicz K, Maione S, Cristino L, Palazzo E, Marabese I, Rossi F, de Novellis V, Di Marzo V (2007) Tonic endovanilloid facilitation of glutamate release in brainstem descending antinociceptive pathways. J Neurosci 27(50):13739–13749. doi:10.1523/jneurosci.3258-07.2007

Sudbury JR, Ciura S, Sharif-Naeini R, Bourque CW (2010) Osmotic and thermal control of magnocellular neurosecretory neurons—role of an N-terminal variant of Trpv1. Eur J Neurosci 32(12):2022–2030. doi:10.1111/j.1460-9568.2010.07512.x

Szabo T, Biro T, Gonzalez AF, Palkovits M, Blumberg PM (2002) Pharmacological characterization of vanilloid receptor located in the brain. Mol Brain Res 98(1–2):51–57

Szallasi A, Blumberg PM (1991) Characterization of vanilloid receptors in the dorsal horn of pig spinal cord. Brain Res 547(2):335–338. http://dx.doi.org/10.1016/0006-8993(91)90982-2

Szolcsányi J, Pintér E (2013) Transient receptor potential vanilloid 1 as a therapeutic target in analgesia. Expert Opin Ther Targets 17(6):641–657. doi:10.1517/14728222.2013.772580

Tominaga M, Caterina MJ, Malmberg AB, Rosen TA, Gilbert H, Skinner K, Raumann BE, Basbaum AI, Julius D (1998) The cloned capsaicin receptor integrates multiple pain-producing stimuli. Neuron 21(3):531–543. http://dx.doi.org/10.1016/S0896-6273(00)80564-4

Tominaga M, Tominaga T (2005) Structure and function of TRPV1. Pflügers Arch Eur J Physiol 451(1):143–150

Tóth A, Blumberg PM, Boczán J (2009) Anandamide and the Vanilloid Receptor (TRPV1). In: Gerald L (ed) Vitamins & Hormones, Vol 81. Academic Press, Burlington pp 389–419. http://dx.doi.org/10.1016/S0083-6729(09)81015-7

Toth A, Boczan J, Kedei N, Lizanecz E, Bagi Z, Papp Z, Edes I, Csiba L, Blumberg PM (2005) Expression and distribution of vanilloid receptor 1 (TRPV1) in the adult rat brain. Mol Brain Res 135(1–2):162–168

Whittington MA, Traub RD (2003) Interneuron diversity series: Inhibitory interneurons and network oscillations in vitro. Trends Neurosci 26(12):676–682

Woo DH, Jung SJ, Zhu MH, Park CK, Kim YH, Oh SB, Lee CJ (2008) Direct activation of transient receptor potential vanilloid 1(TRPV1) by diacylglycerol (DAG). Mol Pain 4:42 1744-8069-4-42 [pii] 10.1186/1744-8069-4-42

Wu Z-Z, Chen S-R, Pan H-L (2005) Transient receptor potential vanilloid type 1 activation down-regulates voltage-gated calcium channels through calcium-dependent calcineurin in sensory neurons. J Biol Chem 280(18):18142–18151. doi:10.1074/jbc.M501229200

Yuan S, Burrell BD (2010) Endocannabinoid-dependent LTD in a nociceptive synapse requires activation of a presynaptic TRPV-like receptor. J Neurophysiol 104(5):2766–2777. doi:10.1152/jn.00491.2010

Yuan S, Burrell BD (2012) Long-term depression of nociceptive synapses by non-nociceptive afferent activity: Role of endocannabinoids, Ca2+, and calcineurin. Brain Res 1460(0): 1–11. http://dx.doi.org/10.1016/j.brainres.2012.04.030

Yuan S, Burrell BD (2013) Endocannabinoid-dependent long-term depression in a nociceptive synapse requires coordinated presynaptic and postsynaptic transcription and translation. J Neurosci 33(10):4349–4358. doi:10.1523/jneurosci.3922-12.2013

Zeng H, Chattarji S, Barbarosie M, Rondi-Reig L, Philpot BD, Miyakawa T, Bear MF, Tonegawa S (2001) Forebrain-specific calcineurin knockout selectively impairs bidirectional synaptic plasticity and working/episodic-like memory. Cell 107(5):617–629

Zhang H, Cang C-L, Kawasaki Y, Liang L-L, Zhang Y-Q, Ji R-R, Zhao Z-Q (2007) Neurokinin-1 receptor enhances TRPV1 activity in primary sensory neurons via PKC{varepsilon}: A novel pathway for heat hyperalgesia. J Neurosci 27(44):12067–12077. doi:10.1523/jneurosci.0496-07.2007

Zschenderlein C, Gebhardt C, von Bohlen und Halbach O, Kulisch C, Albrecht D (2011) Capsaicin-induced changes in LTP in the lateral amygdala are mediated by TRPV1. PLoS ONE 6(1):e16116. doi:10.1371/journal.pone.0016116

Chapter 4
Topical Capsaicin Formulations in the Management of Neuropathic Pain

Mark Schumacher and George Pasvankas

Abstract This chapter reviews the scientific and clinical evidence supporting the use of topical formulations containing the pungent principle of chili peppers—capsaicin, for the treatment of peripheral neuropathic pain. Given the limitations of current oral and parenteral therapies for the management of pain arising from various forms of nerve injury, alternate therapeutic approaches that are not associated with systemic adverse events that limit quality of life, impair function, or threaten respiratory depression are critically needed. Moreover, neuropathic conditions can be complicated by progressive changes in the central and peripheral nervous system, leading to persistent reorganization of pain pathways and chronic neuropathic pain. Recent advances in the use of high-dose topical capsaicin preparations hold promise in managing a wide range of painful conditions associated with peripheral neuropathies and may in fact help reduce suffering by reversing progressive changes in the nervous system associated with chronic neuropathic pain conditions.

4.1 Introduction

Physicians have faced a common dilemma over the ages, how to relieve a patient's pain without doing harm. Fortunately, long before the advent of clinical trials, early physicians successfully used native plant derivatives to provide pain relief. Although

M. Schumacher (✉)
Division of Pain Medicine, Department of Anesthesia and Perioperative Care,
University of California, 513 Parnassus Ave, Box 0427, San Francisco,
CA 94143-0427, USA
e-mail: schumacm@anesthesia.ucsf.edu

G. Pasvankas
Division of Pain Medicine, Department of Anesthesia and Perioperative Care,
University of California, 2255 Post St., MZ Bldg N, San Francisco, CA 94143, USA
e-mail: pasvankasg@anesthesia.ucsf.edu

O. M. E. Abdel-Salam (ed.), *Capsaicin as a Therapeutic Molecule*, Progress in Drug Research 68, DOI: 10.1007/978-3-0348-0828-6_4, © Springer Basel 2014

Table 4.1 Peripheral neuropathic conditions treated with topical capsaicin

Peripheral neuropathic conditions treated with Topical capsaicin
Postherpetic neuralgia (PHN)
Painful diabetic polyneuropathy (PDPN)
HIV-associated distal symmetrical polyneuropathy (HIV-DSPN)
Persistent postsurgical pain

their preparations may have been crude by today's standards, they apparently provided effective pain relief for their time. Use of medicinal plant derivatives from hot chilies in South America dates as far back as 4000 BC. However, much of our modern accounts and written records of chili's irritant properties and medicinal use in the western hemisphere are derived from Aztec culture beginning in the twelfth century. Beyond their irritant use, Aztec physicians also realized chili's usefulness to treat painful maladies such as toothaches—perhaps one of the earliest recorded forms of "nerve pain."

Use of medicinal salves and balms used in ancient times appeared to reemerge in the 1800s with the isolation of the principle agent from hot chili peppers—capsaicin. Building on the realization that the experience of pain is based on specialized nerves, "nociceptors," that respond to noxious stimuli (Sherrington 1906), later Hungarian investigators in the 1940s observed that capsaicin both activates and subsequently inactivates sensory nerves. Following the confirmation of the "nociceptor" hypothesis by Bessou and Perl in 1969, the existence of a "capsaicin receptor" expressed on C-polymodal nociceptors was investigated and importantly the phenomenon of nociceptor "desensitization" due to repetitive exposure to capsaicin was formally investigated (Bessou and Perl 1969; Szolcsanyi and Jancso-Gabor 1975, 1976; Szolcsanyi et al. 1975).

As described in detail in this chapter, it was not until the 1980s that the broader use of topical capsaicin appeared in earnest in the medical literature as a therapy for difficult-to-manage pain syndromes—especially for the treatment of painful conditions associated with nerve injury, such as post-herpetic neuralgia (PHN). Conditions such as PHN describe one of a number of maladies that are associated with sensations of burning, shooting, and/or electrical-quality pain. Unfortunately, attempts to manage such painful conditions with therapies that rely primarily on opioid analgesics have been associated with well-known side effects such as nausea/vomiting, constipation, pruritus and at higher dosing, respiratory depression. Moreover, certain patient populations, such as those with advanced age, multiple medical problems, pulmonary disease, or those with increasing opioid requirements may have an unacceptably high risk of adverse events including urinary retention and life threatening respiratory depression. Such opioid-associated adverse events can rapidly degrade quality of life and level of function, limiting their usefulness in chronic painful conditions involving nerve injury.

This chapter reviews the application of topical formulations containing the pungent principle of chili peppers—capsaicin, for the treatment of neuropathic painful conditions (see Table 4.1). Given the limitations of current oral and parenteral therapies for the management of pain arising from various forms of nerve injury, alternate therapeutic approaches that are not associated with adverse events that limit quality of life, impair function or threaten respiratory depression are critically needed. Moreover, neuropathic events can be complicated by progressive changes in the central nervous system, such as central sensitization leading to persistent reorganization of pain pathways and chronic pain. Recent advances in the use of high-dose topical capsaicin preparations hold promise in managing a wide range of painful conditions associated with nerve injury and may in fact help stop or reverse progressive changes in the nervous system associated with chronic neuropathic pain conditions.

4.2 Neuropathic Pain

Whether noted by clinician or patient, neuropathic pain can be one of the most disabling and challenging medical conditions to effectively manage. This is in part due to the diverse and poorly understood pathophysiological drivers that are associated with persistent neuropathic pain. Of the known sources of painful neuropathic pain, this chapter will focus on a subgroup of those of peripheral origin or manifested in a peripheral site of disease that have shown to be responsive to topical capsaicin. These include infectious (herpes zoster, HIV, metabolic (diabetes), and nerve entrapment/surgical/trauma). Although it is uncertain what specific property these diverse disease states or lesions share that engender the development of persistent painful neuropathic conditions, by definition, pain arising as a direct consequence of a lesion or disease affecting the somatosensory system either peripheral or central, now serves as the current definition of neuropathic pain by the International Association for the Study of Pain—Special Interest Group on Neuropathic Pain (NeuPSIG).

4.2.1 Pathways and Mechanisms

4.2.1.1 Nociceptors: The Site of Capsaicin Action

Since the early observations of Sherrington, who believed that the experience of pain was based on nerves that responded to specific types of noxious stimuli that cause tissue damage, the concept of "nociceptive nerves" and later the term "nociceptor" emerged to describe what we now refer to as primary afferent nociceptors (Sherrington 1906). Nociceptors represent that portion of the peripheral nervous system that is specialized for the detection of noxious stimuli. One of the principle benefits provided by nociceptors is their rapid detection of impending or actual tissue injury. Nociceptors accomplish this by being a part of an integrated system or "pain pathway" beginning with peripheral nociceptive terminals that function to detect multiple noxious stimuli (transduction), the relay of these signals to the central nervous system through the conduction of action potentials (transmission) and finally their interpretation as a harmful or unpleasant experience (perception) (Fields 1990).

Within the peripheral nervous system, somatosensory detection of tissue damaging stimuli (thermal, mechanical, chemical) begins at the peripheral terminals of primary afferent nociceptors whose cell bodies reside primarily in the trigeminal (V) and dorsal root ganglia (DRG). In addition, cranial nerves V (innervation of the majority of the face, conjunctiva, mouth, and dura mater) as well as cranial nerves VII, IX, and X (innervation of the skin of the external ear, and mucous membranes of the larynx and pharynx) also participate in nociception (Carpenter 1985). Likewise, nerve terminals derived from nociceptors residing in spinal dorsal root ganglia (cervical, thoracic, and lumbar) innervate the somatotopic dermatomes of the skin and underlying tissue. Nociceptors derived from dorsal root ganglia then send central processes to laminae I, II, and V of the dorsal horn of the spinal cord and following synaptic connection with second-order dorsal horn neurons, nociceptive information is relayed to higher centers of the brain.

Detection of noxious stimuli of the skin and underlying deep tissues (somatic) has been divided into three modalities: noxious thermal, mechanical, and chemical. The behavioral and physiological responses following the application of one of these three painful modalities have served as the cornerstone for a classification scheme of nociceptors. Within this classification scheme, the threshold for evoking the sensation of pain has been determined in human volunteers with certain external forces applied to the skin such as noxious thermal stimuli (temperatures $\geq$43–45 °C) or intense mechanical stimuli. Criteria for detection of noxious chemical stimuli have also been applied and rely on the sensation of pain in response to certain compounds such as *capsaicin*, the pungent principle ingredient in hot chili peppers and the therapeutic focus of this chapter (Fields 1990).

Primary afferent nociceptors have been further classified based on their axon diameter, conduction velocity, degree of myelination, and more recently, cross-sectional area of neuronal soma. The axons of primary afferent neurons fall into three distinct groups, Aß (large-diameter, 6–22 μm, heavily myelinated with fast conduction velocities (CV) of 33–75 m/sec), Aδ (diameter 2–5 μm, thinly myelinated with CV 5–30 m/sec), and C fibers (diameter 0.3–3 μm, unmyelinated with CV of 0.5–2 m/sec) (Bessou and Perl 1969). Nociceptors activated by multiple noxious stimuli are referred to as "polymodal nociceptors." (McMahon and Koltzenburg 1990) Included in this category are C fiber type mechano-heat nociceptors and at least two types of A fiber type nociceptors: mechano-heat Type I (high heat threshold >49 °C) and mechano-heat Type II, (heat threshold ~43 °C) (Fields 1990). Finally, high threshold mechano-nociceptors that fail to respond to thermal stimuli have been characterized for both C and A fiber types as well as for nociceptors that respond only to noxious chemical stimuli.

The sensation of peripheral neuropathic pain arising from peripheral sites of pathology has been described as arising from both unmyelinated C-type (slowly conducting) nerve fibers associated with sensations of dull, aching, burning, and poorly localized pain as well as thinly myelenated Aδ nerve fibers which are more rapidly conducting and signal sensations of sharp, stabbing, and often well-localized pain. However, despite this elegant classification of nociceptor subtypes, discharge patterns of polymodal nociceptors do not precisely correlate with stimulus-induced pain sensation (Adriaensen et al. 1984). Therefore, central processing of nociceptor impulses must be required for the discrimination of painful sensations. Although not proven, one may hypothesize that the selective destruction and/or functional silencing of a subset of polymodal nociceptors following topical capsaicin treatment, as discussed below, could disrupt the input of peripheral neuropathic pain signal processing of polymodal nociceptors.

Nociceptors also have the ability to adjust their sensitivity following repetitive noxious stimuli or tissue/nerve injury. Sensitization encompasses an increase in spontaneous nociceptor activity, a lowered threshold for activation, and an increase in action potential firing after suprathreshold stimuli (Fields 1990). Together with plasticity changes in the dorsal horn of the spinal cord, sensitization of nociceptors contributes to hyperalgesia. Nociceptor modulation is complex and multiple pathways exist to both detect noxious stimuli and modulate transducing element sensitivity. Under neuropathic conditions this complexity is increased, driven by overlapping biochemical processes—some common to both tissue and nerve injury. Examples of changes more prominent to experimental neuropathic pain models arising from peripheral nociceptor sensitization include increased small-afferent signaling arising from distal sprouting of injured nerves and aberrations in nociceptor channels/receptor expression (sodium and calcium channels, Nerve Growth Factor/NGF receptor-TrkA) in injured and uninjured (adjacent) sensory neurons.

One signaling molecule long associated with experimental neuropathic pain is the trophic factor "nerve growth factor" (NGF). Since its identification by Levi-Montalcini and Calissano, NGF has been distinguished from other neurotrophin family members (brain-derived neurotrophic factor NT-3, and NT-4/5) as being essential for normal nociceptor development and function (Koltzenburg 1999; Lewin and Mendell 1994; McMahon et al. 1995). NGF is synthesized and secreted by a wide variety of tissues including Schwann cells located within sensory ganglion and importantly, in the end-target tissues of nociceptive terminals—epidermal fibroblasts and keratinocytes. NGF is intimately involved in maintaining and modifying the phenotype of the nociceptor population. Adult sensory neurons lose their dependency on NGF for survival but retain expression of its high-affinity receptor TrkA primarily on the small-diameter primary afferent nociceptors (C and Aδ) (Koltzenburg 1999). Tissue and nerve injury are associated with increased NGF production and content at the site of the injury, serving as the driving signal for the associated pain and hyperalgesia (Woolf and Costigan 1999). Therefore, long-term exposure of nociceptive terminals to increased levels of NGF can result in long-term phenotypic changes in the repertoire of nociceptive transducing elements such as the capsaicin receptor. Such changes may lead to aberrations in pain signaling and in turn, may represent a molecular template for sustained peripheral neuropathic pain. Although the focus of this chapter is on peripheral mechanisms of neuropathic pain and its treatment with topical capsaicin, other more central changes associated with models of neuropathic pain also include the loss of the blood brain barrier integrity surrounding the spinal cord, allowing migration of non-neuronal inflammatory cells into the dorsal horn (sensory) of the spinal cord and the DRG. Other changes associated with experimental models of neuropathic pain include activation of dorsal horn microglia that are known to be associated with chronic pain (Watkins et al. 2001).

4.2.2 *Assessment*

Neuropathic pain often goes unrecognized and therefore is under-reported being unsuccessfully treated with agents such as non-steroidal anti-inflammatory drugs (NSAIDS) and/or acetaminophen (Gore et al. 2007). Although there is no "gold standard," pathognomonic sign or symptom for the diagnosis of neuropathic pain, a focused history and sensory exam can often provide clinicians the critical insight for early recognition and subsequent treatment. A combination of signs (hypoesthesia, hyper/hypo-algesia, heat/cold hyperalgesia, allodynia) and symptoms (paraesthesias, sensation of burning, and/or shooting pain) together with the appropriate clinical context increases the likelihood of a reliable diagnosis of neuropathic pain (Haanpaa et al. 2009).

To assist the clinician, standardized screening tools have been developed to provide the practitioner a reliable and importantly, validated approach to forming an accurate diagnosis. Two such tools are the "Leeds assessment of neuropathic symptoms and signs" (LANSS) (Bennett 2001) and the "Douleur Neruopathiques 4 questions" (DN4) (Bouhassira et al. 2005). Although a clinical history may provide a high degree of suspicion about whether a particular patient indeed is suffering from pain of peripheral neuropathic origins, the incidence of neuropathic pain varies geographically. Whereas patients in developing countries with high rates of HIV or trauma due to war may be predisposed to neuropathic pain from these processes, patients from developed countries may be more likely to develop neuropathic pain as a consequence of diabetes or a herpes zoster infection predisposing to PHN (Haanpaa et al. 2009).

4.2.3 *Treatment of Neuropathic Pain*

Evidence-based guidelines for the treatment of painful neuropathic conditions continue to gain strength as additional randomized controlled trials are successfully completed. Expert opinion in the form of guideline recommendations have emerged and in many cases have been updated from societies dedicated to the evidence-based management of neuropathic pain such as NeuPSIG (Special Interest Group on Neuropathic Pain of the International Association for the Study of Pain) (Dworkin et al. 2010, 2007). Therefore, guidelines intended to recommend any therapy as a "first-line" treatment for a particular type of neuropathic pain require that efficacy has been established in multiple randomized clinical trials (RCT) (Oxford Center for Evidence-based Medicine, Grade A) and that these recommendations are consistent with the provider's experience/patient population. Unfortunately, few neuropathic pain therapies including those involving the topical application of capsaicin, fulfill such criteria. Nevertheless, an evolving list of first-line medications have been recommended that include: antidepressants with both norepinephrine and serotonin reuptake inhibition, calcium channel alpha 2 delta ligands (gabapentin and pregabalin), and topical lidocaine (Dworkin et al. 2010). Second-line therapies (which may be considered "first-line" under certain circumstances) include tramadol and opioid analgesics. Finally, so-called "third line" therapies include other anticonvulsants and "low-dose" capsaicin creams, as high-dose capsaicin-based patch studies were just emerging as these guidelines were reported. These recommendations are in line with other international expert groups (Attal et al. 2010). Among a collection of European countries that participated in comparison of their clinical practice guidelines on the treatment of neuropathic pain in cancer patients, all responded that the use of amitriptyline was a first-line recommendation (Piano et al. 2014). Second, the use of gabapentinoids was recommended. Within this report, the clinical practice guidelines across nine countries also included whether the use of capsaicin-containing plasters should be recommended for the treatment of conditions of "local (peripheral) neuropathic pain", presumably having a restricted pattern of distribution (dermatomal or non-dermatomal). Although four of the countries did not provide data, the remaining five countries all recommended that capsaicin-containing plasters should be utilized for the treatment of neuropathic conditions (Piano et al. 2014).

Therefore, providers are faced with a range of choices from pharmacologic therapies of nonopioid and opioid agents, adjuvant analgesics, topical preparations, and interventional techniques such as neuroblockade and intraspinal infusions to recently advancing neurostimulatory techniques. Unfortunately, there is even less evidence in support of interventional approaches to manage pain from neuropathic conditions refractory to pharmacologic interventions. Due to the paucity of RCT data in this area, only weak recommendations so far exist that include the use of epidural injections for herpes zoster, epidural steroid injections for radiculopathy, spinal cord stimulation (SCS) therapy for failed back surgical syndrome, and SCS for complex regional pain syndrome type 1 (CRPS type 1) (Dworkin et al. 2013). More invasive-ablative techniques are also sometimes used under conditions of compassionate care for patients with progressive malignant disease driving neuropathic symptoms (Kanpolat et al. 2009; Meyerson 2001; Turnbull et al. 2011) although these can also be associated with significant risks or unmasking other painful sensations.

As we await additional randomized clinical trials, a step-wise approach for the treatment of neuropathic pain is recommended where a combination of proven medications may represent a superior therapeutic plan. Nevertheless, clinical trials investigating the use of such combination therapies have yet to fully emerge. Just as one considers the application of multiple pharmacologic agents to a particular condition, patients suffering from chronic neuropathic pain will likely benefit from a multimodal or multidisciplinary approach to their pain management. Importantly, multidisciplinary treatment programs compared with conventional treatment are effective in reducing the intensity of the pain reported by the patient for a period of four months to one year (evidence category A2). Although multimodal therapy has been shown to be efficacious for a number of conditions, its superiority over uni-modal therapies has not yet been fully supported in the literature due to the absence of sufficient high quality randomized controlled trials (category D evidence). Nevertheless, it is the recommendation of the American Society of Anesthesiologists—ASA task force in 2010 on practice guidelines for chronic pain management, that "a multimodal strategy be part of the treatment plan for patients with chronic pain" (2010). Moreover, such a multi-modal approach should ensure early recognition and treatment of psychosocial maladies that are critical for long-term success in any treatment plan and goal to improve functional status and overall quality of life.

4.3 The Action of Capsaicin on Primary Afferent Nociceptors

It has long been appreciated that initial applications of capsaicin are painful, but paradoxically, repeated application produces a topical analgesic effect. It has been proposed that a series of overlapping capsaicin-induced effects that include: desensitization, nociceptor dysfunction, neuropeptide depletion, (Cao et al. 1998; Yaksh et al. 1979), and nociceptive terminal destruction (Robbins et al. 1998; Simone et al. 1998) constitute critical elements producing pain relief. However, several aspects of topical capsaicin treatment appear to limit its overall effectiveness and application in clinical practice. The first is the requirement for repeated capsaicin application (up to 4–5 times daily) to establish and maintain an adequate degree of analgesia. Repeated use of capsaicin-containing topical creams leads to the loss of epidermal nerve fibers that can be detected as soon as 3 days following repeated application. In fact, after 3 weeks of capsaicin treatment on the volar forearm 4 times daily, there was an approximately 80 % reduction in epidermal nerve processes. Loss of the epidermal fibers (see Fig. 4.1) was concordant with a reduction in painful sensation to noxious heat and mechanical stimuli (Nolano et al. 1999). Similar findings were observed when capsaicin was injected subcutaneously in volunteers (Simone et al. 1998).

Yet in other clinical studies performed to better quantify the effects of low-dose capsaicin on expression of TRPV1 and neuropeptides in human nociceptive terminals, control human skin biopsies showed abundant immunoreactivity to the neuropeptides SP (substance-P) and CGRP (calcitonin gene related peptide). After 1 day of repeated topical application of capsaicin (five times daily) at a concentration of 0.025 %, a diminution of SP and CGRP immunoreactivity in nerve fibers was observed (Stander et al. 2004). Continuous application of capsaicin for 24 days, 1 and 8 months, respectively, resulted in a decrease of SP and CGRP

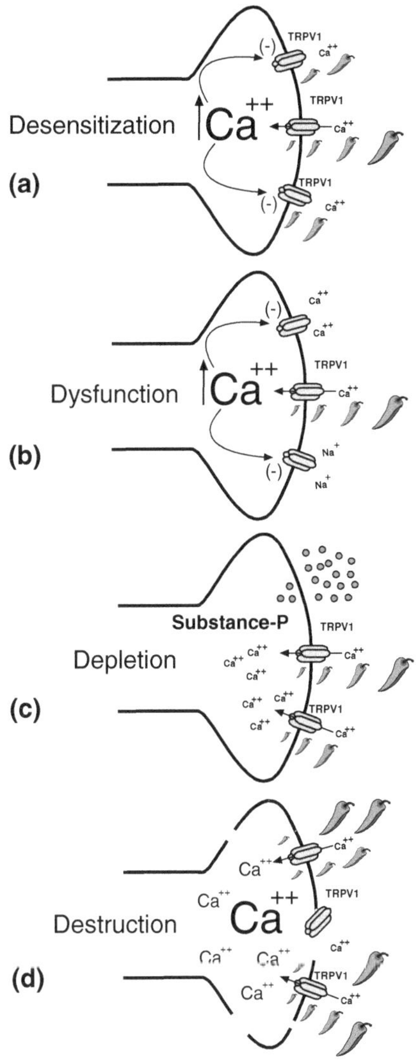

Fig. 4.1 Topical capsaicin-mediated analgesia. Topical application of capsaicin to the skin can produce concentration, dosing interval, and time-dependent changes to underlying sensory nerve terminals expressing the capsaicin receptor (*TRPV1*). As illustrated in panels (**a**–**d**), functional (**a**–**c**) and subsequently structural (**d**) changes in the *TRPV1*-expressing nociceptive terminals occur as a result of the magnitude and duration of *TRPV1* activation. Long-term analgesia may arise from selective destruction and/or functional silencing of a subset of polymodal nociceptors following topical capsaicin treatment disrupting central nociceptive input from peripheral neuropathic pain signal processes. **a** Desensitization is a calcium-dependent phenomenon where application of capsaicin leads to a decrease in inward current response during continued capsaicin application. When capsaicin is applied at repeated intervals, each subsequent response becomes smaller and is often referred to as tachyphylaxis. *TRPV1* may become refractory to the effect of endogenous inflammatory mediators and intracellular secondary messengers. **b** Repeated or prolonged application of capsaicin can also produce nociceptor dysfunction. Under this condition,

◀ which is dependent on the influx and/or excess of store-released calcium, other pain-transducing receptor–channels are inactivated. This may explain analgesic effects beyond the known function of TRPV1. **c** Depletion of neuropeptides (Substance-P, CGRP) from nociceptive terminal is evoked by capsaicin (low- and high-dose) or repeat applications. Substance-P has been show to play a key role in facilitating nociceptive neurotransmission in the dorsal horn of the spinal cord. **d** Destruction of TRPV1-expressing nociceptive terminals has been the most reliable marker correlating the application of capsaicin with analgesia

expression in superficial small nerve fibers of the papillary dermis, whereas, in nerve fibers of the deep dermis, the content of neuropeptides was unchanged. In contrast, the distribution and intensity of TRPV1 staining in nerve fibers and appendage structures was not changed as compared to untreated skin. Seven and 14 days after discontinuation of the capsaicin therapy, immunoreactivity to SP and CGRP was again detectable in small papillary nerve fibers. We, and others, hypothesize that capsaicin directs a dose-dependent effect, with low-dose capsaicin treatments associated with loss of neuropeptides in sensory terminals whereas the repetitive and/or highest capsaicin dosing being the most effective in directing the destruction of nociceptor terminals. What properties of nociceptors allow for their selective inactivation/destruction following capsaicin application?

With the isolation of a cDNA clone encoding a capsaicin-activated ion channel in 1997, the molecular basis of the capsaicin receptor, transient receptor potential cation channel subfamily V member 1 (TRPV1) was finally realized (Caterina et al. 1997). Termed TRPV1, it encodes a nonselective cation channel subunit of approximately 95 kDa that is highly expressed in the small-diameter sensory neurons of dorsal root, trigeminal, and vagal ganglion. Its structure mostly resembles that of members of the Kv 1.2 and store-operated channel family (Caterina et al. 1997). The TRPV1 subunit spans the plasma membrane six times, containing large N- and C-terminal intracellular regions, and is proposed to form tetrameric and/or heteromeric channel complexes (Eilers et al. 2007; Kedei et al. 2001; Kuzhikandathil et al. 2001). It is activated by capsaicin on the intracellular surface in a dose-dependent manner. Once activated, TRPV1 allows for the depolarization of the nociceptor through the conduction of cations. However it is not selective for monovalent cations but rather it preferentially conducts calcium through its channel pore, resulting in an increase in intracellular calcium and cellular depolarization. Thus, TRPV1 can be considered a cellular sensor and when expressed on sensory neurons, can confer specialized properties such as the detection of noxious stimuli and as explained below, detects changes in endogenous signaling molecules associated with tissue injury and inflammation.

Nerve and tissue injury result in the production and release of multiple inflammatory products that have been characterized and identified to directly activate TRPV1. These include products of inflammation and tissue injury such as NGF (Koltzenburg 1999; Mendell et al. 1999) as well as anandamide, the endogenous ligand for the cannabinoid receptor (CB1) (Smart et al. 2000; Julius and Basbaum 2001). Products of the lipoxygenase pathway of arachidonic acid, 12-(S)-hydroperoxyeicosatetranoic acid (12-(S)-HPETE), and leukotriene B4, (LTB_4) have also been found to activate

Table 4.2 Topical capsaicin formulations

Low concentration topical	High concentration topical
Over the counter	Prescription
Multiple formulations including cream, liquid, patch	Patch
Generally at or below 0.15 % capsaicin	8 % capsaicin
Applied by patient at any location	Applied by medical professional in an appropriate clinical venue
Application repeated multiple times daily for anywhere from weeks to indefinite time period	Applied once for one hour, repeated as needed at three month or greater intervals
Does not require pretreatment to the application area	Requires pretreatment with topical local anesthetic to the application area

TRPV1 in vitro (Shin et al. 2002). It has been reported that TRPV1 is expressed on large and small cutaneous nerve fibers in the human dermis and at the epidermal–dermal junction, while intraepidermal nerve fibers only occasionally stained for TRPV1. A similar staining pattern of TRPV1 immunoreactivity was also described in rat skin (Guo et al. 1999). Importantly, TRPV1 and SP are also co-localized in human cutaneous nerve fibers confirming previous reports in rat and mice. Therefore, beyond the ability of capsaicin to disrupt the function of polymodal nociceptors expressing TRPV1, capsaicin-induced inactivation could also result in blockade of endogenous activation of TRPV that is associated with pathophysiologic conditions giving rise to neuropathic pain symptoms.

4.3.1 Painful Neuropathic Conditions Treated with Topical Capsaicin Preparations

4.3.1.1 Overview

Early meta-analysis that included patients suffering from diabetic neuropathy and osteoarthritis concluded that topical capsaicin improved pain when compared with a placebo (Zhang and Li Wan Po 1994), the analysis includes a number of uncontrolled and/or underpowered trials, a concern that has weakened their influence on changing clinical practice over time. Moreover, if one applies a more "rigorous" standard for clinical trials (as exists presently) on trial data prior to 2004, topical capsaicin (0.025 or 0.075 %) showed poor to moderate efficacy in the treatment of either musculoskeletal or neuropathic symptoms (Mason et al. 2004). Coupled with one-third of these study patients experiencing mild to moderate adverse effects such as erythema, irritation, and transient increase in pain, (see Table 4.2) enthusiasm for widespread use of these agents in the absence of concurrent local anesthetic pretreatment appeared to plateau. Therefore, such treatments were considered for so-called "nonresponders" rather than as a first-line treatment option.

To obtain improved patient acceptance and analgesic efficacy using capsaicin-based creams, therapeutic trials have progressively shifted from repeated applications of a combination of local anesthetic pretreatment followed by low-dose capsaicin (Turnbull et al. 2011) to potentially a single application of high-dose topical capsaicin patch. This shift, in part, owes its origin to a case series that included 10 patients suffering from intractable lower extremity pain with neuropathic features. Application of capsaicin (5–10 %) under regional anesthesia resulted in a wide range of posttreatment pain relief (Robbins et al. 1998).

Therefore, the report of Robbins et al. suggested an alternative approach, a single application period of a high-dose capsaicin rather than the onerous task of repeat daily applications of low-dose formulations that are associated with a high dropout rate. Later, a high concentration capsaicin patch (8 %) was devised and its application to the skin for a period of 1–2 h produced longer term changes in epidermal nerve fibers that included loss of staining and reduction of heat sensitization. This illustrated that a short-term application of a high concentration of capsaicin can mimic those changes previously seen under repeat application (3–5 times/day for 1 week) of lower concentration capsaicin cream (Malmberg et al. 2004). Subsequently, a randomized double-blinded study for the treatment of PHN using a 1-hour application of a high-dose capsaicin (8 %) patch was found to provide significant pain relief between study weeks 2–12 (Backonja et al. 2008). However, just as repeated application of low-dose capsaicin creams has found limited acceptance by patients due to application-induced burning and/or irritation, application of a high-dose capsaicin patch must also overcome a similar therapeutic barrier. To address this additional therapeutic barrier, high-dose capsaicin patch administration requires a unique application protocol as compared with low-dose breams and a health care provider (see Table 4.2). Pilot studies indicated that pretreating the proposed application area with 4 % lidocaine jelly for one hour was reported to provide "acceptable" side effects following application of high-dose capsaicin patch, though such treatment was commonly associated with localized pain and erythema (Backonja et al. 2008).

4.4 Safety and Tolerability of High-Dose Capsaicin Patch

Beginning with a series of small, open label studies, more rigorous double-blinded randomized controlled studies focused on the safety and tolerability of high-dose capsaicin-containing patches following prior application of a topical local anesthetic. Importantly, it was studied whether the type of local anesthetic influenced the degree of tolerability of the subsequent capsaicin patch application. In a randomized prospective study of 117 patients suffering from a range of peripheral neuropathies including PHN and diabetic neuropathy, using LMX 4, Topicaine, or Betacaine, with endpoints of average pain score at baseline versus at 2–12 weeks, no significant difference in tolerability was found between the various local anesthetics (Webster et al. 2012). Although no serious adverse events

Table 4.3 Capsaicin application site adverse effects

Capsaicin application site adverse effects
Erythema
Pain
Pruritus
Papules

Adverse reactions occurring in clinical studies in ≥5 % of patients treated with high concentration capsaicin patch and of higher incidence than controls. Symptoms were generally rated as "mild" or "moderate" and generally resolved by postapplication day 0–2

(AE) related to high-dose capsaicin patch treatment were reported, 50–59 % of the study patients reported adverse effects (see Table 4.3), which were primarily local, mild to moderate in severity, and resolved within in 1–2 days. Furthermore, analgesic responses were not significantly different between local anesthetic pretreatment groups. Importantly, patients receiving a longer (90-min) patch application were associated with greater procedural discomfort and greater use of periprocedural analgesics without a proportional increase in analgesic effect. Thus a 60-min application period was largely adopted (Webster et al. 2012). Moreover, these results mirror a smaller study with a focus only on patients with PHN treated topically with lidocaine 2.5 %/prilocaine 2.5 % cream for 60 min before receiving a single 60-min application of topical high concentration capsaicin. Maximum mean change in NPRS score was +3.0 observed at 55-min postpatch application with scores gradually declining to near preanesthetic levels within 85 min of patch removal. However, half of the patients received analgesic medication on the day of treatment (Webster et al. 2011). More broadly, analysis of twelve studies of mixed experimental design and patients with various peripheral painful neuropathies (PHN, HIV-DSPN, and PDN) showed that the maximum increase in pain reporting score ranged from 2.3 to 2.8 with no difference in treatment-associated pain among the different neuropathies (Webster et al. 2012).

Despite the mild to moderate adverse effects described above (localized pain and irritation) topical capsaicin engenders an overall favorable safety profile due to several complementary factors. Capsaicin can be systemically absorbed through the skin as a function of its applied concentration and duration of exposure. When the kinetics of systemic capsaicin absorption were investigated in patients receiving a high-dose capsaicin (8 %) patch for pain arising from either PHN, HIV-associated neuropathy (HIV-AN), or from diabetes mellitus (PDN), patch application to the trunk (PHN) directed the greatest plasma levels (peak 17.8 ng/mL). Conversely, significantly lower plasma concentrations were detected when the patch was applied to the feet (diabetic neuropathy, HIV-AN). Likewise, if application time was increased from 60 to 90 min, the hourly plasma concentration was observed to double (Babbar et al. 2009). Ultimately following absorption, capsaicin is rapidly eliminated by the cytochrome P450 hepatic enzyme system, (Chanda et al. 2008) with a population elimination half-life of 1.64 h (Babbar et al. 2009).

In summary, the application of high-dose capsaicin in the treatment of a diverse range of peripheral neuropathic states results in significant postapplication pain (up to a change of +3 on the NPRS) but treatment-associated pain is independent of underlying neuropathic condition or type of pretreatment local anesthetic. Greater than half of patients appeared to require supplemental analgesics to manage the treatment-associated pain which may be greater with a longer (90-min) application period. Nevertheless, pain associated with patch treatments was relatively transient in duration with the majority of patients returning to baseline pain levels within 2 days and overall without report of severe adverse events. For these reasons, high-dose capsaicin patch therapy has been advanced and investigated for efficacy in the treatment of a number of chronic painful conditions arising from peripheral neuropathic states, but with an apparent majority of studies derived from patients suffering from PHN (Peppin et al. 2011; Simpson et al. 2010).

4.4.1 Postherpetic Neuralgia

PHN is one of the most prevalent painful conditions associated with neuropathy that clinicians may encounter. PHN is driven in the USA by some 800,000 cases of primary herpes zoster infection each year (Schmader 2002). In Germany by comparison, from 2004 to 2009, 403,625 herpes zoster infection cases were estimated per year with approximately 5 % of such cases developing PHN (Ultsch et al. 2013). Following a primary systemic infection, the herpes zoster virus remains dormant in the dorsal root (sensory) ganglion but may become reactivated under conditions of stress, infection, malignancy (especially lymphoma), or immune-suppression resulting in its renewed replication. As a result of increased herpes zoster viral transport to the skin via infected sensory nerves, eruption of painful lesions along dermatomal distributions are manifest resulting in an increased risk of developing PHN after age 55 (Ultsch et al. 2013).

Acute outbreaks of herpes zoster are treated with a combination of medications to suppress viral replication and if needed, to manage painful symptoms. Although pain is well known to be associated with a reactivation (shingles) event, it is when pain and discomfort persist for more than 1 month after the zoster rash has healed that the diagnosis of PHN is typically made. Symptoms can include perceptions of constant burning and gnawing as well as paroxysmal sharp shooting and/or shocking pain either at rest or induced by light tactile stimulation. A combination of antiviral therapy (Acyclovir) and multimodal analgesics (gabapentinoids, TCAs, topical capsaicin preparations, opioids, topical lidocaine preparations) are intended to decrease the duration of outbreak, promote healing, and manage pain. Unfortunately, despite the effective treatment of herpes zoster infection, PHN may still develop resulting in pain that is notoriously difficult to manage—degrading a patient's quality of life.

In response to this therapeutic dilemma, a variety of treatment options have been investigated including the use of topically applied agents, such as capsaicin.

Initially formulated as "low-dose" capsaicin creams, several large, double-blinded, vehicle-controlled studies of patients with chronic PHN-demonstrated efficacy of low-dose capsaicin creams (0.075 %). The authors of these studies suggested that they should be considered as part of the initial plan for PHN pain management (Watson et al. 1993). Given the modest success of low-dose capsaicin, the development of a high-dose capsaicin patch has more recently reinvigorated the idea that high-dose topical capsaicin preparations could one day take their place among first-line treatments of painful symptoms of PHN pain. In support of this effort and as previously introduced, a topical patch capable of delivering high-dose (8 %) capsaicin therapy was subsequently developed.

4.4.1.1 Efficacy of High-Dose Capsaicin Patch Therapy for the Treatment of PHN

Randomized controlled trials: building a case for the therapeutic efficacy of high-dose capsaicin treatment in peripheral neuropathies has required substantial evidence. What must be overcome is not only an analgesia endpoint, but that the increase in pain associated with a single patch treatment can be sufficiently tolerated and be of short duration such that the benefit of a long-term analgesia will outweigh the mild—moderate short-term adverse effects. Therefore, multiple randomized, double-blinded controlled multicenter trials were conducted. NPRS for weeks 2–8 post high-dose capsaicin patch application were compared with a low concentration (0.04 %) control patch. Initial results showed a 29.65 versus 19.9 % reduction of pain intensity in treatment versus control patients during weeks 2–8 and a similar 29.6 versus 19.9 % for weeks 2–12. Importantly, these findings held true regardless of whether or not patients were taking concomitant antineuropathic pain medications (Backonja et al. 2008).

In a dose finding study, 299 PHN patients received high-dose or low-dose capsaicin patch for 30, 60, or 90 min. Although the 30-min group did not meet statistical significance, the 60-min treatment was significant with the largest improvement for patients during weeks 2–8 was following the 90-min treatment (27.8 vs. 17.3 %) (Webster et al. 2010a). Notably, the degree of pain relief for PHN in these studies appeared independent of whether patients were treated within the first 6 months of PHN or later (after 6 months). Whereas, another report suggested a greater overall improvement (including patient satisfaction) in analgesic treatment profile for patients suffering from PHN for greater than 6 months (Webster et al. 2010b).

Beyond individual or multicenter-integrated data studies described previously, meta-analysis of high-dose capsaicin prospective randomized trials have been performed inclusive of PHN, painful diabetic neuropathy, and HIV-associated neuropathy. Such meta-analysis continued to demonstrate a significant decrease in reported pain between high-dose capsaicin patch treatments versus low-dose controls (30.7 % reduction from baseline during weeks 2–12 vs. 22.7 % drop in low-dose control patch). Overall, (all sub groups of neuropathic pain) there was a 30 % reduction achieved in 44 % of high-dose patch versus 34 % control (low-dose patch), however, the overall magnitude of these differences is relatively small—approximately 8–10 %. Such meta-analysis were limited by a study period that was 12 weeks, and a neuropathic pain subgroup cohort that was insufficient in size to detect subgroup treatment benefits (Mou et al. 2013) (Irving et al. 2012). Subsequent meta-analysis was undertaken with a larger number of PHN patients (1313 PHN) studied with high-dose capsaicin patch treatment, and using a 30 % reduction in mean pain intensity score as characterizing a "responder." This analysis revealed a mean of 3.4 days until onset of analgesia, with duration of analgesic response of 5 months (Irving et al. 2012). Furthermore, in an attempt to identify patients that may have gained the greatest benefit from high-dose patch treatment, a study identified five types of "responders:" (1) a population showing worsening of response (i.e., pain increases during treatment) which were 1.5 and 0.8 % of patch versus control; (2) a population showing no analgesic response which were 22.7 % of patch and 39.1 % of control; (3) a population showing a partial or full analgesic response but with a return to pretreatment pain levels within 12 weeks (24.7 % patch vs. 17.6 % control); (4) a population showing a partial analgesic response at week 1 that remained constant during the study period (14.5 % patch and 14.3 % control); and (5) a population that showed an ongoing decline in pain rating during the 12 weeks of the study which were 36.6 % patch and 28.2 % control. Importantly, increasing age and duration of disease as well as concurrent opioid use all were negative predictors of resolution of the pain (Group 5), and generally, no analgesic response to the high-dose capsaicin patch treatment (Group 2) (Martini et al. 2013).

Taking a complementary approach, a systematic review of six studies including 2073 patients was performed by the Cochrane Database through December of 2012 that included RCT and controlled trials of at least 6-week duration. Four studies of 1272 participants for PHN showed numbers needed to treat (NNT) to attain "much improved or very much improved" of 8.8 and 7.0. Serious adverse events were no more common with high-dose treatment than controls nor were the rate of study withdrawals, however the "lack of efficacy" withdrawals were found to be greater in controls—supporting a beneficial effect of the high-dose patch. Overall, the systematic review of high-dose patch treatment for PHN (and HIV-associated neuropathy) generated more participants with high levels of pain relief than control—but the additional proportion of that benefit is not large. Nevertheless, for those who did respond, benefits in sleep, fatigue, depression, and quality of life were also seen (Derry et al. 2013).

4.4.1.2 Summary: Treatment of PHN with High-Dose Capsaicin

PHN can result in severe neuropathic pain and impaired functional status. The majority of oral analgesic treatments for PHN carry the risk of significant systemic side effects. This has been in large part responsible for the interest in topically administered therapies. Prior to the advent of a high-dose capsaicin patch, widespread acceptance of capsaicin in lower concentration forms were limited by unimpressive evidence and compliance with the cumbersome and uncomfortable nature of chronic administration. With the advent of a high-dose patch, a capsaicin treatment option now exists that does not eliminate, but changes and potentially improves upon the limitations of its administration. There is now a modest but growing evidence base including several RCTs, meta-analysis, and systematic review supporting safety and efficacy in the use of high-dose capsaicin patch treatment for PHN. Interestingly, thus far only a single retrospective study has attempted to provide insight as to the financial impact of the use of the high concentration capsaicin patch in the treatment of PHN. Using a model based on monthly analgesic medication cycles, including analgesic dose titration and management of adverse events, the proportion of patients achieving at least a 30 % improvement in PHN pain with outcomes cost per quality-adjusted life-year (QALY) were calculated. Although no head-to-head studies were identified for comparison, they found that the high-dose (8 %) capsaicin patch (and topical lidocaine patch) were significantly more effective than oral analgesic medications prescribed for PHN. The incremental cost-effectiveness ratio for the capsaicin patch overlapped with the topical lidocaine patch and was within the accepted threshold of cost per QALY gained compared to tricyclic antidepressants (TCAs), duloxetine, gabapentin, and pregabalin. However, the frequency of the high-dose capsaicin patch retreatment could significantly impact its cost-effectiveness (Armstrong et al. 2011).

4.4.2 Diabetic Neuropathy

Diabetes mellitus affects more than 14 million people within the USA, and estimates predict that globally, rates will increase to 366 million by 2030 (Wild et al. 2004). Among this cohort, some estimate that between 18 and 24 % may suffer from some form of painful diabetic neuropathy (PDN) and a subset of patients suffering from diabetic polyneuropathy is termed PDPN (Schmader 2002; Spallone and Greco 2013). PDPN is thought to arise from the metabolic and microvessel consequences associated with chronic hyperglycemic exposure, as occurs in diabetes type I or II. PDPN represents the most bothersome of symptoms of diabetic polyneuropathy that develops into a chronic painful condition. Management of the painful neuropathic symptoms associated with PDNP has been difficult given limited choices of therapeutic agents (TCAs, gabapentinoids, topical lidocaine), and often less than 50 % pain reduction or high number-needed-to-treat—NNT.

Given the apparent widespread prevalence and difficulty in managing PDPN, use of preparations containing either low or high concentrations of capsaicin have been investigated. Early randomized studies using relatively low-dose capsaicin preparations (0.075 %) versus a vehicle control four times daily on patients suffering from PDPN, showed a small but statistically significant improvement in pain intensity scores (VAS) and pain relief (The Capsaicin Study Group 1991). More recently the idea that capsaicin-containing topical preparations may, in fact, have a therapeutic advantage in the treatment of diabetic neuropathy was advanced due to over-expression of its natural target—the capsaicin receptor (TRPV1) in an experimental rodent model of diabetes (Rashid et al. 2003). Unfortunately, such a promising idea has not yet been observed to translate into therapeutic outcome. For example, in a noncontrolled, prospective observational study, 91 patients with PDPN were enrolled for single treatment with 1–4 high-dose topical capsaicin patches and pain scores were studied longitudinally over a 12-week period. Approximately one-third (34 %) of patients treated with a single application of the high-dose capsaicin patch showed a rapid and clinically relevant reduction in pain that persisted (70 ± 5 % pain reduction) by week 12. However, an equal percentage either had no improvement or a short-term benefit that peaked at 3 weeks following treatment (Martini et al. 2012). As observed in the treatment of other peripheral neuropathies, high-dose capsaicin patch therapy for PDNP was also associated with a mean increase in reported pain scores of 2.3–2.8 on night two, resulting in 14 % of treated patients requiring additional analgesics to manage their treatment-associated pain (Peppin et al. 2011). Therefore, although some patient's suffering from PDNP may indeed experience significant analgesic benefit, its overall lower response rate has made it problematic to consider high-dose capsaicin patch therapy as a first-line analgesic treatment until more convincing evidence from RCT is reported.

4.4.3 HIV-Associated Painful Neuropathy

Painful peripheral neuropathies as a result of HIV infection represent another therapeutic challenge for both patient and clinician. HIV-associated distal symmetrical polyneuropathy (DSPN), represents perhaps the most common neurologic complication (30–50 %) of HIV-infected patients. Although the mechanism of HIV-DSPN-associated pain remains unclear, it is presumably driven by a combination of cytotoxic HIV-viral protein product(s) and/or is exacerbated by certain antiretroviral therapies (Acharjee et al. 2010; Huang et al. 2013). Such pain can be refractory to standard pharmacologic treatment leading to major morbidity and disability. In response for the need of more effective treatments, early trials again focused on the use of low-dose capsaicin-containing topical preparations but with unsatisfactory results (Paice et al. 2000). With the development of the high-dose (8 %) capsaicin patch, a renewed effort was launched to demonstrate the efficacy of topical capsaicin for the treatment of HIV-DSPN without a detectable change in the perception of warmth, cold, sharp pain, or vibration sensation (Simpson et al. 2008). Although an initial RCT study showed a trend toward better pain relief for these patients, the study failed to meet its primary endpoint (Clifford et al. 2012). Subsequently, the combination of two similarly designed RCT revealed a reduction in pain with application of the high-dose patch treatment for 30 but not 60 min—missing significance due to an unusually high level of pain relief from the low-dose control patch application (Brown et al. 2013). Finally, with study of a greater number of subjects (801 HIV-DSPN patients) with pain of the lower extremities (feet) showed modest pain relief with 41 % of HIV-DSPN patients having a 30 % reduction in symptoms and a mean duration of response of 5 months. Importantly, of those that were followed for the entire 12 months, 10 % had complete resolution of painful symptoms (Mou et al. 2013). Moreover, there was no apparent relationship between the duration of patch application, the number of patch applications or the degree of analgesia achieved. Numbers needed to treat (NNT) to achieve a patient report of "better or much better" was 5.8 and higher NNT for other outcome measures. Adverse events included short-term site swelling and burning sensation with 44 % of the patients requesting oxycodone/acetaminophen following capsaicin patch placement. A small number of patients also experienced itching or coughing (Derry et al. 2013). Given the NNT of HIV-DSPN patients to achieve even a modest analgesic result, use of high-dose capsaicin patch does not appear to be a first-line analgesic treatment for HIV-DSPN although an unpredictable subset of such patients may obtain significant long-term relief of painful symptoms.

4.4.4 Other Painful Conditions with Neuropathic Features

Just as postherpetic neuralgia, diabetic and HIV-associated neuropathies represent distinct disease entities they also share overlapping features of pain and dysfunction of the peripheral nociceptive system. Although less well known, there are a number of other painful conditions with neuropathic features arising from diverse pathophysiology. Of these, the more commonly known include: trigeminal neuralgia, complex regional pain syndrome type-II (causalgia) and persistent postsurgical pain. Paradoxically, despite sharing apparently similar mechanistic origins (partial nerve injury) they differ widely in terms of their therapeutic response to pharmacologic and interventional therapies but all are known to be difficult to effectively manage and generally resistant to opioid based analgesic strategies. Perhaps due to their complexity and relative scarcity, there does not appear to be any controlled studies for the treatment of trigeminal neuralgia or CRPS-II with topical capsaicin—except perhaps a case report of the successful treatment of PHN in the trigeminal (V1) distribution with a high-dose capsaicin patch (Sayanlar et al. 2012).

In contrast, the use of topical capsaicin for the management of postoperative incisional pain includes a series of case reports (McPartland 2002; Rayner et al. 1989; Weintraub et al. 1990). Controlled trials for the treatment of persistent postsurgical pain following mastectomy has been pursued with reasonable success and later in part confirmed by an open label trial (Dini et al. 1993; Watson and Evans 1992). Capsaicin-based topical applications were also investigated with a controlled trial on postsurgical neuropathic pain in cancer patients with the use of 0.075 % cream applied four times daily. Impressively, 53 versus 17 % (placebo control) of patients experienced a significantly greater pain relief while using topical capsaicin (Ellison et al. 1997). As concern of persistent postsurgical pain syndromes grow, additional trials utilizing capsaicin-containing preparations should be forthcoming.

4.5 Conclusions

As our understanding of the molecular basis of pain transduction has advanced, propelled with the isolation of the capsaicin receptor (TRPV1), there has been a renewed effort to leverage these discoveries to develop more effective treatment for persistent painful conditions. Despite the historic use of topical preparations containing capsaicin, the recent combination of neurobiology, biotechnology, and advances in clinical trial design has allowed concentrated forms of capsaicin to be safely applied to manage painful neuropathic conditions. Of the painful conditions described in this chapter, the strongest evidence exists for the use of high-dose capsaicin for the management of painful PHN. However, as with other therapeutic options for the treatment of painful neuropathic conditions, there appear to be patient responders and non-responders suffering from PHN and a range of other neuropathic conditions. Fortunately, there appears no advantage, nor disadvantage, of such patients taking concurrent anti-neuropathic/analgesic medications while undergoing high-dose capsaicin patch treatment. For those patients fortunate to receive analgesic benefit from a single application of the high-dose capsaicin patch, there is the potential of long-lasting relief of painful symptoms without the requirement of continued daily topical application. Nevertheless, analgesic response rates for peripheral neuropathic painful conditions tend to average approximately 30 % and rarely if ever exceed 50 %. Moreover, the magnitude of analgesic effect is typically modest (10–30 %). Beyond PHN, other painful neuropathic conditions sensitive to the analgesic effects of topical capsaicin (with decreasing level of evidence) include HIV-associated painful neuropathy (DSPN), painful diabetic neuropathy and postsurgical neuropathic pain. In these cases, there is not yet adequate evidence to support capsaicin-based topical therapies as first-line treatments. However, for some patients who are intolerant of standard pharmacologic approaches for the treatment of peripheral neuropathic pain syndromes, topical capsaicin preparations continue to offer a rational and often successful option—largely free of systemic side effects such as sedation, altered mental status, or risks of dependence and addiction.

Acknowledgments Thanks to Morgen Ahearn for her editorial assistance.

References

The Capsaicin Study Group (1991) Treatment of painful diabetic neuropathy with topical capsaicin. A multicenter, double-blind, vehicle-controlled study. Arch Intern Med 151:2225–2229

American Society of Anesthesiologists Task Force on Chronic Pain Management and the American Society of Regional Anesthesia and Pain Medicine (2010) Practice guidelines for chronic pain management: an updated report by the American Society of Anesthesiologists Task Force on Chronic Pain Management and the American Society of Regional Anesthesia and Pain Medicine. Anesthesiology 112:810–833

Acharjee S, Noorbakhsh F, Stemkowski PL, Olechowski C, Cohen EA, Ballanyi K, Kerr B, Pardo C, Smith PA, Power C (2010) HIV-1 viral protein R causes peripheral nervous system injury associated with in vivo neuropathic pain. Faseb J 24:4343–4353

Adriaensen H, Gybels J, Handwerker HO, Van Hees J (1984) Nociceptor discharges and sensations due to prolonged noxious mechanical stimulation–a paradox. Hum Neurobiol 3:53–58
Armstrong EP, Malone DC, McCarberg B, Panarites CJ, Pham SV (2011) Cost-effectiveness analysis of a new 8 % capsaicin patch compared to existing therapies for postherpetic neuralgia. Curr Med Res Opin 27:939–950
Attal N, Cruccu G, Baron R, Haanpaa M, Hansson P, Jensen TS, Nurmikko T (2010) EFNS guidelines on the pharmacological treatment of neuropathic pain: 2010 revision. Eur J Neurol 17:9
Babbar S, Marier JF, Mouksassi MS, Beliveau M, Vanhove GF, Chanda S, Bley K (2009) Pharmacokinetic analysis of capsaicin after topical administration of a high-concentration capsaicin patch to patients with peripheral neuropathic pain. Ther Drug Monit 31:502–510
Backonja M, Wallace MS, Blonsky ER, Cutler BJ, Malan P Jr, Rauck R, Tobias J (2008) NGX-4010, a high-concentration capsaicin patch, for the treatment of postherpetic neuralgia: a randomised, double-blind study. Lancet Neurol 7:1106–1112 Epub 2008 Oct 1130
Bennett M (2001) The LANSS Pain Scale: the Leeds assessment of neuropathic symptoms and signs. Pain 92:147–157
Bessou P, Perl ER (1969) Response of cutaneous sensory units with unmyelinated fibers to noxious stimuli. J Neurophysiol 32:1025–1043
Bouhassira D, Attal N, Alchaar H, Boureau F, Brochet B, Bruxelle J, Cunin G, Fermanian J, Ginies P, Grun-Overdyking A, Jafari-Schluep H, Lanteri-Minet M, Laurent B, Mick G, Serrie A, Valade D, Vicaut E (2005) Comparison of pain syndromes associated with nervous or somatic lesions and development of a new neuropathic pain diagnostic questionnaire (DN4). Pain 114:29–36
Brown S, Simpson DM, Moyle G, Brew BJ, Schifitto G, Larbalestier N, Orkin C, Fisher M, Vanhove GF, Tobias JK (2013) NGX-4010, a capsaicin 8 % patch, for the treatment of painful HIV-associated distal sensory polyneuropathy: integrated analysis of two phase III, randomized, controlled trials. AIDS Res Ther 10:5
Cao YQ, Mantyh PW, Carlson EJ, Gillespie AM, Epstein CJ, Basbaum AI (1998) Primary afferent tachykinins are required to experience moderate to intense pain. Nature 392:390–394
Carpenter MB (1985) Core text of neuroanatomy, 3rd edn. Williams & Wilkins, Baltimore
Caterina MJ, Schumacher MA, Tominaga M, Rosen TA, Levine JD, Julius D (1997) The capsaicin receptor: a heat-activated ion channel in the pain pathway. Nature 389:816–824
Chanda S, Bashir M, Babbar S, Koganti A, Bley K (2008) In vitro hepatic and skin metabolism of capsaicin. Drug Metab Dispos 36:670–675 Epub 2008 Jan 2007
Clifford DB, Simpson DM, Brown S, Moyle G, Brew BJ, Conway B, Tobias JK, Vanhove GF (2012) A randomized, double-blind, controlled study of NGX-4010, a capsaicin 8 % dermal patch, for the treatment of painful HIV-associated distal sensory polyneuropathy. J Acquir Immune Defic Syndr 59:126–133
Derry S, Sven-Rice A, Cole P, Tan T, Moore RA (2013) Topical capsaicin (high concentration) for chronic neuropathic pain in adults. Cochrane Database Syst Rev 2:CD007393
Dini D, Bertelli G, Gozza A, Forno GG (1993) Treatment of the post-mastectomy pain syndrome with topical capsaicin. Pain 54:223–226
Dworkin RH, O'Connor AB, Audette J, Baron R, Gourlay GK, Haanpaa ML, Kent JL, Krane EJ, Lebel AA, Levy RM, Mackey SC, Mayer J, Miaskowski C, Raja SN, Rice AS, Schmader KE, Stacey B, Stanos S, Treede RD, Turk DC, Walco GA, Wells CD (2010) Recommendations for the pharmacological management of neuropathic pain: an overview and literature update. Mayo Clin Proc 85:S3–S14
Dworkin RH, O'Connor AB, Backonja M, Farrar JT, Finnerup NB, Jensen TS, Kalso EA, Loeser JD, Miaskowski C, Nurmikko TJ, Portenoy RK, Rice AS, Stacey BR, Treede RD, Turk DC, Wallace MS (2007) Pharmacologic management of neuropathic pain: evidence-based recommendations. Pain 132:237–251
Dworkin RH, O'Connor AB, Kent J, Mackey SC, Raja SN, Stacey BR, Levy RM, Backonja M, Baron R, Harke H, Loeser JD, Treede RD, Turk DC, Wells CD (2013) Interventional management of neuropathic pain: NeuPSIG recommendations. *Pain* 154:2249–2261

Eilers H, Lee SY, Hau CW, Logvinova A, Schumacher MA (2007) The rat vanilloid receptor splice variant VR.5′sv blocks TRPV1 activation. NeuroReport 18:969–973
Ellison N, Loprinzi CL, Kugler J, Hatfield AK, Miser A, Sloan JA, Wender DB, Rowland KM, Molina R, Cascino TL, Vukov AM, Dhaliwal HS, Ghosh C (1997) Phase III placebo-controlled trial of capsaicin cream in the management of surgical neuropathic pain in cancer patients. J Clin Oncol 15:2974–2980
Fields HL (1990) Pain syndromes in neurology. Butterworths-Heinemann Ltd, London
Gore M, Dukes E, Rowbotham DJ, Tai KS, Leslie D (2007) Clinical characteristics and pain management among patients with painful peripheral neuropathic disorders in general practice settings. Eur J Pain 11:652–664
Guo A, Vulchanova L, Wang J, Li X, Elde R (1999) Immunocytochemical localization of the vanilloid receptor 1 (VR1): relationship to neuropeptides, the P2X3 purinoceptor and IB4 binding sites. Eur J Neurosci 11:946–958
Haanpaa ML, Backonja MM, Bennett MI, Bouhassira D, Cruccu G, Hansson PT, Jensen TS, Kauppila T, Rice AS, Smith BH, Treede RD, Baron R (2009) Assessment of neuropathic pain in primary care. Am J Med 122:S13–S21
Huang W, Calvo M, Karu K, Olausen HR, Bathgate G, Okuse K, Bennett DL, Rice AS (2013) A clinically relevant rodent model of the HIV antiretroviral drug stavudine induced painful peripheral neuropathy. Pain 154:560–575
Irving G, Backonja M, Rauck R, Webster LR, Tobias JK, Vanhove GF (2012) NGX-4010, a capsaicin 8 % dermal patch, administered alone or in combination with systemic neuropathic pain medications, reduces pain in patients with postherpetic neuralgia. Clin J Pain 28:101–107
Julius D, Basbaum AI (2001) Molecular mechanisms of nociception. Nature 413:203–210
Kanpolat Y, Ugur HC, Ayten M, Elhan AH (2009) Computed tomography-guided percutaneous cordotomy for intractable pain in\ malignancy. Neurosurgery 64:187–193; discussion 193–184
Kedei N, Szabo T, Lile JD, Treanor JJ, Olah Z, Iadarola MJ, Blumberg PM (2001) Analysis of the native quaternary structure of vanilloid receptor 1. J Biol Chem 276:28613–28619
Koltzenburg M (1999) The changing sensitivity in the life of the nociceptor. Pain Suppl 6:S93–S102
Kuzhikandathil EV, Wang H, Szabo T, Morozova N, Blumberg PM, Oxford GS (2001) Functional analysis of capsaicin receptor (vanilloid receptor subtype 1) multimerization and agonist responsiveness using a dominant negative mutation. J Neurosci 21:8697–8706
Lewin GR, Mendell LM (1994) Regulation of cutaneous C-fiber heat nociceptors by nerve growth factor in the developing rat. J Neurophysiol 71:941–949
Malmberg AB, Mizisin AP, Calcutt NA, von Stein T, Robbins WR, Bley KR (2004) Reduced heat sensitivity and epidermal nerve fiber immunostaining following single applications of a high-concentration capsaicin patch. Pain 111:360–367
Martini C, Yassen A, Olofsen E, Passier P, Stoker M, Dahan A (2012) Pharmacodynamic analysis of the analgesic effect of capsaicin 8 % patch (Qutenza) in diabetic neuropathic pain patients: detection of distinct response groups. J Pain Res 5:51–59
Martini CH, Yassen A, Krebs-Brown A, Passier P, Stoker M, Olofsen E, Dahan A (2013) A novel approach to identify responder subgroups and predictors of response to low- and high-dose capsaicin patches in postherpetic neuralgia. *Eur J Pain*
Mason L, Moore RA, Derry S, Edwards JE, McQuay HJ (2004) Systematic review of topical capsaicin for the treatment of chronic pain. Bmj 328:991. Epub 2004 Mar 2019
McMahon SB, Bennett DL, Priestley JV, Shelton DL (1995) The biological effects of endogenous nerve growth factor on adult sensory neurons revealed by a trkA-IgG fusion molecule. Nat Med 1:774–780
McMahon SB, Koltzenburg M (1990) Novel classes of nociceptors: beyond Sherrington. Trends Neurosci 13:199–201
McPartland JM (2002) Use of capsaicin cream for abdominal wall scar pain. Am Fam Physician 65:2211; author reply 2212

Mendell LM, Albers KM, Davis BM (1999) Neurotrophins, nociceptors, and pain. Microsc Res Tech 45:252–261
Meyerson BA (2001) Neurosurgical approaches to pain treatment. Acta Anaesthesiol Scand 45:1108–1113
Mou J, Paillard F, Turnbull B, Trudeau J, Stoker M, Katz NP (2013) Efficacy of Qutenza(R) (capsaicin) 8% patch for neuropathic pain: a meta-analysis of the Qutenza Clinical Trials Database. Pain 154:1632–1639
Nolano M, Simone DA, Wendelschafer-Crabb G, Johnson T, Hazen E, Kennedy WR (1999) Topical capsaicin in humans: parallel loss of epidermal nerve fibers and pain sensation. Pain 81:135–145
Paice JA, Ferrans CE, Lashley FR, Shott S, Vizgirda V, Pitrak D (2000) Topical capsaicin in the management of HIV-associated peripheral neuropathy. J Pain Symptom Manage 19:45–52
Peppin JF, Majors K, Webster LR, Simpson DM, Tobias JK, Vanhove GF (2011) Tolerability of NGX-4010, a capsaicin 8% patch for peripheral neuropathic pain. J Pain Res 4:385–392
Piano V, Verhagen S, Schalkwijk A, Hekster Y, Kress H, Lanteri-Minet M, Burgers J, Treede RD, Engels Y, Vissers K (2014) Treatment for Neuropathic Pain in Patients with Cancer: Comparative Analysis of Recommendations in National Clinical Practice Guidelines from European Countries. Pain Pract Official J World Inst Pain 14:1–7
Rashid MH, Inoue M, Bakoshi S, Ueda H (2003) Increased expression of vanilloid receptor 1 on myelinated primary afferent neurons contributes to the antihyperalgesic effect of capsaicin cream in diabetic neuropathic pain in mice. J Pharmacol Exp Ther 306:709–717
Rayner HC, Atkins RC, Westerman RA (1989) Relief of local stump pain by capsaicin cream. Lancet 2:1276–1277
Robbins WR, Staats PS, Levine J, Fields HL, Allen RW, Campbell JN, Pappagallo M (1998) Treatment of intractable pain with topical large-dose capsaicin: preliminary report. Anesth Analg 86:579–583
Sayanlar J, Guleyupoglu N, Portenoy R, Ashina S (2012) Trigeminal postherpetic neuralgia responsive to treatment with capsaicin 8 % topical patch: a case report. J Headache Pain 13:587–589
Schmader KE (2002) Epidemiology and impact on quality of life of postherpetic neuralgia and painful diabetic neuropathy. Clin J Pain 18:350–354
Sherrington CS (1906) The integrative action of the nervous system. C. Scribner's Sons, New York
Shin J, Cho H, Hwang SW, Jung J, Shin CY, Lee SY, Kim SH, Lee MG, Choi YH, Kim J, Haber NA, Reichling DB, Khasar S, Levine JD, Oh U (2002) Bradykinin-12-lipoxygenase-VR1 signaling pathway for inflammatory hyperalgesia. Proc Natl Acad Sci U S A 99:10150–10155
Simone DA, Nolano M, Johnson T, Wendelschafer-Crabb G, Kennedy WR (1998) Intradermal injection of capsaicin in humans produces degeneration and subsequent reinnervation of epidermal nerve fibers: correlation with sensory function. J Neurosci 18:8947–8959
Simpson DM, Brown S, Tobias J (2008) Controlled trial of high-concentration capsaicin patch for treatment of painful HIV neuropathy. Neurology 70:2305–2313
Simpson DM, Gazda S, Brown S, Webster LR, Lu SP, Tobias JK, Vanhove GF (2010) Long-term safety of NGX-4010, a high-concentration capsaicin patch, in patients with peripheral neuropathic pain. J Pain Symptom Manage 39:1053–1064
Smart D, Gunthorpe MJ, Jerman JC, Nasir S, Gray J, Muir AI, Chambers JK, Randall AD, Davis JB (2000) The endogenous lipid anandamide is a full agonist at the human vanilloid receptor (hVR1). Br J Pharmacol 129:227–230
Spallone V, Greco C (2013) Painful and painless diabetic neuropathy: one disease or two? Curr Diab Rep 13:533–549
Stander S, Moormann C, Schumacher M, Buddenkotte J, Artuc M, Shpacovitch V, Brzoska T, Lippert U, Henz BM, Luger TA, Metze D, Steinhoff M (2004) Expression of vanilloid receptor subtype 1 in cutaneous sensory nerve fibers, mast cells, and epithelial cells of appendage structures. Exp Dermatol 13:129–139
Szolcsanyi J, Jancso-Gabor A (1975) Sensory effects of capsaicin congeners I. Relationship between chemical structure and pain-producing potency of pungent agents. Arzneimittelforschung 25:1877–1881

Szolcsanyi J, Jancso-Gabor A (1976) Sensory effects of capsaicin congeners. Part II: Importance of chemical structure and pungency in desensitizing activity of capsaicin-type compounds. Arzneimittelforschung 26:33–37

Szolcsanyi J, Jancso-Gabor A, Joo F (1975) Functional and fine structural characteristics of the sensory neuron blocking effect of capsaicin. Naunyn Schmiedebergs Arch Pharmacol 287:157–169

Turnbull JH, Gebauer SL, Miller BL, Barbaro NM, Blanc PD, Schumacher MA (2011) Cutaneous nerve transection for the management of intractable upper extremity pain caused by invasive squamous cell carcinoma. J Pain Symptom Manage 42:126–133

Ultsch B, Koster I, Reinhold T, Siedler A, Krause G, Icks A, Schubert I, Wichmann O (2013) Epidemiology and cost of herpes zoster and postherpetic neuralgia in Germany. Eur J Health Econ 14:1015–1026

Watkins LR, Milligan ED, Maier SF (2001) Glial activation: a driving force for pathological pain. Trends Neurosci 24:450–455

Watson CP, Evans RJ (1992) The postmastectomy pain syndrome and topical capsaicin: a randomized trial. Pain 51:375–379

Watson CP, Tyler KL, Bickers DR, Millikan LE, Smith S, Coleman E (1993) A randomized vehicle-controlled trial of topical capsaicin in the treatment of postherpetic neuralgia. Clin Ther 15:510–526

Webster LR, Malan TP, Tuchman MM, Mollen MD, Tobias JK, Vanhove GF (2010a) A multicenter, randomized, double-blind, controlled dose finding study of NGX-4010, a high-concentration capsaicin patch, for the treatment of postherpetic neuralgia. J Pain Official J Am Pain Soc 11:972–982

Webster LR, Nunez M, Tark MD, Dunteman ED, Lu B, Tobias JK, Vanhove GF (2011) Tolerability of NGX-4010, a capsaicin 8 % dermal patch, following pretreatment with lidocaine 2.5 %/prilocaine 2.5 % cream in patients with post-herpetic neuralgia. BMC Anesthesiol 11:25

Webster LR, Peppin JF, Murphy FT, Tobias JK, Vanhove GF (2012) Tolerability of NGX-4010, a capsaicin 8% patch, in conjunction with three topical anesthetic formulations for the treatment of neuropathic pain. J Pain Res 5:7–13

Webster LR, Tark M, Rauck R, Tobias JK, Vanhove GF (2010b) Effect of duration of postherpetic neuralgia on efficacy analyses in a multicenter, randomized, controlled study of NGX-4010, an 8 % capsaicin patch evaluated for the treatment of postherpetic neuralgia. BMC Neurol 10:92

Weintraub M, Golik A, Rubio A (1990) Capsaicin for treatment of post-traumatic amputation stump pain. Lancet 336:1003–1004

Wild S, Roglic G, Green A, Sicree R, King H (2004) Global prevalence of diabetes: estimates for the year 2000 and projections for 2030. Diabetes Care 27:1047–1053

Woolf CJ, Costigan M (1999) Transcriptional and posttranslational plasticity and the generation of inflammatory pain. Proc Natl Acad Sci U S A 96:7723–7730

Yaksh TL, Farb DH, Leeman SE, Jessell TM (1979) Intrathecal capsaicin depletes substance P in the rat spinal cord and produces prolonged thermal analgesia. Science 206:481–483

Zhang WY, Li Wan Po A (1994) The effectiveness of topically applied capsaicin. A meta-analysis. Eur J Clin Pharmacol 46:517–522

Chapter 5
Capsaicin-Based Therapies for Pain Control

Howard Smith and John R. Brooks

Abstract The TRPV1 receptor is known to play a role in nociceptive transmission in multiple organ systems, usually in response to the pain of inflammation. TRPV1 antagonism has so far shown limited benefit in antinociception. Capsaicin, a TRPV1 agonist, has been shown to induce a refractory period in the nerve terminal expressing TRPV1 and even, in sufficient dosing, to create long-term nerve terminal defunctionalization. This has led to research into topical capsaicin as a treatment for multiple painful conditions. The majority of work has focused on musculoskeletal pain and neuropathic pain and has revealed that although low-dose topical capsaicin has limited effectiveness as an analgesic, high-dose capsaicin, when tolerated, has the potential for long-term analgesia in certain types of neuropathic pain.

5.1 Introduction

There exist many chronic painful conditions for which the search for effective therapies is still underway. These conditions include painful musculoskeletal conditions, migraine headache, biliary and pancreatic pain, the pain associated with cancer, and multiple forms of neuropathic pain; from diabetic neuropathy to postherpetic neuralgia, among others (Nilius 2007; Immke and Gavva 2006). Depending on the specific condition, research into new forms of pain treatment have come about due to various reasons including the need for more effective

H. Smith · J. R. Brooks (✉)
Department of Anesthesiology, Albany Medical College, 47 New Scotland Avenue, MC-131, Albany, NY 12208, USA
e-mail: brooksj1@mail.amc.edu

O. M. E. Abdel-Salam (ed.), *Capsaicin as a Therapeutic Molecule*, Progress in Drug Research 68, DOI: 10.1007/978-3-0348-0828-6_5, © Springer Basel 2014

treatments, for potential "adjunctive" treatments, or even the need to decrease overall pill or opioid burden and improve patient adherence (Derry and Moore 2009).

The vanilloid compound capsaicin, found in various chili peppers, has long been known to produce a hot, burning, stinging sensation, whether on ingestion of spicy food or when applied to the skin (Caterina et al. 1997; Premkumar and Abooj 2013; Immke and Gavva 2006; Nilius 2007). As somewhat of a paradox, capsaicin has also been known to provide superficial pain relief despite, again, an initial unpleasant sensation. Although this has been known for a century, the molecular target and mechanism for capsaicin's effects have only relatively recently been investigated and brought to light. Modern scientific technique has allowed for a more complete characterization of not only capsaicin and its action but also of its target—the TRPV1 receptor—itself and the class of receptors to which it belongs (Caterina et al. 1997). More and more light is being shed on the TRP receptors and their various roles throughout the body.

Perhaps as a logical evolution, topical capsaicin-based therapies have been developed and tested in the hope that, for certain painful conditions, a new, reliable form of pain relief may be available to patients suffering from these conditions (Haanpää and Treede 2012). Various forms of topical capsaicin have been studied. The purposes of this chapter are (1) to review TRPV1 and its nociceptive role both in general and in various painful conditions, (2) to briefly review current research into potential TRPV1 antagonists and their role in antinociception, and (3) to review the current research and recommendations regarding topical capsaicin and pain relief, as well as to briefly discuss future research directions.

5.2 Capsaicin and TRPV1: Structure and Function

The scientific community has long been indirectly aware of the ligand-gated ion channel known as the Transient Receptor Potential cation channel, subfamily V, member 1 (TRPV1) through early observations of the antinociceptive properties of the compound—and TRPV1 agonist—known as capsaicin. Modern knowledge of TRPV1 began with its initial characterization using cloning techniques in 1997 (Caterina et al. 1997; Premkumar and Abooj 2013). It was the first receptor of its class to be discovered and has subsequently been the subject of numerous molecular characterization studies which have led to the elucidation of its varied roles in a number of nociceptive and nonnociceptive processes (Nilius 2007; Cao et al. 2013; Khairatkar-Joshi and Szallasi 2009; Immke and Gavva 2006). Knowledge of TRPV1 additionally spawned research into the TRPV class of receptors as a whole and, since its discovery, there have been a number of additional TRPV receptors discovered and studied in various degrees of detail (Premkumar and Abooj 2013).

TRPV1 is a tetrameric, nonselective channel permeable to cations, especially calcium (Wong and Gavva 2009). Original patch-clamp studies (Bevan and Szolcsányi 1990) showed TRPV1 to open in response to capsaicin, producing a slow inward depolarizing current. Extensive work by numerous authors has shown

TRPV1 to be expressed in small-diameter sensory neurons, both centrally and peripherally (Premkumar and Abooj 2013; Immke and Gavva 2006). The TRPV1 receptor has been found in the nociceptive, distal ends of Aδ and C fibers. These small-diameter fibers are involved in the transmission of nociceptive impulses from the periphery, implying a role for TRPV1 in pain transmission. However the receptor has also been found at the synapse of the dorsal root (and trigeminal) ganglion and their central second-order neuronal targets (Premkumar and Abooj 2013). Additionally, research has shown TRPV1 to be a polymodal receptor, displaying activation in the presence not only of vanilloids like capsaicin, but of elevated temperatures and acidity (Immke and Gavva 2006) as well as a broad range of other mediators including but not limited to adenosine, arachidonic acid metabolites, anandamide, and resiniferatoxin (Premkumar and Abooj 2013). This points to TRPV1 playing more of a role in the pain of inflammatory and/or thermal insult rather than generalized nociception as a whole.

Further supporting the potential role of TRPV1 in inflammatory pain is a study linking the TRPV1 receptor to the immune response in humans. In a study by Hutchinson et al. (2013), injection of low-dose endotoxin and subsequent activation of toll-like receptor 4 (TLR-4) was associated with an increase in the allodynia, flare, and hyperalgesia of capsaicin dermal injection over control subjects injected with capsaicin and no endotoxin. Additionally, an increase in the cytokine IL-6 was observed after endotoxin injection. The precise mechanisms of the effects of endotoxin on TRPV1 sensitivity have not been clearly delineated. Several mechanisms have been proposed, including (1) a direct TLR-4 interaction with endotoxin in the periphery with subsequent direct sensitization of TRPV1, (2) an endotoxin-induced cytokine cascade with direct, peripheral sensitization of TRPV1, and (3) an endotoxin-induced cytokine cascade with subsequent "central sensitization" via the TRPV1 receptor. Given that there was observed an increase in "allodynia", largely thought to be a central phenomenon, it appears likely based on this study that there is at least a component of endotoxin-induced cytokine cascade and subsequent centrally-directed sensitization (Hutchinson et al. 2013). Regardless of mechanism, the linking of an immune stimulus, an increase in inflammatory mediators/biomarkers, and TRPV1 activity lends a significant amount of support to the role of TRPV1 in pain associated with inflammation and the immune response in general (Hutchinson et al. 2013). Equally important is the identification of a potential target—TRPV1—for modifying neurohumoral-related pain (Hutchinson et al. 2013).

Antagonist studies using the compound capsazepine have further confirmed a role for the receptor in inflammatory pain (Immke and Gavva 2006). In addition, a reduction in the thermal pain associated with inflammation in knockout mice (Davis et al. 2000) also suggested that TRPV1 is involved in inflammatory pain. Immke and Gavva (2006) describe several other knockout studies that have also been helpful in exploring the role or roles this receptor plays in nociception. TRPV1 is widely believed to contribute to thermal homeostasis in not only experimental animal models such as the rat and dog, but in humans as well. As will be discussed later, this discovery was an unexpected result of TRPV1 antagonism studies (Wong and Gavva 2009).

Interestingly, multiple studies have shown that the different TRPV1 agonists work in concert to modulate the receptor's activity; for example, the presence of one agonist sensitizes the receptor to the effect of a second agonist (Nagy et al. 2004). Multiple inflammatory mediators, including bradykinin, prostaglandins, ATP, and glutamate, also have the ability to sensitize the receptor. This observation points to TRPV1 as a receptor at the convergence of multiple biochemical processes (Immke and Gavva 2006). In the typical inflammatory milieu, with multiple mediators present, it seems that TRPV1 responds with greater, longer lasting, even tonic activation. This potentially robust response is presumably one of the reasons TRPV1 has been such a desirable target for the relief of pain in certain conditions.

The compound capsaicin, known formally by its IUPAC name (E)-N-[(4-hydroxy-3-methoxyphenyl)methyl]-8-methylnon-6-enamide, is an alkylamide with the chemical formula $C_{18}H_{27}NO_3$. It is found in pepper-bearing plants of the genus capsicum. First isolated in 1816, it is a compound long known to the scientific community. Capsaicin, then, possesses both a lipophilic (fatty acid) moiety and a vanilloid moiety (Tominaga and Tominaga 2005). Capsaicin interacts with several key amino acid residues of the TRPV family of cation channels- Tyr 511 and Ser 512 in particular (Tominaga and Tominaga 2005). Furthermore, Immke and Gavva (2006) describe a vanilloid-binding pocket comprising the third and fourth transmembrane portions of the protein. It is thought that the lipophilic portion of the capsaicin molecule may bind to transmembrane domains on the channel-lipid interface of the receptor and that the vanilloid component of the molecule interacts with cytosolic residues, thus cross-linking transmembrane domains (Tominaga and Tominaga 2005). It appears as well that several of these residues are critical not only for agonist binding but for antagonist binding as well. Thus it is believed that TRPV1 agonists and antagonists occupy overlapping regions in the same vanilloid-binding site (Immke and Gavva 2006). Other sites on the TRPV1 receptor have also been described as having the ability to bind ligands, such as protons, and activate the receptor (Immke and Gavva 2006).

Although the role of capsaicin in nociception and antinociception is the topic of this chapter, it is interesting to note that capsaicin is being investigated with regard to possible roles outside the realm of pain management. For instance, it is believed to play a role in inducing apoptosis in breast tumors. A study by Chang et al. (2011) found capsaicin to induce S-phase cell cycle arrest and accompanying apoptosis in two different human breast cancer cell lines; this effect is believed by the authors to occur through a mitochondrial-mediated pathway. Although, again, outside the scope of this chapter, it is important to note just how potentially broad the role of capsaicin in modern medicine is capable of being.

5.3 TRPV1 and Its Role in Nociception

The role of the TRPV1 receptor in a variety of locations and pain modalities has been the subject of much research and effort. The location of TRPV1 at both peripheral nociceptive nerve terminals and the primary central synapse of those same nociceptive nerves suggest TRPV1 as a potential mediator of neuropathic pain. This has been undoubtedly borne out in the literature. It is the peripheral location of TRPV1 that has spawned research into its targeting in the relief of such pain. As will be discussed in detail later, multiple studies have shown that topical TRPV1 agonism via capsaicin has been able to successfully modulate neuropathic pain, confirming TRPV1's involvement in these pathologic conditions (Haanpää and Treede 2012; McCleane 2003).

TRPV1 has been implicated in the pain associated with pancreatitis as well. Schwartz et al. (2011) induced pancreatitis in the mouse and found that pancreatic inflammation led to an upregulation of TRPV1 in the pancreas and an increase in the activity of afferent nociceptive neurons originating within the pancreas. Additionally, Schwartz found that TRPV1 antagonism was effective in reducing pancreatic inflammation and pain-associated behaviors (Schwartz et al. 2011). Indeed, a review by Liddle (2007) describes numerous other studies that have additionally shown (1) the presence of TRPV1 in pancreatic nociceptive neurons, (2) the upregulation of these receptors in pancreatitis, (3) the contribution of multiple inflammatory mediators found in pancreatitis to TRPV1 activation, and (4) the amelioration of experimental pancreatic pain with TRPV1 antagonism. Of additional note, Zhu et al. (2011) have shown that nerve growth factor one (NGF-1) contributes to TRPV1 expression and activity in chronic pancreatitis.

TRPV1 has additionally been demonstrated to have involvement in joint pain from both osteoarthritis and rheumatoid arthritis. TRPV1 is expressed in synovial fibroblasts in both these painful joint conditions (Engler et al. 2007). Terenzi et al. (2013) showed TRPV1 activation by neuropeptides in rheumatoid synovial fibroblasts. A Cochrane Review by Richards et al. (2012) demonstrated the topical capsaicin may be at least somewhat efficacious in treating pain in patients with rheumatoid arthritis. Even in muscle, TRPV1 activation contributes to nociception and its activation appears to be involved in chronic muscular pain (Ro et al. 2009).

TRPV1's expression in the dura (Huang et al. 2012) and in extracranial arteries (Cianchetti 2010) have made it a potential target in migraine. Capsaicin jelly displayed effectiveness in reducing migraine pain in some patients with arterial pain during migraine attacks (Cianchetti 2010). Summ et al. (2011) however failed to demonstrate success of TRPV1 antagonism in preventing trigeminal-mediated nociception in rat models of migraine. Indeed, work by Lambert et al. (2009) demonstrated that although TRPV1 antagonism may play a role in suppressing sensitization in certain trigeminal pathologies including transformed migraine, TRPV1 antagonism alone was not effective at ameliorating symptoms of primary migraine. Taken together, the current body of work suggests that more has to be done to elucidate TRPV1's exact role in migraine.

TRPV1 has additionally been shown to play a role in multiple other areas of human pathophysiology, including work that demonstrates its activation in cough and other respiratory pathways (Adcock 2009). A review by Takemura et al. (2008) describes TRPV1's presence in the lung and potential for mediating inflammatory lung illnesses; however, more work admittedly needs to be done in this arena. TRPV1 has been investigated in other various roles of everything from visceral pain, to cancer pain, and even to acupuncture.

5.4 TRPV1 Antagonists and Antinociception

With the role of TRPV1 in multiple modalities of nociception well documented, it would seem a logical expectation that TRPV1 antagonism would aid in antinociception, an expectation that has, to varying degrees, played out in research. The hope of researchers has long been to develop an effective analgesic or analgesics based around the TRPV1 channel, which has been so extensively linked to peripheral nociceptors. Numerous small molecules have been investigated for their potential use as antihyperalgesics, especially in, but not limited to, the setting of inflammatory-type pain (Wong and Gavva 2009). The first TRPV1 antagonist, capsazepine, has been used in numerous in vivo and in vitro pharmacology studies (Nagy et al. 2004).

A review by Wong and Gavva (2009) details multiple TRPV1 antagonists that have been investigated and have shown varying degrees in efficacy with regard to their ability to attenuate thermal and inflammatory hyperalgesia. The existing compounds, according to Wong, appear to show maximum efficacy when they possess the ability to block three distinct modes of TRPV1 activation: capsaicin, acidity, and heat (Wong and Gavva 2009). This relates to TRPV1's proposed physiologic role in sensing thermal- and inflammatory-related nociception in the periphery. Additionally, Cui et al. (2006) showed that CNS penetration is also important for TRPV1 antagonists to display an acceptable antinociceptive profile. These findings have served as the backdrop for the development of clinical TRPV1 antagonists.

One such antagonist, ABT-102, was investigated in a double-blind, randomized, controlled clinical trial among healthy volunteers. The study showed that ABT-102 was effective in increasing heat-pain thresholds and reduced painfulness of suprathreshold oral and cutaneous heat (Rowbotham et al. 2011). Subjects' ability to sense injurious levels of heat, however, was not impaired (Rowbotham et al. 2011). In addition, Chizh et al. (2007) investigated the proposed antagonist SB-705498 in a randomized, controlled, single blind, crossover study in healthy volunteers. Similar to ABT-102, SB-705498 increased the heat-pain threshold versus placebo, although this increase was not seen in capsaicin-sensitized skin. Additionally, capsaicin-evoked flair was decreased in patients given SB-705498 (Chizh et al. 2007).

An important reported side effect of TRPV1 antagonism is hyperthermia in multiple animal models, suggesting that TRPV1 does play a role in thermoregulation in addition to its role in nociception (Wong and Gavva 2009). Indeed, although not all antagonist studies have reported or observed hyperthermia in humans, multiple studies have (Gavva et al. 2008). This includes, among others, a molecule initially investigated in phase-one clinical trials, AMG-517 (Gavva et al. 2008). The phase-one trial of AMG-517 was stopped due to undesirable levels of hyperthermia in volunteers and as a result the efficacy of this drug is not fully elucidated (Wong and Gavva 2009).

Studies investigating other TRPV1 antagonists, as well as potential ways to minimize the risk of hyperthermia in humans, are ongoing. However much research is instead focusing on TRPV1 agonists such as capsaicin based on their ability to activate, and then desensitize, TRPV1 and potentially ablate TRPV1-expressing neurons, thus providing an antagonist-like effect without the risk of the hyperthermia seen in trials of AMG-517 (Wong and Gavva 2009).

5.5 Topical Capsaicin and Analgesia

Much of the research into capsaicin-based therapy has focused on topical capsaicin and its potential to treat various painful conditions. Topical therapy has the advantage of being able to be applied directly over the painful region and therefore has the potential to deliver direct, targeted therapy. Furthermore, topical therapy can reduce overall pill burden and may be easier for patients to take, thus promoting adherence. Capsaicin is proposed, as discussed earlier, to act as an agonist at the TRPV1 receptor and produce a refractory state with regard to receptor activity and therefore produce antinociception. Repeated doses have been proposed to lead to "defunctionalization" of the nerve and an overall long-term reduction of pain. Defunctionalization is a broad term that describes a number of cellular physiologic processes that ultimately result in a loss of nerve function as opposed to the outright degeneration or destruction of the nerve terminal itself. It is thought to be due to a number of cellular and molecular changes induced by tonic and TRPV1 activation, temporary loss of membrane potential, impaired cellular transport, and reversible retraction of nerve fiber endings (Anand and Bley 2011). Also seen alongside defunctionalization is a depletion of Substance P, although this is now thought to be merely an association and not causative (Anand and Bley 2011).

The potentially beneficial effects of capsaicin-based therapy must be weighed against potential drawbacks. Capsaicin therapy is associated with pain described often as stinging or burning, as well as erythema (Haanpää and Treede 2012). These side effects can be presumably quite undesired in patients already experiencing pain significant enough to warrant therapy in the first place. Regardless, the obvious aforementioned benefits of both capsaicin and topical therapy have kept interest in this area alive. Capsaicin-based topical therapy has long been in existence and has long been the subject of research. Multiple modalities of pain have been investigated with regard to their potential to be alleviated by topical capsaicin-based TRPV1 activation, including musculoskeletal pain, diabetic neuropathy, postherpetic neuralgia, and other forms of chronic neuropathic pain. Capsaicin-based creams have been studied in different concentrations as well in an attempt to find the most efficacious dose producing the least adverse effects. As we will soon discuss in further detail, topical capsaicin has been investigated in three different concentrations: 2, 0.025, and 0.075 %, considered "low dose," and 1, 8 %, considered "high dose."

5.5.1 Preclinical Data

Preclinical work into TRPV1 and capsaicin as they pertain to potential antinociception has already been briefly discussed. To resummarize, TRPV1 knockout models in the mouse have demonstrated the role of TRPV1 in not only peripheral nociception, but thermoregulation as well (Haanpää and Treede 2012). TRPV1 antagonism appears to mimic the effects of TRPV1 knockout, both in mice and in humans (Haanpää and Treede 2012). This potential for hyperthermia in humans has been a significant roadblock to advances in TRPV1 antagonism (Haanpää and Treede 2012). In contrast, studies using TRPV1 agonists such as capsaicin and risiniferatoxin have shown an ability to inactivate TRPV1 and even cause longer-term nerve defunctionalization in specific nerves expressing the TRPV1 receptor (Haanpää and Treede 2012). Thus, TRPV1 agonism has emerged from preclinical work as a promising therapeutic option for patients in whom chronic pain is in part contributed to by TRPV1 activation, be it physiologic or pathologic.

5.5.2 *Topical Capsaicin and Musculoskeletal Pain*

A meta-analysis by Mason et al. (2004) investigated the efficacy of 0.025 % one of the two concentrations referred to as "low dose" capsaicin. It was an update to prior work done on the effectiveness of capsaicin in musculoskeletal conditions. Three double-blind placebo-controlled trials involved patients with musculoskeletal conditions. The relative benefit from topical capsaicin 0.025 % compared with placebo was 1.5 with a number needed to treat of 8.1 (Mason et al. 2004). Thus, this particular concentration of topical capsaicin appears to show limited efficacy in patients with musculoskeletal conditions. Additionally, one-third of patients experienced adverse effects of capsaicin on application. The authors were unable to directly compare topical capsaicin to topical NSAIDs in the relief of musculoskeletal pain; however, indirect comparisons noted by the authors suggest capsaicin to be less efficacious (Mason et al. 2004).

5.5.3 *Topical Capsaicin and Neuropathic Pain*

Neuropathic pain, a broad term describing pain arising from lesions of sensory nerves themselves, affects a large number of people with an often-significant reduction in overall quality of life. It is typically characterized by pain and sensation-related symptoms as hypersensitivity, burning, numbness, or tonic, unrelenting pain. Neuropathic pain can result from a number of conditions, including but not limited to diabetes, trigeminal neuralgia, HIV, herpes zoster, medical treatments, and trauma. These patients often have difficulty finding effective treatment regimens and there has been much research into optimizing care for people living with chronic neuropathic pain (Dworkin et al. 2010). Traditional treatment for neuropathic pain has involved tricyclic antidepressants, gabapentin, Selective serotonin reuptake inhibitors (SSRIs), serotonin and noradrenaline reuptake inhibitors (SNRIs), and even opioids. Topical capsaicin is being investigated with regard to whether it can provide safe, effective relief in different neuropathic pain conditions including diabetic neuropathy, fibromyalgia, and trigeminal neuralgia (Dworkin et al. 2010). Interest in capsaicin in neuropathic pain has, not surprisingly, come about as a result of our knowledge of TRPV1 and its location on peripheral nerves, as well as the ability of capsaicin to not only provide pain relief but to cause degradation of the nerve with repeated exposures.

5.5.4 Capsaicin (Low Dose) and Neuropathic Pain

Topical capsaicin has been available for some time in a low dose, i.e., less than 1 %, form for some time. Many studies have been published in an attempt to evaluate its efficacy and safety. Again, it is important to note that "low-dose capsaicin" here actually refers to two different concentrations: 0.025 and 0.075 %.

The aforementioned systematic review by Mason et al. (2004) looked not only at 0.025 % topical capsaicin in the treatment of chronic musculoskeletal pain, but at 0.075 % (still considered low dose) topical capsaicin in the treatment of chronic neuropathic pain. Six double-blind, randomized, placebo-controlled trials were analyzed. It was found in the studies analyzed, that low-dose topical capsaicin has a number needed to treat (NNT) of 5.7 with, as mentioned previously, a significant rate of capsaicin-related adverse effects (Mason et al. 2004). Therefore, similar to its conclusion on capsaicin for musculoskeletal pain, low-dose topical capsaicin is not an effective treatment for chronic neuropathic pain, although it still may be considered in refractory cases or patients in which the magnitude of pain is sufficiently great to warrant a search for multiple or adjuvant therapies (Mason et al. 2004).

In 2010, the National Institute of Health and Clinical Excellence in the UK (NICE) published guidelines for the treatment of neuropathic pain in adults. The guidelines described currently recommended treatment options for neuropathic pain, from first to third order. In general, duloxetine or amitriptyline were recommended as first-line agents, followed by pregabalin as a second-line agent, and tramadol or a lidocaine patch were recommended as third-line agents (NICE 2010). Capsaicin failed to earn a recommendation as either a first-, second-, or third-line agent (NICE 2010). Interestingly, though, guidelines published by Dworkin et al. (2010) do list topical low-dose capsaicin as a third-line agent in the treatment of chronic neuropathic pain. Although current capsaicin use, as will be detailed below, focuses on higher doses, the inclusion of capsaicin in this set of guidelines stands in contrast to the NICE guidelines and implies potential benefits to topical capsaicin despite limited and mixed clinical data (Dworkin et al. 2010).

More recently, a Cochrane review published by Derry and Moore in (2012) attempted to evaluate the available literature in an attempt to assess whether low-dose topical capsaicin was indeed a viable option for patients with neuropathic pain. The review included seven studies of 1,600 patients in total. Each of the studies evaluated 0.075 % topical capsaicin. Neuropathic conditions involved included distal painful polyneuropathy, HIV neuropathy, postherpetic neuralgia, postsurgical cancer pain, diabetic neuropathy, and postmastectomy pain. The studies focused on pain that was at least moderate in nature and, in most cases, unresponsive or poorly responsive to other therapies. Studies were all randomized, controlled, and double-blinded and of at least 6 weeks' duration.

Derry and Moore made two key conclusions in their review. First, they concluded that the available data regarding 0.075 % (low dose) capsaicin is limited; indeed the number of studies and participants they were able to use in their review was deemed relatively suboptimal (Derry and Moore 2012). This appears somewhat surprising given that low-dose capsaicin cream is already used with some frequency. This paucity of data, however, is borne out in reviews by Mason et al. (2004) and the NICE guidelines (2010). In several studies, data were too small in amount to perform meaningful statistical analyses (Derry and Moore 2012).

However, the Cochrane review by Derry and Moore (2012), based on the existing data available, did conclude that low-dose topical capsaicin was likely ineffective as a treatment for multiple modalities of chronic neuropathic pain in adults. The review additionally concluded that further treatment into low-dose capsaicin for this purpose was likely to be largely unproductive (Derry and Moore 2012). Interestingly enough, the 2012 Cochrane review was an update to a 2009 review by the same authors. The 2009 review, looking at both high and low-dose capsaicin, concluded that topical application could in fact be effective in some patients (Derry et al. 2009). However, using stricter inclusion criteria in 2012, the authors arrived at a different conclusion when it comes to low-dose capsaicin. As will be discussed shortly, however, higher doses of capsaicin delivered topically are currently being investigated, research that has been fueled largely by the seeming ineffective nature of low-dose capsaicin in neuropathic pain.

Of additional note, a randomized controlled trial by Casanueva et al. (2013) investigated low dose again, 0.075 %- capsaicin in the treatment of fibromyalgia, a chronic, painful condition thought to arise as a result of primary nervous system pathology. The study included 126 patients receiving either their usual fibromyalgia treatment or their usual treatment with the addition of topical capsaicin. The study found that patients with severe fibromyalgia did show short-term improvement after the addition of topical capsaicin to their previously established treatment regimen (Casanueva et al. 2013). Outcomes measured included not only pain scores but overall quality of life assessments as well. Thus, although the majority of available data do seem to suggest that low-dose capsaicin for neuropathic or musculoskeletal pain is not an effective treatment option, there are some data to suggest that, in some patients (depending on individual factors such as disease type or severity), low-dose capsaicin may be a reasonable therapeutic option when others have failed to provide sufficiently complete pain relief and quality of life improvement.

5.5.5 High-Dose Topical Capsaicin and Neuropathic Pain

While there exist low dose, 0.075 % formulations of capsaicin, there exists a much higher dosing option: 8 %. This formulation, commonly referred to in the literature as high dose, has also been the subject of much study. This has been driven, in part, by the lack of convincing evidence for low-dose capsaicin's efficacy as an analgesic.

Application of high-dose capsaicin carries with it a unique problem. While low-dose capsaicin was associated with occasional skin irritation and discomfort that was often a barrier to its effective use, 8 % capsaicin causes significant, nearly universal skin symptoms that are painful and make its use, in and of itself, incredibly undesirable to patients (Derry and Moore 2012). In fact, an early study with doses up to 10 % warranted the use of regional anesthesia to allow patients to tolerate the treatment (Robbins et al. 1998)! *Currently, it is accepted practice for 8 % application to be accompanied by pretreatment with a local anesthetic or other medication to facilitate tolerability.* Interestingly, it seems that although low-dose application requires multiple dosings at predetermined intervals, high-dose capsaicin requires a single application (Derry and Moore 2012). Thus, although apparently far more irritating than its low-dose counterpart, high-dose capsaicin at least spares its patients from multiple painful applications.

Webster et al. (2012) investigated the pretreatment of patients with local anesthetic prior to application of 8 % capsaicin. They enrolled 117 patients in a study in which, in addition to a 60 or 90 min high-dose capsaicin treatment, they received one of three possible local anesthetics. Oral oxycodone was also given on an as needed basis to all participants during application and participants could take oral hydrocodone/acetaminophen for 5 days posttreatment (Webster et al. 2012).

While the study ultimately found no statistically significant differences between the three topical anesthetics used in the study in terms of overall tolerability of the high-dose capsaicin treatment, what the study also found is important to note. That is, while no differences existed between types of pretreatment, pretreatment *itself* allowed significant tolerability of the application (Webster et al. 2012). More than 90 % of the treatment was completed by most patients and they reported up to 30 % reductions in neuropathic pain up to 12 weeks after the application. Thus we see that, although the type of pretreatment does not matter much, pretreatment in and of itself allows tolerability of a treatment that appears, at least from this study, to be effective in long-term reductions in neuropathic pain among patients suffering from this constellation of painful illnesses (Webster et al. 2012). As an additional note, another study by Webster et al. (2011) showed success in 8 % patch tolerability following pretreatment with 2.5 % lidocaine/2.5 % prilocaine, further supporting the notion that not only is 8 % capsaicin able to be tolerated following pretreatment, but ultimately it is pretreatment itself and not the specific type that facilitates application of high-dose capsaicin.

As part of their updated review on topical capsaicin, Derry and Moore (2012) dedicated a separate review to high-dose delivery, reflecting both (1) the increased amount of research into the subject and (2) the apparent difference on potential for therapeutic effect versus its low-dose cousin. High dose differs, again, because of its potential for a single application over 12 weeks and the potential for quick sensory neuronal degradation; the tradeoff again being the requirement for pretreatment to facilitate tolerability (Derry and Moore 2012). Six studies of a total of over 2,000 patients were included in the review; all were randomized, controlled (with 0.04 % capsaicin as a control), and double-blinded. Results included pain scores at various intervals posttreatment, ranging from 2 to 12 weeks. Patients' specific neuropathies included HIV neuropathy and postherpetic neuralgia. These two conditions, it seems, are the most studied in the literature for 8 % capsaicin and the two most common conditions for which high-dose capsaicin is currently being prescribed (Derry and Moore 2012). Studies were of at least 6 weeks' duration, as in the review of low-dose capsaicin.

The Cochrane review found that in both HIV neuropathy and postherpetic neuralgia, 8 % topical capsaicin was significantly more effective than "placebo" (0.04 % capsaicin) in providing 30–50 % reductions in pain scores in the weeks following treatment (Derry and Moore 2012). These data stand in stark contrast to those for low-dose capsaicin, where the little evidence available failed to show a significant benefit for that particular formulation. Furthermore, the data behind 8 % capsaicin is high quality and points to not only pain relief but also an improvement in overall quality-of-life indicators including improved sleep and reduced fatigue and depression (Derry and Moore 2012). These data also appear to support those from a previous review (Derry et al. 2009) in which a limited amount of data from only two available studies were used to suggest a potential benefit from 8 % application despite the obvious need for further investigation into that formulation as a potential therapy in adult neuropathic pain.

The application of high-dose capsaicin was obviously not without its side effects, as could be expected since there were significant side effects with even low-dose application (Derry and Moore 2012). Side effects of treatment included pain, erythema, pruritis, and even edema that tended to resolve shortly after the treatment (Derry and Moore 2012). Finally, the studies included in this review did pretreat their participants with local anesthetic; this is a technique that is largely accepted as being necessary to facilitate adherence to treatment in light of such a high dose of a compound known to induce pain all by itself (Webster et al. 2012).

Current guidelines for the treatment of postherpetic neuralgia, based on the available evidence, have included 8 % topical capsaicin as either a second- or third-line agent (Argoff 2011). Ultimately, capsaicin, and therefore TRPV1 agonism in general, has found to be most beneficial in the form of high-dose capsaicin, applied topically, in patients with postherpetic neuralgia who have failed at least one line of therapeutic options (Argoff 2011). Additionally, a case report by Sayanlar et al. (2012) describes the efficacious use of 8 % capsaicin in the treatment of post-herpetic trigeminal neuralgia in a 64-year-old woman. She reportedly experienced pain relief even 1 year after treatment (Sayanlar et al. 2012), which is a significant amount of time especially considering the end points for Derry and Moore's Cochrane reviews (2009, 2012) went only as far as 12 weeks. The results of this case report suggest that, although high-dose capsaicin as been studied mainly in nontrigeminal postherpetic neuralgia, it may be effective in the trigeminal variety as well (Sayanlar et al. 2012).

Currently, 8 % topical capsaicin is FDA-approved for the treatment of postherpetic neuralgia. It has not yet been FDA-approved for uses in other neuropathies or other painful conditions. In fact, an open-label study was performed by Simpson et al. (2008) in which 12 volunteers received high-dose topical capsaicin for painful HIV neuropathy. All 12 experienced some reduction in pain, with a subset even responding with a greater than 50 % reduction in pain (Simpson et al. 2008). This pain reduction often persisted over 12 weeks post-application. Although the results of this study showed promise, a newer, larger, randomized controlled study by Clifford et al. (2012) failed to show any difference in pain reduction with regard to capsaicin and HIV neuropathy. Ultimately, based on the available evidence, the FDA has not approved capsaicin for the treatment of HIV neuropathy.

High-dose capsaicin is commercially available topically as a patch (Qutenza© 2009). Qutenza© is, again, FDA-approved for the treatment of postherpetic neuralgia. Each patch contains 179 mg of capsaicin. It must be applied by a physician and may be cut into an appropriate shape prior to its use. Up to four patches may be used at a time. The skin is pretreated with a local anesthetic and the patch applied. It is kept in place for 60 min while any acute pain that results is treated on an as-needed basis. After a 60 min treatment, it need not be reapplied for 3 months. Common side effects typically include skin erythema, pruritis, pain, papules, and a transient increase in blood pressure (Qutenza© 2009).

5.6 Future Directions

It appears from the available data that, while low-dose capsaicin is generally ineffective as an analgesic in either musculoskeletal or multiple forms of chronic neuropathic pain in adults, high-dose capsaicin has shown efficacy in certain forms of chronic neuropathic pain. A logical evolution in research into investigation of TRPV1 agonism, then, most likely ought to focus on either 8 % topical capsaicin in musculoskeletal pain or forms of chronic neuropathic pain *not* yet investigated, be it diabetic peripheral neuropathy, or distal painful polyneuropathy.

Another research target may lie in a different TRPV1 agonist, resiniferatoxin. A review by Brederson et al. (2013) details work done with regard to resiniferatoxin and its potential role in analgesia and antinociception. The compound is being studied in animal models and has demonstrated the ability to (1) prevent surgically-induced neuropathic pain when injected perineurally and (2) (potentially) permanently ablate localized chronic pain when injected either into a specific ganglion or even intrathecally (Brederson et al. 2013). Additionally, resiniferatoxin has shown the ability to provide multidermatome cancer pain relief when injected intrathecally in dogs with osteosarcoma; there is even a trial underway in a human volunteer (Brederson et al. 2013). Taken together, it appears that resiniferatoxin has the potential to play a significant role in the alleviation of certain types of chronic pain.

Finally, one specific type of neuropathic pain—opioid-induced hyperalgesia—deserves mention. It is a form of neuropathic pain thought to result from chronic use of opioid pain medications, such as morphine. Although the mechanism of the development of pain seems to involve the opioid's interaction with toll-like receptor four (TLR-4, Li 2012), research has also shown that TRPV1 may in fact play a mediating role as well. Rodent TRPV1 knockout studies by Vardanyan et al. (2009) has suggested that TRPV1 is involved in the development of neuropathic pain in chronic opioid use. Of course, more work needs to be done. However, it is

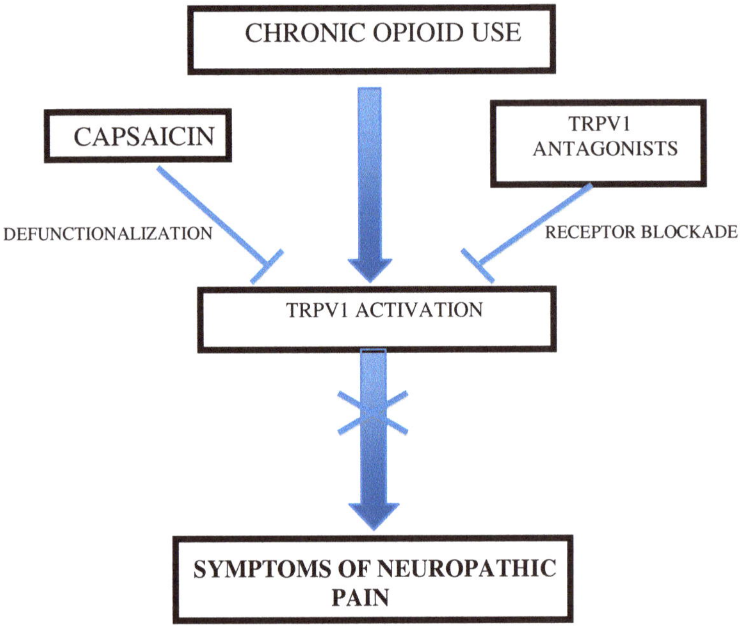

Fig. 5.1 Potential for TRPV1 modulation to reduce pain related to opioid-induced hyperalgesia. Either capsaicin-based defunctionalization or outright TRPV1 antagonism may be useful in alleviating this subset of chronic pain

conceivable that TRPV1 manipulation (see Fig. 5.1), whether it be defunctionalization via capsaicin or outright antagonism, may provide pain relief in this subset of patients with chronic neuropathic pain.

Further investigation into TRPV1 antagonists may continue to yield fruitful results; however, work must be done to investigate further the potential of that drug class to induce hyperthermia in humans in the hope of mitigating that potentially deleterious effect and thus removing a major roadblock to the therapeutic potential of TRPV1 antagonists as a whole.

5.7 Summary and Conclusions

Capsaicin has long held a place in our understanding of nociception and antinociception, even significantly predating our knowledge of its molecular mechanism and the molecular biology of its target, the TRPV1 receptor (Prekumar and Abooj 2013). The growing body of research into transient receptor-potential vanilloid receptors has yielded an understanding of a class of receptor that is involved in multiple types of nociception across multiple organ systems, with additional roles in physiologic processes such as the inflammatory response and thermoregulation in the mammalian organism (Nilius 2007). It is of no surprise, given the diversity of TRPV1 location and functions, that it has emerged as a potential therapeutic target in multiple painful conditions in which the desire for either more effective therapies or therapies that might reduce overall opioid, or even pill, burden has fostered the search for available, effective, and safe therapeutic options (Derry et al. 2009).

TRPV1 antagonists have been investigated; the premise behind investigation being that they may provide effective antinociception by interfering with an otherwise nociceptive ion channel. The major roadblock in this route of therapy remains the class' potential for inducing hyperthermia in humans. Thus TRPV1 antagonism, while a logical next step in theory, has to date yet to pan out in terms of being a safe therapeutic option (Wong and Gavva 2009, Chizh et al. 2007).

TRPV1 agonism, such as that produced by capsaicin and resiferatoxin, produces a predictable initial painful stimulus followed by a refractory state at the receptor. Over time, this leads to degeneration of the receptor itself and an overall reduction in capacity for nociceptive input (Derry and Moore 2012). While the TRPV1 receptor has been traditionally thought of as mediating inflammatory pain through its interaction with the inflammatory milieu produced by any number of stimuli, the ability to reduce the functional capacity for peripheral sensory nerve activity has led to research into TRPV1 agonism as a potential treatment for musculoskeletal and, more frequently, multiple forms of chronic neuropathic pain, from diabetic neuropathy to postherpetic neuralgia among several others.

Research into TRPV1 agonism has taken the form of application of topical capsaicin in one of two forms: low dose (0.075 %) and high dose (8 %). Commercial preparations of both these doses are available currently. The available data point to three main conclusions: (1) that low-dose topical capsaicin does not seem to be particularly effective at treating chronic musculoskeletal pain especially compared with topical NSAID treatment, (2) low-dose capsaicin does not appear to be effective at treating multiple forms of chronic neuropathic pain in adults, although this conclusion is limited by a relative lack of evidence, and finally that (3) high-dose capsaicin does appear to be safe and effective in the treatment of HIV neuropathy and postherpetic neuralgia in adults (Derry and Moore 2012). Topical capsaicin is not without its drawbacks, however. While not appearing to put patients at a significant risk of systemic effects, local pain and erythema have the potential to limit the use of topical capsaicin in the arena of pain treatment (Wong and Gavva 2009); certainly the *creation* of pain appears counterintuitive in patients with whom pain is already a significant problem and a significant limitation to an acceptable quality of life. However, especially in the case of high-dose capsaicin, long-term pain reduction may be worth the short-term painful effects of drug administration. Furthermore, pretreatment with local anesthetics and pre and posttreatment with oral opioids appears to reduce overall discomfort and dissatisfaction to the point where adherence is optimized and long-term effects may be realized (Wong and Gavva 2009). This is no small achievement, especially given the propensity of these patient populations to not only experience suboptimal pain control and a significant pill burden.

Certainly, more work needs to be done. Overall evidence for or against topical capsaicin is limited. Furthermore, the effectiveness of 8 % capsaicin has only been shown in two specific types of neuropathy. The potential for high-dose application to provide relief in not only other types of chronic neuropathy (distal painful polyneuropathy, trigeminal neuralgia, cancer-related pain, and others) but also in other painful conditions including migraine and musculoskeletal pain should prompt further research into high-dose applications of capsaicin, both alone and in conjunction with other more established therapies. While more work obviously needs to be done, the available evidence points to the conclusion that, in sufficient doses, TRPV1 agonism with capsaicin can be used as an effective analgesic, at least in certain types of adult chronic neuropathic pain.

References

Adcock JJ (2009) TRPV1 receptors in sensitisation of cough and pain reflexes. Pulm Pharmacol Ther 22:65–70. doi:10.1016/j.pupt.2008

Anand P, Bley K (2011) Topical capsaicin for pain management: therapeutic potential and mechanisms of action of the new high-concentration capsaicin 8 % patch. Br J Anaesth 107:490–502. doi:10.1093/bja/aer260

Argoff CE (2011) Review of current guidelines on the care of postherpetic neuralgia. Postgrad Med 123:134–142. doi:10.3810/pgm.2011.09.2469

Bevan S, Szolcsányi J (1990) Sensory neuron-specific actions of capsaicin: mechanisms and applications. Trends Pharmacol Sci 11:330–333

Brederson JD, Kym PR, Szallasi A (2013) Targeting TRP channels for pain relief. Eur J Pharmacol doi:pii: S0014 2999(13)00173 8. 10.1016/j.ejphar.2013.03.003

Cao E, Cordero-Morales JF, Liu B, Qin F, Julius D (2013) TRPV1 channels are intrinsically heat sensitiveand negatively regulated by phosphoinositide lipids. Neuron 77:667–679. doi:10.1016/j.neuron.2012.12.016

Casanueva B, Rodero B, Quintial C, Llorca J, González-Gay MA (2013) Short term efficacy of topical capsaicin therapy in severely affected fibromyalgia patients. Rheumatol Int 33(10):2665–2670

Caterina MJ, Schumacher MA, Tominaga M, Rosen TA, Levine JD, Julius D (1997) The capsaicin receptor: a heat-activated ion channel in the pain pathway. Nature 389:816–824

Chang HC, Chen ST, Chien SY, Kuo SJ, Tsai HT, Chen DR (2011) Capsaicin may induce breast cancer cell death through apoptosis-inducing factor involving mitochondrial dysfunction. Hum Exp Toxicol 30:1657–1665. doi:10.1177/0960327110396530

Chizh BA, O'Donnell MB, Napolitano A, Wang J, Brooke AC, Aylott MC, Bullman JN, Gray EJ, Lai RY, Williams PM, Appleby JM (2007) The effects of the TRPV1 antagonist SB-705498 on TRPV1 receptor mediated activity and inflammatory hyperalgesia in humans. Pain 132:132–141

Cianchetti C (2010) Capsaicin jelly against migraine pain. Int J Clin Pract 64:457–459. doi:10.1111/j.1742-1241.2009.02294.x

Clifford DB, Simpson DM, Brown S (2012) A randomized, double-blind, controlled study of NGX-4010, a capsaicin 8 % Dermal patch, for the treatment of painful HIV-associated distal sensory polyneuropathy. J Acquir Immune Defic Syndr 59:126–133. doi:10.1097/QAI.0b013e31823e31f7

Cui M, Honore P, Zhong C, Gauvin D, Mikusa J, Hernandez G, Chandran P, Gomtsyan A, Brown B, Bayburt EK, Marsh K, Bianchi B, McDonald H, Niforatos W, Neelands TR, Moreland RB, Decker MW, Lee CH, Sullivan JP, Faltynek CR (2006) TRPV1 receptors in the CNS play a key role in broad-spectrum analgesia of TRPV1 antagonists. J Neurosci 26:9385–9393

Davis JB, Gray J, Gunthorpe MJ, Hatcher JP, Davey PT, Overend P, Harries MH, Latcham J, Clapham C, Atkinson K, Hughes SA, Rance K, Grau E, Harper AJ, Pugh PL, Rogers DC, Bingham S, Randall A, Sheardown SA (2000) Vanilloid receptor-1 is essential for inflammatory thermal hyperalgesia. Nature 405:183–187

Derry S, Moore RA (2012) Topical capsaicin (low concentration) for chronic neuropathic pain in adults. Cochrane Database Syst Rev 9:CD010111. doi:10.1002/14651858.CD010111

Derry S, Lloyd R, Moore RA, McQuay HJ (2009) Topical capsaicin for chronic neuropathic pain in adults. Cochrane Database Syst Rev (4):CD007393. doi:10.1002/14651858.CD007393.pub2

Dworkin RH, O'Connor AB, Audette J, Baron R, Gourlay GK, Haanpää ML, Kent JL, Krane EJ, LeBel AA, Levy RM, Mackey SC, Mayer J, Miaskowski C, Raja SN, Rice ASC, Schmader KE, Stacey B, Stanos S, Treede RD, Turk DC, Walco CA, Wells CD (2010) Recommendations for the pharmacological management of neuropathic pain: an overview and literature update. Mayo Clin Proc 85:S3–S14. doi:10.4065/mcp.2009.0649

Engler A, Aeschlimann A, Simmen BR, Michel BA, Gay RE, Gay S, Sprott H (2007) Expression of transient receptor potential vanilloid 1 (TRPV1) in synovial fibroblasts from patients with osteoarthritisand rheumatoid arthritis. Biochem Biophys Res Commun 359:884–888

Gavva NR, Treanor JJS, Garami A, Fang L, Surapaneni S, Akrami A, Alvarez F, Bak A, Darling M, Gore A, Jang GR, Kesslak JP, Ni L, Norman MH, Palluconi G, Rose MJ, Salfi M, Tan E, Romanovsky AA, Banfield C, Davar G (2008) Pharmacological blockade of the vanilloid receptor TRPV1 elicits marked hyperthermia in humans. Pain 136:202–210. doi:10.1016/j.pain.2008.01.024

Haanpää M, Treede RD (2012) Capsaicin for neuropathic pain: linking traditional medicine and molecular biology. Eur Neurol 68:264–275. doi:10.1159/000339944

Huang D, Li S, Dhaka A, Story GM, Cao YQ (2012) Expression of the transient receptor potential channels TRPV1, TRPA1 and TRPM8 in mouse trigeminal primary afferent neurons innervating the dura. Mol Pain 8:66. doi:10.1186/1744-8069-8-66

Hutchinson MR, Buijs M, Tuke J, Kwok YH, Gentgall M, Williams D, Rolan P (2013) Low-dose endotoxin potentiates capsaicin-induced pain in man: Evidence for a pain neuroimmune connection. Brain Behav Immun pii:S0889–1591(13)00131-1. doi:10.1016/j.bbi.2013.03.002

Immke David C, Gavva Narender R (2006) The TRPV1 receptor and nociception. Semin Cell Dev Biol 17:582–591

Khairatkar-Joshi N, Szallasi A (2009) TRPV1 antagonists: the challenges for therapeutic targeting. Trends Mol Med 15:14–22. doi:10.1016/j.molmed.2008.11.004

Lambert GA, Davis JB, Appleby JM, Chizh BA, Hoskin KL, Zagami AS (2009) The effects of the TRPV1 receptor antagonist SB-705498 on trigeminovascular sensitisation and neurotransmission. Naunyn Schmiedebergs Arch Pharmacol 380:311–325. doi:10.1007/s00210-009-0437-5

Li Q (2012) Antagonists of toll like receptor 4 maybe a new strategy to counteract opioid-induced hyperalgesia and opioid tolerance. Med Hypotheses 79:754–756. doi:10.1016/j.mehy.2012.08.021

Liddle RA (2007) The role of transient receptor potential vanilloid 1 (TRPV1) channels in pancreatitis. Biochim Biophys Acta 1772:869–878

Mason L, Moore RA, Derry S, Edwards JE, McQuay HJ (2004) Systematic review of topical capsaicin for the treatment of chronic pain. BMJ 328:991

McCleane G (2003) Pharmacological management of neuropathic pain. CNS Drugs 17:1031–1043

Nagy I, Sántha P, Jancsó G, Urbán L (2004) The role of the vanilloid (capsaicin) receptor (TRPV1) in physiology and pathology. Eur J Pharmacol 500:351–369

Nilius B (2007) TRP channels in disease. Biochim Biophys Acta 1772:805–812

NICE Clinical Guideline 96 (2010) Neuropathic pain: The pharmacological management of neuropathic pain in adults in non-specialist settings. Issued: March 2010. National Institute for Health and Clinical Excellence. http://www.nice.org.uk/guidance/CG96. Accessed 24 April 2013

Premkumar LS, Abooj M (2013) TRP channels and analgesia. Life Sci 92:415–424. doi:10.1016/j.lfs.2012.08.010

Qutenza Prescribing Information (2009) Copyright 2009 NeurogesX

Richards BL, Whittle SL, Buchbinder R (2012) Neuromodulators for pain management in rheumatoid arthritis. Cochrane Database Syst Rev 1:CD008921. doi:10.1002/14651858.CD008921.pub2

Ro JY, Lee JS, Zhang Y (2009) Activation of TRPV1 and TRPA1 leads to muscle nociception and mechanical hyperalgesia. Pain 144:270–277. doi:10.1016/j.pain.2009.04.021

Robbins WR, Staats PS, Levine J, Fields HL, Allen RW, Campbell JN, Pappagallo M (1998) Treatment of intractable pain with topical large-dose capsaicin: preliminary report. Anesth Analg 86(3):579–583

Rowbotham MC, Nothaft W, Duan WR, Wang Y, Faltynek C, McGaraughty S, Chu KL, Svensson P (2011) Oral and cutaneous thermosensory profile of selective TRPV1 inhibition by ABT-102 in a randomized healthy volunteer trial. Pain 152:1192–1200. doi:10.1016/j.pain.2011.01.051

Sayanlar J, Guleyupoglu N, Portenoy R, Ashina S (2012) Trigeminal postherpetic neuralgia responsive to treatment with capsaicin 8 % topical patch: a case report. J Headache Pain 13:587–589. doi:10.1007/s10194-012-0467-0

Schwartz ES, Christianson JA, LA Jun-Ho XC, Davis BM, Albers KM, Gebhart GF (2011) Synergistic role of TRPV1 and TRPA1 in pancreatic pain and inflammation. Gastroenterology 140:1283–1291. doi:10.1053/j.gastro.2010.12.033

Simpson DM, Estanislao L, Brown SJ, Sampson J (2008) An open-label pilot study of high-concentration capsaicin patch in painful HIV neuropathy. J Pain Symptom Manage 35:299–306

Summ O, Holland PR, Akerman S, Goadsby PJ (2011) TRPV1 receptor blockade is ineffective in different in vivo models of migraine. Cephalalgia 31:172–180. doi:10.1177/0333102410375626

Takemura M, Quarcoo D, Niimi A, Dinh QT, Geppetti P, Fischer A, Chung KF, Groneberg DA (2008) Is TRPV1 a useful target in respiratory diseases? Pulm Pharmacol Ther 21:833–839. doi:10.1016/j.pupt.2008.09.005

Terenzi R, Romano E, Manetti M, Peruzzi F, Niacci F, Matucci-Cerinic M, Guiducci S (2013) Neuropeptides activate TRPV1 in rheumatoid arthritis fibroblast-like synoviocytes and foster IL-6 and IL-8 production. Ann Rheum Dis 72(6):1107–1109

Tominaga M, Tominaga T (2005) Structure and function of TRPV1. Pflugers Arch 451:143–150

Vardanyan A, Wang R, Vanderah TW, Ossipov MH, Lai J, Porreca F, King T (2009) TRPV1 receptor in expression of opioid-induced hyperalgesia. J Pain 10:243–252. doi:10.1016/j.jpain.2008.07.004

Webster LR, Nunez M, Tark MD, Dunteman ED, Lu B, Tobias JK, Vanhove GF (2011) Tolerability of NGX-4010, a capsaicin 8 % dermal patch, following pretreatment with lidocaine 2.5 %/prilocaine 2.5 % cream in patients with postherpetic neuralgia. BMC Anesthesiol 11:25. doi:10.1186/1471-2253-11-25

Webster LR, Peppin JF, Murphy FT, Tobias JK, Vanhove GF (2012) Tolerability of NGX-4010, a capsaicin 8 % patch, in conjunction with three topical anesthetic formulations for the treatment of neuropathic pain. J Pain Res 5:7–13. doi:10.2147/JPR.S25272

Wong GY, Gavva NR (2009) Therapeutic potential of vanilloid receptor TRPV1 agonists and antagonists as analgesics: recent advances and setbacks. Brain Res Rev 60:267–277. doi:10.1016/j.brainresrev.2008.12.006

Zhu Y, Colak T, Shenoy M, Liu L, Pai R, Li C, Mehta K, Pasricha PJ (2011) Nerve growth factor modulates TRPV1 expression and function and mediates pain in chronic pancreatitis. Gastroenterology 141:370–377. doi:10.1053/j.gastro.2011.03.046

Chapter 6
Intranasal Capsaicin in Management of Nonallergic (Vasomotor) Rhinitis

Umesh Singh and Jonathan A. Bernstein

Abstract Capsaicin is a selective transient receptor potential vanilloid 1 (TRPV1) ion channel agonist and has been demonstrated to reduce nerve conduction of nociceptive C fibers in the trigeminal nerve without affecting conduction in Aδ fibers. This chapter reviews the classification of chronic rhinitis subtypes, the prevalence and epidemiology of nonallergic rhinitis (NAR), postulated pathophysiology and mechanisms of NAR including the role of transient receptor potential (TRP) ion channels and discusses the potential therapeutic benefits of capsaicin in the treatment of chronic rhinitis subtypes, specifically NAR. Evidence supports that hypersensitivity of TRP ion channels on sensory afferent neurons innervating nasal mucosa is responsible for inducing NAR symptoms. These symptoms, characterized as excessive nasal glandular secretion, nasal congestion, and headache, are mediated through neuropeptide release during axonal and parasympathetic reflexes which are initiated by a spectrum of nonspecific irritants that activate TRP channels. Rational approaches to treat the pathophysiology of NAR would be to develop therapies with selective TRPV1 agonist activity like capsaicin that target desensitization of TRP ion channels on sensory afferent nerves.

6.1 Introduction

Capsicum, or therapeutic peppers, have been used for thousands of years to treat a wide variety of ailments and are included in the traditional medicine practices of India, China, Japan, and Korea. Cayenne pepper or *Capsicum* is included the

U. Singh · J. A. Bernstein (✉)
Department of Internal Medicine, Division of Immunology/Allergy Section, University of Cincinnati College of Medicine, 3255 Eden Avenue, Suite 350, ML#563, Cincinnati, OH 45267-0563, USA
e-mail: jonathan.bernstein@uc.edu

U. Singh · J. A. Bernstein
Bernstein Allergy Group, Inc, Cincinnati, OH, USA

O. M. E. Abdel-Salam (ed.), *Capsaicin as a Therapeutic Molecule*, Progress in Drug Research 68, DOI: 10.1007/978-3-0348-0828-6_6, © Springer Basel 2014

German Pharmacopeia, Commission E monographs and approved in the US as an OTC topical analgesic. *Capsicum* tincture and oleoresin were formerly in the official United States Pharmacopeia and National Formulary as a carminative, stimulant, and rubefacient (Leung and Foster 1996; Taber 2005).

In modern times, there have been over 40 clinical trials on capsaicin for the treatment of sinusitis, allergic (AR) and nonallergic rhinitis (NAR), cough, and headache. Investigational studies using capsaicin for the treatment of NAR have been most promising (Tran et al. 2011). Capsaicin (C18H27NO3, MW: 305.41) is known to be a selective TRPVI ion channel agonist and has been demonstrated to reduce nerve conduction of nociceptive C fibers in the trigeminal nerve without affecting conduction in Aδ fibers (Docherty et al. 2013).

Studies investigating the health effects of capsaicin continue to expand and there is now an emerging body of research that has elucidated how this novel compound may exert its therapeutic benefits. This chapter will review the classification of chronic rhinitis subtypes, the prevalence and epidemiology of NAR, postulated pathophysiology, and mechanisms of NAR including the role of TRP ion channels and discuss the potential therapeutic benefits of capsaicin in the treatment of chronic rhinitis subtypes, specifically NAR.

6.2 Classification and Definition of Chronic Rhinitis Subtypes

Chronic rhinitis is defined as persistent inflammation of the mucosal membranes lining the nasal cavity, characterized by symptoms including nasal congestion, rhinorrhea, sneezing, and itching with or without post-nasal drainage (Bernstein 2013a; Schroer and Pien 2012). Broadly defined, rhinitis can be divided into inflammatory and noninflammatory rhinitis. Inflammatory rhinitis includes seasonal (SAR) or perennial allergic rhinitis (PAR) and nonallergic rhinitis eosinophilic syndrome (NARES), whereas noninflammatory rhinitis includes vasomotor rhinitis (VMR) and other NAR conditions such as rhinitis medicamentosa, gustatory rhinitis, and hormonally-induced rhinitis. If one includes all of the NAR conditions into one category (i.e., NARES and VMR) then developing a common phenotype becomes more difficult to establish (Bernstein et al. 2012). To complicate matters further, patients with AR or NAR often exhibit significantly increased symptoms in response to irritant triggers, leading clinicians to postulate another rhinitis subtype termed "mixed rhinitis" which is the coexistence of an AR and NAR component (Bernstein 2010). NAR conditions are diagnoses by exclusion. To establish a definitive diagnosis of NAR, all other NAR syndromes should first be properly considered and excluded (Shah and McGrath 2012; Scarupa and Kaliner 2009; Settipane and Lieberman 2001). A diagnosis of NAR requires negative specific IgE responses by skin or serologic testing, the absence of localized specific IgE in the nose ("entopic" rhinitis), exclusion of an infectious etiology, and the absence of a structural problem such as nasal septal deviation, osteomeatal complex disease, and/or nasal polyps. Furthermore, symptoms are frequently triggered by irritant triggers such as tobacco smoke, solvents, perfumes/fragrances as well as temperature and/or barometric pressure changes but recognition of nonallergic triggers is not characteristic of all NAR patients (Tran et al. 2011; Bernstein et al. 2012). Differentiation of the nonallergic conditions, VMR and NARES, is limited to the presence or absence of eosinophilia in the nasal passages (Ito 1993; Bernstein 2009). Therefore, VMR is truly a noninflammatory, nonallergic condition whereas NARES is an inflammatory, nonallergic condition. It should be emphasized that symptoms and physical findings are not pathognomonic for AR as patients with NAR often manifest similar features. Therefore, proper diagnostic testing is essential to accurately classify these disorders.

The management of chronic NAR can be very challenging for physicians and extremely frustrating for patients. Many people with this chronic condition are inadequately diagnosed (Ledford 2003). Previously, chronic rhinitis and sinusitis conditions were lumped into the "catch all" diagnosis of VMR (relating to dysfunction of nerves and muscles that cause the blood vessels to constrict or dilate). More recent studies indicate that neural or autonomic dysregulation of the nasal mucosa may be an important cause of NAR (van Rijswijk and Gerth van Wijk 2006; Bernstein 2013b). However, since the mechanism(s) of NAR is still incompletely understood, some experts, now refer to these (NAR) conditions as Idiopathic (unknown cause) rhinitis (IR), to emphasize the lack of understanding the underlying cause(s) of this disorder (van Rijswijk and Gerth van Wijk 2006). In addition, to further emphasize the significant morbidity associated with rhinitis, the term "rhinosinusitis" instead of sinusitis has been adopted, which more accurately reflects the importance of correctly diagnosing and treating chronic rhinitis disorders to prevent complications such as sinusitis. Sinusitis is almost always accompanied by concurrent nasal airway inflammation, and in many cases sinusitis is preceded by rhinitis symptoms (Sedaghat et al. 2012). Although the term rhinosinusitis is believed to more accurately describe the spectrum of infectious and inflammatory conditions previously grouped under the term sinusitis, most patients with the VMR form of NAR do not have persistent sinus mucosal swelling or obstruction of the osteomeatal complexes if recognized and treated appropriately (Settipane and Lieberman 2001).

6.3 Prevalence and Epidemiology of NAR

It is estimated that more than 70 million people suffer from rhinitis in the United States frequently complicated by sinusitis each year, and that about 36.2 ($\pm$0.3) million people visit their physician each year due to chronic sinusitis (Lee and Bhattacharyya 2011). Rhinitis ("inflammation of the nose") and sinusitis ("inflammation of the sinuses") causes significant burden of disease which significantly impairs patient's quality of life and their daily functioning (Meltzer et al. 2009).

The incidence of NAR in the general population is estimated to be 2–4 % (Bousquet et al. 2001), but among chronic rhinitis sufferers it is approximately 25 % (Settipane 2008). Other studies have reported that NAR affects up to 22 million Americans annually (Settipane and Kaliner 2013). However, large population studies have yet to be conducted to determine the true prevalence or incidence of PAR or NAR disorders. One cross-sectional survey found that the diagnosis of AR ranged between 43 and 83 %, whereas the prevalence of NAR ranged between 17 and 52 % (Shah and McGrath 2012; Scarupa and Kaliner 2009; Bernstein 2009). The National Rhinitis Classification Task Force questionnaire survey evaluated 975 patients with chronic rhinitis and is one of the few studies that attempted to identify the prevalence of mixed rhinitis (MR), defined as the presence of patients experience symptoms in response to AR and nonallergic triggers. They found that 34 % of these patients met the criteria for MR (Settipane and Lieberman 2001; Bernstein 2010).

6.4 Clinical Presentation of NAR

NAR can present with or without known triggers. Nonallergic triggers typically include symptoms in response to odors and chemical irritants and to weather changes (i.e., temperature and barometric pressure changes). However, since NAR is a diagnosis of exclusion there is no specific test available to confirm the diagnosis of non- allergic conditions. It has been previously reported that patients who present with new onset symptoms later in life (age >45 years), have no family history of allergies, no seasonality of their symptoms or symptoms around cats, dogs, or furry animals and increased symptoms around strong odors such as perfumes and fragrances, have more than 98 % likelihood of having a diagnosis of NAR that will correlate with an allergy specialist's diagnosis of NAR after allergy skin testing (Bernstein et al. 2012; Bernstein 2009, 2013b). Typically, patients suffering from NAR may have tried multiple treatments without benefit, including second generation antihistamines and nasal corticosteroids. In addition, these patients often undergo fiberoptic endoscopic nasal surgery in an attempt to gain symptom relief with often unsatisfactory or incomplete results.

6.5 Innervation and Blood Supply to the Nasal Mucosa

The surface of the nasal cavity is primarily composed of respiratory epithelium with numerous seromucous acinar glands, blood vessels, and nerves within the lamina propria. Nasal cavity resistance is directly influenced by swelling of nasal mucosa. The alternating variations of nasal engorgement with airflow restriction from one side of the nasal passages to the other, that occurs normally every 1–5 h, comprises the nasal cycle which is due to variations in sympathetic tone to the vascular tissue in the nasal mucosa (Mirza et al. 1997).

Trigeminal nerve branches innervate blood vessels and mucous membrane of nasal cavities. Branches of the ophthalmic and maxillary divisions of the trigeminal nerve are responsible for mediating general sensations such as touch, pain, and temperature from the nasal mucosa to the central nervous system. The superficial trigeminal nerve fibers in the epithelium are more sensitive to noxious irritant stimuli. The nasal mucosal glands are also innervated by autonomic fibers that control cyclical and reactive vascular activity (Cassano et al. 2012).

The nasal blood vessels are supplied by sympathetic postganglionic fibers whereas the secretomotor supply to the nasal mucous glands are innervated by postganglionic parasympathetic fibers, derived from the pterygopalatine ganglion, which are distributed through branches of the maxillary nerves. Interactions of sensory, parasympathetic, and sympathetic nervous systems innervating nasal mucosa regulate mucosal glandular secretion as well as blood flow within the nasal mucosal vasculature.

6.6 Proposed Rhinitis Pathophysiology for Nonallergic Rhinitis

The most widely accepted mechanism for NAR patients has been an autonomic imbalance between the sympathetic and parasympathetic nervous system resulting in parasympathetic hyperactivity leading to nasal congestion, rhinorrhea, and postnasal drainage (Bernstein 2013b; Harlor et al. 2012; Devillier et al. 1988). Nasal congestion and rhinorrhea are primarily due to engorgement of vascular anastomoses and caverns in the submucosa and increased glandular secretions from goblet cells in serous and mucous glands. Inhaled irritants can stimulate Type C nociceptive sensory nerves. Activation of these nerve endings release neuropeptides, e.g., Substance P (SP) and Calcitonin G-Related Peptide (CGRP), through an axonal response system as an immediate protective mucosal defense mechanism against these noxious irritants (antidromic reflex) (Fig. 6.1) (Norlander et al. 1996; Baraniuk 1992, 2001; Kavut et al. 2013). These reflexes increase glandular secretions (mostly in NAR) and also cause plasma extravasation (mostly in AR) leading to mucosal edema. Increased glandular secretions, as opposed to fluid transudation from blood vessels, has been postulated to represent a primary pathophysiologic characteristic of NAR (Norlander et al. 1996).

In addition, SP and other mediators (e.g., acetylcholine) released through central parasympathetic reflexes, activate neurokinin1 and acetylcholine or muscarinic receptors, respectively. The coexistence of an acetycholine peptide may increase the secretory response to acetylcholine (ACh) resulting in increased submucosal glandular secretion (Baraniuk 2001; Tai and Baraniuk 2002; Lindh and Hokfelt 1990). Sympathetic activities mediated by neuropeptide Y (NPY) and norepinephrine maintain nasal patency by causing vasoconstriction leading to decongestion of the nasal mucosa. Collectively, these autonomic responses constitute what is referred to as the orthodromic response (Baraniuk 2001). Over activity of these axonal (antidromic)

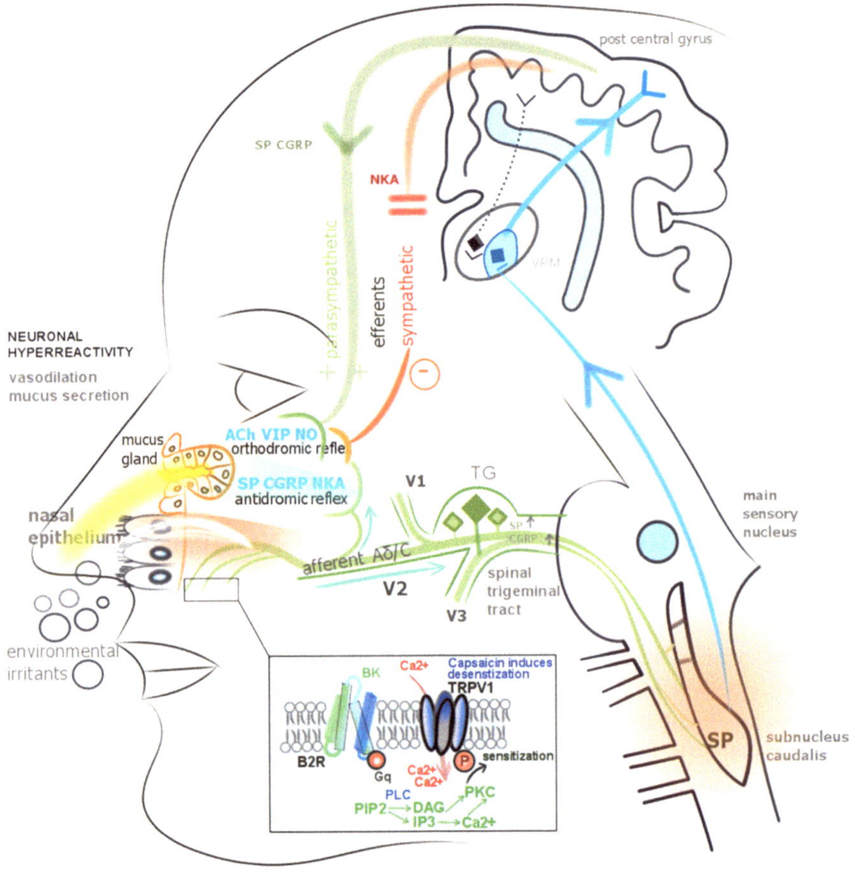

Fig. 6.1 Outlines the hypothetical mechanisms of AR, NAR, or MR and the role of capsaicin in TRPV1 desensitization in such clinical conditions. Stimulation of maxillary division of trigeminal nerves (*V2*) is initiated by environmental irritants, and hypersensitivity of TRPV1 on these nerve fibers is mediated by inflammatory mediators such as bradykinin (BK) acting on bradykinin receptors (*B2R*) in case of allergic rhinitis. Specific involvement of BK in mediating TRPV1 sensitization to irritants in NAR have not been demonstrated in previous studies. Increased glandular secretion or plasma protein exudation occurs specifically in NAR or AR respectively, that are possibly mediated by locally activated antidromic reflexes causing neuropeptide release or through autonomic imbalance causing parasympathetic over activity

reflexes suppress or dampen these sympathetic activities allowing parasympathetic activity to be more prominent resulting in increased nasal congestion (Baraniuk 1992; Baraniuk and Kaliner 1991). Reduction in the nasal luminal cross-sectional area as an index of increased nasal obstruction and mucus secretions, both induced by parasympathetic over stimulation, have been demonstrated to be predictive of nasal nonspecific hyper-responsiveness (Kim and Jang 2012).

6.7 Role of Transient Receptor Potential Ion Channels in NAR Pathophysiology

There are several protective reflexes initiated by trigeminal sensory afferent nerves, such as sneezing, cough, mucus secretion, and bronchoconstriction that are essential for expelling or neutralizing irritants and allergens from the respiratory system. Transient Receptor Potential (TRP) ion channels, such as TRPV1 (vanilloid) and the TRPA1 (ankyrin), on non-myelinated C fibers of trigeminal sensory nerves that innervate the nasal mucosa, are sensors of inhaled irritants (Geppetti et al. 2010). The vanilloid subtype, TRPV1, is an integrative, multigated ion channel widely expressed in human nasal epithelium and neuronal tissue and is known to be activated typically by capsaicin, protons and heat (Szolcsányi and Sándor 2012; Cao et al. 2013; Brauchi et al. 2006; Myers et al. 2008). This channel is believed to be important in a spectrum of important physiological functions that are inhibited in cell or animal models that have TRPV1 gene deletion (White et al. 2011; Szolcsányi 2008). On the other hand, development of nasal hyper-responsiveness to environmental factors that may initiate symptoms of rhinitis may be caused by TRPV1 hyperactivity (Lambert et al. 2013). Neuropeptides such as SP and CGRP secreted as a result of stimulation of these afferent nerves cause vasodilatation, increased vascular permeability, and glandular secretion that can explain many of the symptoms associated with chronic rhinitis (Pfaar et al. 2009). It is also known that TRP channel activation is also highly regulated by neuropeptides such as SP and CGRP (Chung et al. 2008).

TRPV1 channels interact and regulate other colocalized TRP channels (e.g., TRPA1) and ion channels (e.g., Na^+ channels) (Raisinghani et al. 2011). Intracellular cascades triggered by other G-protein coupled receptors such as bradykinin receptors (B2R) have been demonstrated to further sensitize these channels. (Szolcsányi and Pintér 2013; Mizumura et al. 2005).

Changes in the regulatory mechanisms that control TRPV1 channel function can result in pathologic alteration of its activity. N-glycosylation of the TRPV1 channel affects pharmacokinetics (EC50) and dose–response curves of TRPV1 agonists (Wirkner et al. 2005). Thus, any pathological alteration in TRPV1 glycosylation may cause TRPV1 channel hyper-responsiveness (Veldhuis et al. 2012). TRPV1 N-glycosylation facilitates TRPV1 pore dilation and therefore significantly reduces agonist-induced desensitization of these channels. Pore dilation confers resistance to channel desensitization or conformational changes to desensitized state. Interestingly, glycosylation end products have been found to be elevated in patients with AR (Di Lorenzo et al. 2013), but such changes have not been investigated for NAR.

6.8 Capsaicin Regulation of TRPV1 Channel Gating

Capsaicin-gated TRPV1 conductance is regulated by calcium in a concentration and voltage dependent manner by causing hyperpolarizing shifts in the voltage dependence of these channels (Aneiros et al. 2011; Blanchard and

Kellenberger 2011). Capsaicin-induced TRPV1 activation hydrolyzes the membrane phosphatidylinositol 4, 5-bisphosphate PIP2 and its subsequent depletion has been shown to occur in parallel with TRPV1 ion channel activation (Akopian et al. 2007). Recovery of the channel from the desensitized state is determined by replenishment of PIP2 in the cell membrane (Liu et al. 2005). It has been demonstrated that TRPV1 desensitization to repeated applications of capsaicin (tachyphylaxis) is prevented by ATP or PIP2, while calmodulin was necessary for sustaining tachyphylaxis (Lishko et al. 2007). Interestingly, another study has shown that PIP2 along with PIP4 inhibits TRPV1 leading investigators to conclude that the phosphoinositide turnover contributes to thermal hyperalgesia by blocking inhibition of the channel (Cao et al. 2013). In addition, PKC and PKA mediated phosphorylation sensitizes TRPV1 channels by promoting downstream changes in channel activation that enhances the channel opening time rather than by a direct action of phosphorylation on the capsaicin binding site (Brauchi et al. 2006; Samways and Egan 2011; Studer and McNaughton 2010; Garcia-Sanz et al. 2007). Novel proteins associated with GABA receptors have been identified to be associated with TRPV1 signaling complex. These proteins increase trafficking and surface expression of TRPV1, besides modulating channel gating and sensitivity (Lainez et al. 2010).

6.9 Mechanism of Action of Capsaicin in NAR

Surgical denervation of sensory or autonomic nerves as well as treatment with intranasal capsaicin has been demonstrated to reduce glandular secretions and mucosal permeability and therefore relieve symptoms of NAR (Norlander et al. 1996; Baraniuk 1992; Baraniuk and Kaliner 1991). Capsaicin has been shown to reduce mucosal permeability without affecting tight junction of the nasal mucosal epithelium (Jeon et al. 1995). It causes sensory neurons important for relaying pain signals from the nasal cavity to become hyposensitive. As these cells become less hyper-reactive, neurogenic pain signals are significantly reduced. Capsaicin also depletes SP stores in nerve cells. Because SP may dilate nasal blood vessels and increase secretions from mucosal membranes, the depletion of SP stores in nerve cells by capsaicin can also relieve chronic painful sinus conditions. This observation is supported by previous studies that demonstrated that capsaicin-induced TRPV1 desensitization decreases the number of CGRP and SP immune reactive cells, without causing axonal degeneration of urinary bladder nerve fibers in animal models (Avelino and Cruz 2000). Analogous mechanisms may explain observed neuropeptide depletion induced by capsaicin in nasal mucosal glands (Blom et al. 1997). Repeated intranasal capsaicin application has been shown to reduce nasal vascular responses in patients with rhinitis which correlates with reduction of the CGRP-like immunoreactivity in nasal biopsies (Lacroix et al. 1991). Several other potential mechanisms of action for capsaicin continue to be investigated which may further help elucidate the mechanism(s) for underlying complex disorders such as NAR and headache.

6.10 Clinical Trials Investigating the Health Benefits of Capsaicin

Double-blind, placebo-controlled studies have demonstrated that capsaicin provides both significant short- and long-term reduction of symptoms in NAR patients. More recently published controlled trials have demonstrated that capsaicin can be safely administered without having to anesthetize the nose and causes no significant adverse effects (Blom et al. 1997, 1998; Bernstein et al. 2011a, b). Capsaicin and its derivatives have also been demonstrated in controlled studies to reduce the frequency and severity of cluster, migraine, and tension headaches (Fusco et al. 2003).

Table 6.1 summarizes some of the important clinical trials investigating the effects of capsaicin in AR, NAR, or MR as well as on headache and sinusitis. Clinical trials investigating the therapeutic benefit of capsaicin on patients with AR did not find significant effect in reducing nasal hyper-reactivity or in improving rhinorrhea (Gerth Van Wijk et al. 2000). However, some of these trials were able to demonstrate that increased plasma protein extravasation or leucocyte infiltration is neurally mediated through sensory afferents nerves innervating the nasal mucosa (Sanico et al. 1997, 1998a, b). In contrast, a number of clinical trials have described significant therapeutic efficacy and safety of chronic usage of local capsaicin formulations, when used to treat NAR and MR compared to placebo therapies (Bernstein et al. 2011a, b; Ciabatti and D'Ascanio 2009; Zheng et al. 2000; Filiaci et al. 1994, 1996; Rinder 1996; Marabini et al. 1991). Because all of these trials implemented different study designs and dosing regimens, the ability to compare primary endpoints is significantly limited (Table 6.1) (Bernstein et al. 2011a, b; Filiaci et al. 1996; Marabini et al. 1991; Van Rijswijk et al. 2003; Latimer and Poston 1976).

A randomized double blinded placebo-controlled study by Bernstein et al. reported significant improvement in total nasal symptom scores as well as non-nasal symptoms including headaches, sinus pressure, and pain in patients with a significant component of NAR improved significantly, with repeated administration of a locally applied low concentration capsaicin formulation for 2 weeks compared to a placebo (Bernstein et al. 2011a, b). Capsaicin has also been recently demonstrated to improve clinical symptoms in idiopathic rhinitis by down regulating over-expression of TRP ion channels (e.g., TRPV1 and TRPA1) (Van Gerven et al. 2013).

Other placebo-controlled trials by Blom et al. investigated the therapeutic benefit of capsaicin compared to placebo on nasal biopsies and immunohistochemistry among nonallergic noninfectious rhinitis patients (Blom et al. 1997, 1998). Capsaicin significantly improved the symptom visual analog score for nasal congestion and rhinorrhea without affecting cellular homeostasis or immunocompetent cells (Blom et al. 1997, 1998). Local application of capsaicin was demonstrated to exert this clinical effect without affecting eosinophilic cationic protein (ECP) levels in nasal lavage fluid or altering nasal symptoms produced by specific allergen provocation. Furthermore, capsaicin did not alter levels of $CD1^+$, $CD25^+$, $CD3^+$, $CD68^+$, $BMK13^+$, IgE^+, tryptase$^+$, and chymase$^+$ cells in pan-neurogenic staining of nasal mucosa of NAR patients compared to controls (Blom et al. 1998).

Table 6.1 Summary of clinical trials investigating the effects of capsaicin in patients with allergic, nonallergic, mixed rhinitis

Clinical trials investigating effect of capsaicin in patients with allergic rhinitis				
Study	Design	Endpoints	Results	Conclusion
Alenmyr et al. (2012) PMID: 21951314	RDBPCCO; studied the effect of synthetic TRPV1 blocker (SB-705498) on daily allergen challenges in patients with seasonal AR	TNSS, nPIF, ECP	TRPV1 blocking dosage of SB-705498 did not improve TNSS, nPIF, ECP	TRPV1 is not a key mediator of the symptoms in allergic rhinitis
Gerth Van Wijk et al. (2000) PMID: 11122219	RDBPC; evaluated efficacy of repeated capsaicin application to patients with HDM nasal allergy; $N = 26$	Nasal reactivity to HDM (measured by nasal symptoms, albumin + LT levels in NLF), responsiveness to histamine (before and 6 weeks after trt.), VASS, RQL	No significant effect of capsaicin on nasal reactivity to HDM, on VAS or RQL 6 weeks or 3 months after treatment; small effect on the area of the curve (AUC) of histamine dose response curves ($P = 0.03$)	Capsaicin lacks therapeutic effect in perennial allergic rhinitis
Sanico et al. (1998a) PMID: 9537786	Determined if AR and NAR is characterized by sensory neuronal hyper-responsiveness; PAR, NAR, healthy controls were stimulated with TRPV1 agonist capsaicin	Nasal symptoms, glandular secretion and plasma extravasation measured by lactoferrin and albumin levels in NLF respectively	Capsaicin-sensitive nerve stimulation caused similar increases in nasal symptom scores, lactoferrin in all groups but increased albumin levels significantly only in PAR	Hyper-responsiveness of sensory nerve fibers is characteristic of PAR causing increased permeability to albumin in nasal vasculature

(continued)

Table 6.1 (continued)

Clinical trials investigating effect of capsaicin in patients with allergic rhinitis				
Study	Design	Endpoints	Results	Conclusion
Sanico et al. (1998b) PMID: 9475863	Determined whether increased nasal vascular permeability in AR is neuronally mediated. AR volunteers pretreated with atropine or placebo before capsaicin	NLF volume and lysozyme, albumin and fibrinogen content	Atropine or lidocaine pretreatment reduced capsaicin-induced lavage volume and lysozyme content but not albumin and fibrinogen content	Plasma protein extravasation into nasal mucosa in AR is neutrally mediated
Sanico et al. (1997) PMID: 9389293	RDBPC; determined whether neuronal stimulation induces dose-dependent inflammatory changes in human upper airway; $N = 10$ AR patients; Capsaicin 1, 10, 100 μg sprayed into nasal cavity	NLF collected at different time intervals; endpoints-NSS, NLF leucocyte counts, albumin, lysozyme levels	High doses of capsaicin (10, 100 μg) increased leucocyte count, albumin and lysozyme levels at 0.5, 1 and 4 h after application	Nasal sensory nerve stimulation increases leucocyte infiltration and plasma protein extravasation in AR patients
Roche et al. (1995) PMID: 7697245	RDBPC; Studied the effect of colchicine on the nasal response to capsaicin (10^(−9) to 3 × 10^(−5) M in AR; $N = 16$, 8 AR and 8 controls	Nasal airflow conductance (rhinometry), volume of nasal secretions, NLF cytology	Capsaicin-induced increase in elastase in NLF in AR patients was attenuated by colchicine treatment	Colchicine (known to inhibit microtubular axonal transport of peptides) prevents inflammatory response (increase in neutrophil elastase) due to nasal sensory neuronal irritation in AR

(continued)

Table 6.1 (continued)

Clinical trials investigating effect of capsaicin in patients with nonallergic rhinitis				
Study	Design	Endpoints	Results	Conclusion
Van Gerven et al. (2013) PMID: 24139494	RC (Parallel study); N=14 cases (Idiopathic rhinitis), 12 controls (healthy); before and after CDA provocation on and off treatment (with Capsaicin) comparison of VAS and TRES, nasal fluids and biopsy collection, measurement of nPIF	ΔVAS; ΔNHR; nasal fluid SP, expression of TRP channels and mast cell marker	For cases, VAS, TRES, NHR, nPIF, TRPV1/A2 channel expression and SP levels decreased between 4-12 wks. post-treatment	TRPV1-substance P signaling is increased in IR; the corresponding symptoms are significantly reduced by Capsaicin which reduces the TRP channel expression in nasal mucosa without affecting hNECs
Bernstein et al. (2011a, b) PMID: 21802026	RDBPC; $N = 20$ (cases), 22 (controls); compared efficacy and safety of capsaicin nasal spray (ICX72) with placebo in subjects with NAR	ΔTNSS (from baseline to end of study i.e. 2 weeks), ISS	ICX72 improved TNSS ($p < 0.01$), ISS ($p < 0.01$), nasal congestion, sinus pain, sinus pressure, headache; no difference in adverse effects (vs. controls)	Repeated intranasal capsaicin use safely and rapidly improves symptoms in NAR
Blom et al. (1998) PMID: 9824407	Placebo-controlled; NANIR Cases treated with capsaicin every 2nd/3rd day × 7 treatments. at baseline, 2 week, 3, 9 month after treatment.; endpoints-immunocompetent cell densities and neural tissue density in the nasal mucosa	Nasal biopsy and immunohistochemistry	Nasal symptoms improved significantly in capsaicin treated group. Number of immunocompetent cells or neural tissue density did not significantly differ between treated and control groups	Capsaicin nasal spray reduces nasal symptoms without affecting cellular homeostasis or immunocompetent cells

(continued)

Table 6.1 (continued)

Clinical trials investigating effect of capsaicin in patients with nonallergic rhinitis

Study	Design	Endpoints	Results	Conclusion
Kuhn et al. (1997) PMID: 9292182	RPC; Animal study; application of capsaicin or placebo	Substance P in nasal secretion measured before and after capsaicin application	Significant differences in nasal secretion SP between capsaicin treated and control rats	Nasal mucous SP levels following irritant nasal stimulus change after intranasal capsaicin treatment in VMR
Blom et al. (1997) PMID: 9249272	RPC; $N = 25$ NANIPER patients	VASS, LT, PGD2, and tryptase levels in NLF before, during and after capsaicin treatment	Significant and prolonged reduction in VASS in capsaicin treated group. No difference in LT, PGD2, and tryptase levels	Capsaicin has no effect on inflammatory mediators; pathogenesis of NANIPER does not involve inflammatory cells
Filiaci et al. (1996) PMID: 8882755	RD: $N = 15$ patients affected by aspecific nasal hyper-reactivity; determined whether local capsaicin treatment, 1/week, × 5 weeks, improved hyper-reactivity and nasal polyposis	Nasal symptoms, polyp size, nasal cytology	Capsaicin treatment improved symptoms, nasal hyper-reactivity and polyp size	Capsaicin improves aspecific nasal hyper-reactivity and polyposis
Filiaci et al. (1994) PMID: 7892815	Randomized controlled; determined whether capsaicin reduced nasal reactivity in VMR; $N = 10$ VMR patients, were treated with capsaicin (30 μM, 1/week × 5 weeks)	NSS (baseline and after non-specific provocation)	Improvement in symptoms and reduction of nasal resistance and aspecific hyper-reactivity within 2 weeks of capsaicin treatment; benefits lasted 6 months	Capsaicin reduces nasal reactivity in VMR

(continued)

Table 6.1 (continued)

Clinical trials investigating effect of capsaicin in patients with nonallergic rhinitis				
Study	Design	Endpoints	Results	Conclusion
Marabini et al. (1991) PMID: 1859650	Studied effects of capsaicin (15 g, tid, × 3 day) on nasal mucosa in VMR patients	NSS and nasal secretion	Acute effects induced by capsaicin such as pain and secretion of nasal fluid subsided at last capsaicin application	Beneficial effect of capsaicin is due to its desensitization (functional blockade) of nerve endings of sensory neurons in VMR patients

Clinical trial investigating effect of capsaicin in patients with mixed rhinitis				
Study	Design	Endpoints	Results	Conclusion
Ciabatti and D'Ascanio (2009) PMID: 19012048	Randomized placebo-controlled; $N = 208$; evaluated efficacy and safety of capsaicin nasal sprays (1, 2 or 4 μg/puff × 3 days) in IR	pre and post treatment nasal symptoms	Reduced frequency of IR symptoms with 4 μg/puff tid × 3 day; no significant difference in side effects (vs. controls)	Local capsaicin spray is effective and safe treatment for IR
Van Rijswijk et al. (2003) PMID: 12859554	RDBPCCO; Efficacy of alternative capsaicin regimen $N = 15$ (case), 15 (control)	VASS for nasal symptoms, rhinorrhea, nasal blockage	VASS decreased significantly and rapidly with capsaicin applied five times/day at 1 h intervals × 1 day; reduction in nasal hyperreactivity 9 months after treatment; no difference in side effects (vs. placebo)	Intranasal capsaicin is safe for IR; five treatments of capsaicin in a day is better or equally effective as five treatments over 2 weeks

(continued)

Table 6.1 (continued)

Clinical trial investigating effect of capsaicin in patients with mixed rhinitis				
Study	Design	Endpoints	Results	Conclusion
Rajakulasingam et al. (1992) PMID: 1317373	RDBPC; Effect of capsaicin (3 × 10^(−5) M) on nasal airway resistance and plasma protein exudation in nasal mucosa was determined	Nasal airway resistance, NLF albumin levels	No significant changes in nasal airway resistance or plasma protein exudation with capsaicin were measured	No vascular effects of capsaicin on human nasal mucosa

Clinical trial investigating effect of capsaicin in patients with headaches				
Study	Design	Endpoints	Results	Conclusion
Fusco et al. (1994) PMID: 7708405	RDBPC; $N = 52$ patients with episodic cluster headaches and 18 with chronic cluster headache (CH); ascertained the difference in efficacy of treatment with nasal capsaicin depending on side of application	symptomatic improvement	Difference between effects of contralateral and ipsilateral capsaicin treatment was significant in both episodic and chronic sufferers of cluster headache	Repeated capsaicin application was effective in cluster headache
Marks et al. (1993) PMID: 8495452	RDBPC; determined whether nasal application of capsaicin is effective in aborting cluster headache attacks; capsaicin applied ipsilateraly × 7 day, headache severity recorded for 15 day	decrease in headache severity	Headache severity significantly reduced in capsaicin treated group between 8 and 15 days; episodic CH benefited more	Intranasal capsaicin applied ipsilaterally provides therapeutic benefit in CH

(continued)

Table 6.1 (continued)

Clinical trial investigating effect of capsaicin on sinusitis				
Study	Design	Endpoints	Results	Conclusion
Zheng et al. (2000) PMID: 10779188	RDBPC; evaluated the effect of capsaicin on the intensity of nasal obstruction and rhinorrhea and recurrence of nasal polyps post polypectomy; $n = 51$ nasal polyposis patients, 22 controls; patients treated with capsaicin 1/week. × 5 weeks	Nasal airway resistance; Rhinorrhea using VAS; Clinical staging of polyp; all parameters recorded before and after treatment	Marked reduction of nasal airway resistance post polypectomy by capsaicin; no significant reduction in rhinorrhea	Capsaicin reduces polyps and nasal obstruction and is therefore cheaper alternative to corticosteroids for post polypectomy management
May et al. (1998) PMID: 9514561	Experimental study; $n = 7$ healthy volunteers; capsaicin applied to right forehead stimulated Cr. N. V (div. 1)	rCBF measured using PET	Increased rCBF found bilaterally in the insula, cingulate cortex, cavernous sinus and cerebellum;	Increased activation in cavernous sinus suggests that it is probably involved in sensory input through trigeminal n

(continued)

Table 6.1 (continued)

Study	Design	Endpoints	Results	Conclusion
Clinical trial investigating effect of capsaicin on sinusitis				
Rinder (1996) PMID: 8800374			Vanilloid receptors in pig nasal mucosa differ from those in their dorsal horn; Capsaicin evoked vasodilation in pig nasal mucosa indicates activation of sensory nerves; Capsaicin desensitization of the human nasal mucosa attenuated subjective pain response and reduction of cross-sectional area of nasal cavity induced by proton (VR1 activator); Capsazepine did not reduce capsaicin and LA-evoked vasodilation in pig nasal mucosa; CGRP receptor antagonist reduced capsaicin-induced vascular effects in pig mucosa	Nasal secretion induced by VR1 activation are mediated through CGRP release

RDBPC(CO) randomized double blinded placebo-controlled (cross over); *TRPV1* transient receptor potential vanilloid 1; *(T)NSS* (*Total*) nasal symptom Score; *nPIF* nasal peak inspiratory flow; *ECP* seosinophilic cationic protein; *ISS* individual symptom scores; *IR* idiopathic rhinitis; *VASS* Visual analog scale scores for nasal symptoms; *HDM* house dust mite; *LT* leukotriene; *RQL* Rhinitis quality of life; *NANIR* nonallergic noninfectious rhinitis; *PAR* perennial allergic rhinitis; *NAR* nonallergic rhinitis; *NLF* nasal lavage fluid; *VMR*: Vasomotor Rhinits; *rCBF* regional cerebral blood flow; *PET* positron emission tomography

These findings imply that NAR does not involve alterations in a number of immunocompetent cells or modulation of neural tissue density and indicate that capsaicin's effectiveness in treating either NAR, MR, or AR may be attributable to a mechanism(s) unrelated to traditional AR inflammatory pathways (Baudoin et al. 2000).

The inability of these studies to demonstrate a significant effect of capsaicin on inflammatory effector cells, supports an alternative mechanistic pathway of capsaicin in NAR which is most likely neurogenic (Blom et al. 1997; 1998; Rajakulasingam et al. 1992). Stimulation of ophthalmic branch of the trigeminal nerve has been shown to alter vascular flow in the insula and cavernous sinus (May et al. 1998; Marks et al. 1993) and therefore it has been postulated that stimulation of hyper-reactive sensory nerves fibers in the maxillary division of the trigeminal nerve may cause overstimulation of the parasympathetic autonomic nervous system causing headaches, frequently experienced by patients with NAR or MR. It is also known that the insular region of the brain regulates autonomic nervous activity. Specifically, sympathetic activity is controlled by the right insula and parasympathetic activity is controlled by the left insula (Vanneste and De Ridder 2013). Therefore, hyper-reactivity of the maxillary branch of the trigeminal nerve may affect vascular supply in the insular regions possibly leading to autonomic imbalance causing increased parasympathetic over activity and hypersecretion by nasal mucous glands.

6.11 Capsaicin's Ability to Desensitize Trigeminal Afferent C fiber TRPV1 Channels May Explain its Therapeutic Benefits in NAR

Although the therapeutic efficacy of capsaicin in AR or NAR does not appear to involve modulation of classic inflammatory pathways, it has been suggested that it may relieve symptoms of histamine-induced nasal congestion, sneezing, and rhinorrhea by blocking the histamine/PLA2/LPO/TRPV1 pathway (Gerth Van Wijk et al. 2000; Kim et al. 2004; Riechelmann et al. 1993). Histamine can activate TRPV1 in sensory neurons through the intracellular pathway involving phospholipase A2 and lipoxygenase (Kim et al. 2004). In vitro cell studies have demonstrated that Azelastine, an antihistamine agent approved by the FDA for the treatment of NAR can activate and subsequently desensitize TRPV1 (Bernstein et al. 2011a, b; Horak and Zieglmayer 2009; Singh et al. 2014). Therefore, the antihistaminergic activity of Azelastine may be due to its direct or indirect effect on desensitizing TRPV1. Similar mechanism may also account for antihistaminergic effects of capsaicin observed in mice models (Gijbels et al. 2000).

TRPV1 has six trans membrane (TM) domains. The hydrophobic outer pore of the channel is formed between fifth and sixth TM domains (TM5-TM6 linker). During gating, the domain of the channel constituting the pore, undergoes significant conformational rearrangement. The outer pore region is critical for gating of TRPV channels. Capsaicin-induced desensitization of TRPV1 ion channels may also involve conformational changes in the outer pore region that determine the balance between these channels in the opened and closed state (Myers et al. 2008). This effect results in blocking nasal sensory nerve stimulation which results in decreased nasal hyper-responsiveness (Changani et al. 2013; Georgalas and Jovancevic 2012). Therefore it has been proposed that capsaicin works through a feedback mechanism that confers cellular protection against toxic Ca^{2+} overload following channel activation (Vyklicky et al. 2008).

6.12 Current Treatment Options for NAR Indicate an Unmet Need for Novel Therapies

Pharmacotherapy for AR and NAR differs dramatically. However, since there are currently no specific treatments for NAR patients, most of the therapies we currently use to treat this condition are also used to treat AR. Only a few studies have been conducted on well-characterized patients with NAR conditions (VMR and NARES). Nasal corticosteroids have been reported to be effective in NAR with or without anticholinergic agents and fluticasone proprionate has previously been approved by the FDA for NAR (Tran et al. 2011; Bernstein 2013b). Azelastine is a topical antihistamine approved by the FDA for treatment of SAR and NAR. Studies have demonstrated that Azelastine is very effective in alleviating symptoms of nonallergic VMR (Bernstein 2007). In addition to its H1-receptor antagonist activity, Azelastine has also marked anti-inflammatory actions, which include inhibition of leukotrienes, bradykinin, SP, and vasointestinal peptide (Bernstein 2007). Adjunctive agents used to treat symptoms of NAR include first generation antihistamines because of their anticholinergic activity, intranasal anticholinergic agents which have been demonstrated to relieve severe rhinorrhea and/or post-nasal drainage associated with NAR and topical saline which has been shown to reduce symptoms of post-nasal drainage, sneezing, and congestion in some NAR patients (Bernstein 2013b; Huang and Govindaraj 2013).

Alternative therapies have been proposed for treatment of NAR including intranasal capsaicin as discussed. Recently, the intranasal application of CO_2 which has been shown to attenuate trigeminal nociception mediated by TRP channel activity has been found to reduce symptoms in patients with AR but has not yet been studied in NAR patients. Because of the colocalization of TRPM8 with TRPV1 ion channels in trigeminal nerve fibers, TRPM8 antagonists in conjunction with agents such as capsaicin that desensitize TRPV1 ion channels, merit consideration for therapeutic trials in NAR (Keh et al. 2011). Second generation TRPV1 antagonists and capsinoids (capsaicin TRPV1 activity without the burning sensation) which do not exhibit the side effects of hyperthermia and risk of brain injury may also have therapeutic advantages in the future treatment of NAR (Szolcsányi and Sándor 2012).

6.13 Conclusion

Hypersensitivity of TRP ion channels on sensory afferent neurons innervating nasal mucosa may be responsible for inducing NAR symptoms. Excessive nasal glandular secretion through neuropeptides released during axonal and parasympathetic reflexes are initiated by a spectrum of nonspecific irritants acting on these highly reactive TRP channels. Activation of TRP channels resulting in increased blood flow to the cerebral circulation can lead to other symptoms such as headaches which are frequent complaints of NAR patients. Consequently, rational approaches to treat the pathophysiology of NAR would be to develop therapies such as selective TRPV1 agonists like capsaicin that target desensitization of TRP ion channels on sensory afferent nerves.

References

Akopian AN, Ruparel NB, Jeske NA, Hargreaves KM (2007) Transient receptor potential TRPA1 channel desensitization in sensory neurons is agonist dependent and regulated by TRPV1-directed internalization. J Physiol 583(Pt 1):175–193

Aneiros E, Cao L, Papakosta M, Stevens EB, Phillips S, Grimm C (2011) The biophysical and molecular basis of TRPV1 proton gating. EMBO J 30(6):994–1002

Avelino A, Cruz F (2000) Peptide immunoreactivity and ultrastructure of rat urinary bladder nerve fibers after topical desensitization by capsaicin or resiniferatoxin. Auton Neurosci 86(1–2):37–46

Baraniuk JN (1992) Sensory, parasympathetic, and sympathetic neural influences in the nasal mucosa. J Allergy Clin Immunol 90(6 Pt 2):1045–1050

Baraniuk JN (2001) Neurogenic mechanisms in rhinosinusitis. Curr Allergy Asthma Rep 1(3):252–261

Baraniuk JN, Kaliner M (1991) Neuropeptides and nasal secretion. Am J Physiol 261(4 Pt 1): L223–L235

Baudoin T, Kalogjera L, Hat J (2000) Capsaicin significantly reduces sinonasal polyps. Acta Otolaryngol 120(2):307–311

Bernstein JA (2007) Azelastine hydrochloride: a review of pharmacology, pharmacokinetics, clinical efficacy and tolerability. Curr Med Res Opin 23(10):2441–2452

Bernstein JA (2009) Characteristics of Nonallergic Vasomotor Rhinitis. 2009 World Allergy Organization; licensee BioMed Central Ltd, London

Bernstein JA (2010) Allergic and mixed rhinitis: epidemiology and natural history. Allergy Asthma Proc 31(5):365–369

Bernstein JA (2013a) Nonallergic rhinitis: therapeutic options. Curr Opin Allergy Clin Immunol 13(4):410–416

Bernstein JA (2013b) Nonallergic rhinitis: therapeutic options. Curr Opin Allergy Clin Immunol 13(4):399–409

Bernstein JA, Davis BP, Picard JK, Cooper JP, Zheng S, Levin LS (2011a) A randomized, double-blind, parallel trial comparing capsaicin nasal spray with placebo in subjects with a significant component of nonallergic rhinitis. Ann Allergy Asthma Immunol 107(2):171–178

Bernstein JA, Hastings L, Boespflug EL, Allendorfer JB, Lamy M, Eliassen JC (2011b) Alteration of brain activation patterns in nonallergic rhinitis patients using functional magnetic resonance imaging before and after treatment with intranasal azelastine. Ann Allergy Asthma Immunol 106(6):527–532

Bernstein JA, Salapatek AM, Lee JS, Nelson V, Wilson D, D'Angelo P, Tsitoura D, Murdoch R, Patel D (2012) Provocation of nonallergic rhinitis subjects in response to simulated weather conditions using an environmental exposure chamber model. Allergy Asthma Proc 33(4):333–340

Blanchard MG, Kellenberger S (2011) Effect of a temperature increase in the non-noxious range on proton-evoked ASIC and TRPV1 activity. Pflugers Arch 461(1):123–139

Blom HM, Van Rijswijk JB, Garrelds IM, Mulder PG, Timmermans T, Van Wijk RG (1997) Intranasal capsaicin is efficacious in nonallergic, noninfectious perennial rhinitis. A placebo-controlled study. Clin Exp Allergy 27(7):796–801

Blom HM, Severijnen LA, Van Rijswijk JB, Mulder PG, Van Wijk RG, Fokkens WJ (1998) The long-term effects of capsaicin aqueous spray on the nasal mucosa. Clin Exp Allergy 28(11):1351–1358

Bousquet J, Demoly P, Michel FB (2001) Specific immunotherapy in rhinitis and asthma. Ann Allergy Asthma Immunol 87(1 Suppl 1):38–42

Brauchi S, Orta G, Salazar M, Rosenmann E, Latorre R (2006) A hot-sensing cold receptor: C-terminal domain determines thermosensation in transient receptor potential channels. J Neurosci 26(18):4835–4840

Cao E, Cordero-Morales JF, Liu B, Qin F, Julius D (2013) TRPV1 channels are intrinsically heat sensitive and negatively regulated by phosphoinositide lipids. Neuron 77(4):667–679

Cassano M, Russo L, Del Giudice AM, Gelardi M (2012) Cytologic alterations in nasal mucosa after sphenopalatine artery ligation in patients with vasomotor rhinitis. Am J Rhinol Allergy 26(1):49–54

Changani K, Hotee S, Campbell S, Pindoria K, Dinnewell L, Saklatvala P, Thompson SA, Coe D, Biggadike K, Vitulli G, Lines M, Busza A, Denyer J (2013) Effect of the TRPV1 antagonist SB-705498 on the nasal parasympathetic reflex response in the ovalbumin sensitized guinea pig. Br J Pharmacol 169(3):580–589

Chung MK, Guler AD, Caterina MJ (2008) TRPV1 shows dynamic ionic selectivity during agonist stimulation. Nat Neurosci 11(5):555–564

Ciabatti PG, D'Ascanio L (2009) Intranasal Capsicum spray in idiopathic rhinitis: a randomized prospective application regimen trial. Acta Otolaryngol 129(4):367–371

Devillier P, Dessanges JF, Rakotosihanaka F, Ghaem A, Boushey HA, Lockhart A, Marsac J (1988) Nasal response to substance P and methacholine in subjects with and without allergic rhinitis. Eur Respir J 1(4):356–361

Docherty RJ, Ginsberg L, Jadoon S, Orrell RW, Bhattacharjee A (2013) TRPA1 insensitivity of human sural nerve axons after exposure to lidocaine. Pain 154: 1569–1577

Di Lorenzo G, Minciullo PL, Leto-Barone MS, La Piana S, La Porta G, Saija A, Gangemi S (2013) Differences in the behavior of advanced glycation end products and advanced oxidation protein products in patients with allergic rhinitis. J Investig Allergol Clin Immunol 23(2):101–106

Filiaci F, Zambetti G, Ciofalo A, Luce M, Masieri S, Lovecchio A (1994) Local treatment of aspecific nasal hyper-reactivity with capsaicin. Allergol Immunopathol (Madr) 22(6):264–268

Filiaci F, Zambetti G, Luce M, Ciofalo A (1996) Local treatment of nasal polyposis with capsaicin: preliminary findings. Allergol Immunopathol (Madr) 24(1):13–18

Fusco BM, Barzoi G, Agro F (2003) Repeated intranasal capsaicin applications to treat chronic migraine. Br J Anaesth 90(6):812

Fusco BM, Marabini S, Maggi CA, Fiore G, Geppetti P (1994) Preventative effect of repeated nasal applications of capsaicin in cluster headache. Pain 59(3):321–325

Garcia-Sanz N, Valente P, Gomis A, Fernandez-Carvajal A, Fernandez-Ballester G, Viana F, Belmonte C, Ferrer-Montiel A (2007) A role of the transient receptor potential domain of vanilloid receptor I in channel gating. J Neurosci 27(43):11641–11650

Gerth Van Wijk R, Terreehorst IT, Mulder PG, Garrelds IM, Blom HM, Popering S (2000) Intranasal capsaicin is lacking therapeutic effect in perennial allergic rhinitis to house dust mite. A placebo-controlled study. Clin Exp Allergy 30(12):1792–1798

Georgalas C, Jovancevic L (2012) Gustatory rhinitis. Curr Opin Otolaryngol Head Neck Surg 20(1):9–14

Geppetti P, Patacchini R, Nassini R, Materazzi S (2010) Cough: the emerging role of the TRPA1 channel. Lung 188(Suppl 1):S63–S68
Gijbels MJ, Elliott GR, HogenEsch H, Zurcher C, van den Hoven A, Bruijnzeel PL (2000) Therapeutic interventions in mice with chronic proliferative dermatitis (cpdm/cpdm). Exp Dermatol 9(5):351–358
Harlor EJ, Greene JS, Considine C (2012) Traumatic unilateral vasomotor rhinitis. Ear Nose Throat J 91(11):E4–E6
Horak F, Zieglmayer UP (2009) Azelastine nasal spray for the treatment of allergic and nonallergic rhinitis. Expert Rev Clin Immunol 5(6):659–669
Huang A, Govindaraj S (2013) Topical therapy in the management of chronic rhinosinusitis. Curr Opin Otolaryngol Head Neck Surg 21(1):31–38
Ito K (1993) Diagnosis of NARES by methacholine nasal provocative test. Nihon Jibiinkoka Gakkai Kaiho 96(5):818–826
Jeon S, Kim N, Hwang E, Hong S, Min YG(1995) Horseradish peroxidase permeability across rat nasal mucosa in selective stimulation of substance P innervation with capsaicin. Ann Otol Rhinol Laryngol 104(11):895–898
Kavut AB, Kalpaklioglu F, Atasoy P (2013) Contribution of neurogenic and allergic ways to the pathophysiology of nonallergic rhinitis. Int Arch Allergy Immunol 160(2):184–191
Keh SM, Facer P, Yehia A, Sandhu G, Saleh HA, Anand P (2011) The menthol and cold sensation receptor TRPM8 in normal human nasal mucosa and rhinitis. Rhinology 49(4):453–457
Kim YH, Jang TY (2012) Nasal obstruction and rhinorrhea reflect nonspecific nasal hyperreactivity as evaluated by cold dry air provocation. Acta Otolaryngol 132(10):1095–1101
Kim BM, Lee SH, Shim WS, Oh U (2004) Histamine-induced Ca(2+) influx via the PLA(2)/lipoxygenase/TRPV1 pathway in rat sensory neurons. Neurosci Lett 361(1–3):159–162
Kuhn FA, Gonzalez S, Rodriguez M, Siller CC, Zachariou V, Goldstein BD (1997) Capsaicin's effect on rat nasal mucosa substance P release: experimental basis for vasomotor rhinitis treatment. Am J Rhinol 11(4):313–316
Lacroix JS, Buvelot JM, Polla BS, Lundberg JM (1991) Improvement of symptoms of nonallergic chronic rhinitis by local treatment with capsaicin. Clin Exp Allergy 21(5):595–600
Lainez S, Valente P, Ontoria-Oviedo I, Estevez-Herrera J, Camprubi-Robles M, Ferrer-Montiel A, Planells-Cases A (2010) GABAA receptor associated protein (GABARAP) modulates TRPV1 expression and channel function and desensitization. FASEB J 24(6):1958–1970
Lambert EM, Patel CB, Fakhri S, Citardi MJ, Luong A (2013) Optical rhinometry in nonallergic irritant rhinitis: a capsaicin challenge study. Int Forum Allergy Rhinol 3(10):795–800
Latimer BW, Poston P (1976) Multi-state, multi-service corporate model. Top Health Care Financ 2(4):25–37
Ledford D (2003) Inadequate diagnosis of nonallergic rhinitis: assessing the damage. Allergy Asthma Proc 24(3):155–162
Lee LN, Bhattacharyya N (2011) Regional and specialty variations in the treatment of chronic rhinosinusitis. Laryngoscope 121(5):1092–1097
Leung AY, Foster S (1996) Encyclopedia of common natural ingredients used in food, drugs, and cosmetics. 2nd ed. New York, Wiley
Lindh B, Hokfelt T (1990) Structural and functional aspects of acetylcholine peptide coexistence in the autonomic nervous system. Prog Brain Res 84:175–191
Lishko PV, Procko E, Jin X, Phelps CB, Gaudet R (2007) The ankyrin repeats of TRPV1 bind multiple ligands and modulate channel sensitivity. Neuron 54(6):905–918
Liu B, Zhang C, Qin F (2005) Functional recovery from desensitization of vanilloid receptor TRPV1 requires resynthesis of phosphatidylinositol 4, 5-bisphosphate. J Neurosci 25(19):4835–4843
Marabini S, Ciabatti PG, Polli G, Fusco BM, Geppetti P (1991) Beneficial effects of intranasal applications of capsaicin in patients with vasomotor rhinitis. Eur Arch Otorhinolaryngol 248(4):191–194
Marks DR, Rapoport A, Padla D, Weeks R, Rosum R, Sheftell F, Arrowsmith F (1993) A double-blind placebo-controlled trial of intranasal capsaicin for cluster headache. Cephalalgia 13(2):114–116

May A, Kaube H, Buchel C, Eichten C, Rijntjes M, Juptner M, Weiller C, Diener HC (1998) Experimental cranial pain elicited by capsaicin: a PET study. Pain 74(1):61–66
Meltzer EO, Blaiss MS, Derebery MJ, Mahr TA, Gordon BR, Sheth KK, Simmons AL, Wingertzahn MA, Boyle JM (2009) Burden of allergic rhinitis: results from the pediatric allergies in America survey. J Allergy Clin Immunol 124(3 Suppl):S43–S70
Mirza N, Kroger H, Doty RL (1997) Influence of age on the 'nasal cycle'. Laryngoscope 107(1):62–66
Mizumura K, Sugiur T, Koda H, Katanosaka K, Kumar BR, Giron R, Tominaga M (2005) Pain and bradykinin Receptors–sensory transduction mechanism in the nociceptor terminals and expression change of bradykinin receptors in inflamed condition. Nihon Shinkei Seishin Yakurigaku Zasshi 25(1):33–38
Myers BR, Bohlen CJ, Julius D (2008) A yeast genetic screen reveals a critical role for the pore helix domain in TRP channel gating. Neuron 58(3):362–373
Norlander T, Bolger WE, Stierna P, Uddman R, Carlsoo B (1996) A comparison of morphological effects on the rabbit nasal and sinus mucosa after surgical denervation and topical capsaicin application. Eur Arch Otorhinolaryngol 253(4–5):205–213
Pfaar O, Raap U, Holz M, Hormann K, Kilmek L (2009) Pathophysiology of itching and sneezing in allergic rhinitis. Swiss Med Wkly 139(3–4):35–40
Raisinghani M, Zhong L, Jeffry JA, Bishnoi M, Pabbidi RM, Pimentel F, Cao DS, Evans MS, Premkumar LS (2011) Activation characteristics of transient receptor potential ankyrin 1 and its role in nociception. Am J Physiol Cell Physiol 301(3):C587–C600
Rajakulasingam K, Polosa R, Lau LC, Church MK, Holgate ST, Howarth PH (1992) Nasal effects of bradykinin and capsaicin: influence on plasma protein leakage and role of sensory neurons. J Appl Physiol 72(4):1418–1424
Riechelmann H, Davris S, Bader D (1993) Treatment of perennial nonallergic rhinopathy with capsaicin. HNO 41(10):475–479
Rinder J (1996) Sensory neuropeptides and nitric oxide in nasal vascular regulation. Acta Physiol Scand Suppl 632:1–45
Roche N, Lurie A, Authier S, Dusser DJ (1995) Nasal response to capsaicin in patients with allergic rhinitis and in healthy volunteers: effect of colchicine. Am J Respir Crit Care Med 151(4):1151–1158
Samways DS, Egan TM (2011) Calcium-dependent decrease in the single-channel conductance of TRPV1. Pflugers Arch 462(5):681–691
Sanico AM, Atsuta S, Proud D, Togias A (1997) Dose-dependent effects of capsaicin nasal challenge: in vivo evidence of human airway neurogenic inflammation. J Allergy Clin Immunol 100(5):632–641
Sanico AM, Philip G, Proud D, Naclerio RM, Togias A (1998a) Comparison of nasal mucosal responsiveness to neuronal stimulation in nonallergic and allergic rhinitis: effects of capsaicin nasal challenge. Clin Exp Allergy 28(1):92–100
Sanico AM, Atsuta S, Proud D, Togias A (1998b) Plasma extravasation through neuronal stimulation in human nasal mucosa in the setting of allergic rhinitis. J Appl Physiol 84(2):537–543
Scarupa MD, Kaliner MA (2009) Nonallergic rhinitis, with a focus on vasomotor rhinitis: clinical importance, differential diagnosis, and effective treatment recommendations. World Allergy Organ J 2(3):20–25
Schroer B, Pien LC (2012) Nonallergic rhinitis: common problem, chronic symptoms. Cleve Clin J Med 79(4):285–293
Sedaghat AR, Gray ST, Wilke CO, Caradonna DS (2012) Risk factors for development of chronic rhinosinusitis in patients with allergic rhinitis. Int Forum Allergy Rhinol 2(5):370–375
Settipane RA (2008) Special focus: allergy and asthma–introduction. Med Health R I 91(6):160
Settipane RA, Kaliner MA (2013) Chapter 14: Nonallergic rhinitis. Am J Rhinol Allergy 27 Suppl 1:48–51
Settipane RA, Lieberman P (2001) Update on nonallergic rhinitis. Ann Allergy Asthma Immunol 86(5):494–507; quiz 507–508

Shah R, McGrath KG (2012) Chapter 6: Nonallergic rhinitis. Allergy Asthma Proc 33 Suppl 1:S19–21

Singh U, Bernstein JA, Kristin L, Haar LH, Jones KW (2014) Azelastine Desensitization If TRPV1: A Potential Mechanism Explaining Its Therapeutic Effect In Non-Allergic Rhinitis. Am J Rhinol Allergy

Studer M, McNaughton PA (2010) Modulation of single-channel properties of TRPV1 by phosphorylation. J Physiol 588(Pt 19):3743–3756

Szolcsányi J (2008) Hot target on nociceptors: perspectives, caveats and unique features. Br J Pharmacol 155(8):1142–1144

Szolcsányi J, Pintér E (2013) Transient receptor potential vanilloid 1 as a therapeutic target in analgesia. Expert Opin Ther Targets 17(6):641–657

Szolcsányi J, Sándor Z (2012) Multisteric TRPV1 nocisensor: a target for analgesics. Trends Pharmacol Sci 33(12):646–655

Taber, Tabers Dictionary 20 E Pda CD-ROM. 2005: F a Davis Company

Tai CF, Baraniuk JN (2002) Upper airway neurogenic mechanisms. Curr Opin Allergy Clin Immunol 2(1):11–19

Tran NP, Vickery J, Blaiss MS (2011) Management of rhinitis: allergic and nonallergic. Allergy Asthma Immunol Res 3(3):148–156

Van Gerven L, Alpizar YA, Wouters MM, Hox V, Hauben E, Jorissen M, Boeckxstaens G, Talavera K, Hellings PW (2013) Capsaicin treatment reduces nasal hyperreactivity and transient receptor potential cation channel subfamily V, receptor 1 (TRPV1) overexpression in patients with idiopathic rhinitis. J Allergy Clin Immunol

Van Rijswijk JB, Boeke EL, Keizer JM, Mulder PG, Blom HM, Fokkens WJ (2003) Intranasal capsaicin reduces nasal hyper-reactivity in idiopathic rhinitis: a double-blind randomized application regimen study. Allergy 58(8):754–761

van Rijswijk JB, Gerth van Wijk R (2006) Capsaicin treatment of idiopathic rhinitis: the new panacea? Curr Allergy Asthma Rep 6(2):132-137

Vanneste S, De Ridder D (2013) Brain areas controlling heart rate variability in tinnitus and tinnitus-related distress. PLoS ONE 8(3):e59728

Veldhuis NA, Lew MJ, Abogadie FC, Poole DP, Jennings EA, Ivanusic JJ, Eilers H, Bunnett NW, Mclntyre P (2012) N-glycosylation determines ionic permeability and desensitization of the TRPV1 capsaicin receptor. J Biol Chem 287(26):21765–21772

Vyklicky L, Novakova-Tousova K, Benedikt J, Samad A, Touska F, Vlachova V (2008) Calcium-dependent desensitization of vanilloid receptor TRPV1: a mechanism possibly involved in analgesia induced by topical application of capsaicin. Physiol Res 57(Suppl 3):S59–S68

White JP, Urban L, Nagy I (2011) TRPV1 function in health and disease. Curr Pharm Biotechnol 12(1):130–144

Wirkner K, Hognestad H, Jahnel R, Hucho F, Illes P (2005) Characterization of rat transient receptor potential vanilloid 1 receptors lacking the N-glycosylation site N604. Neuro Rep 16(9):997–1001

Zheng C, Wang Z, Lacroix JS (2000) Effect of intranasal treatment with capsaicin on the recurrence of polyps after polypectomy and ethmoidectomy. Acta Otolaryngol 120(1):62–66

Chapter 7
Capsaicin as an Anti-Obesity Drug

Felix W. Leung

Abstract Laboratory studies support a role of capsaicin as an anti-obesity agent. Intestinal mucosal afferent nerves appear to play a role in controlling adipose tissue distribution between visceral and subcutaneous sites. Activation of the transient receptor potential vanilloid-1 channels by capsaicin prevents adipogenesis. A neurogenic mechanism modulates the regulation of fat metabolism by transient receptor potential vanilloid-1-sensitive sensory nerves. A neural pathway enables the selective activation of the central network that regulates brown adipose tissue sympathetic nerve activity in response to a specific stimulation of gastrointestinal transient receptor potential channels. Dietary capsaicin reduces metabolic dysregulation in obese/diabetic mice by enhancing expression of adiponectin and its receptor. The effects of capsaicin in adipose tissue and liver are related to its dual action on peroxisome proliferator-activated receptor alpha and transient receptor potential vanilloid-1 expression/activation. Local desensitization of the abdominal capsaicin-sensitive fibers attenuates the hypometabolic adaptation to food deprivation. Truncal vagotomy leads to significant reductions in both diet-induced weight gain and visceral abdominal fat deposition. Vagal de-afferentation leads to a more modest, but clinically and statistically significant, reduction in visceral abdominal fat. Thermogenesis and lipid metabolism-related proteins are altered upon capsaicin treatment in white adipose tissue. Capsaicin induces apoptosis and inhibits adipogenesis in preadipocytes and adipocytes. Epidemiologic data show that

Disclosure: The author has no conflict of interest to declare.

F. W. Leung (✉)
111G, Division of Gastroenterology, Sepulveda Ambulatory Care Center, VAGLAHS,
16111 Plummer Street, Sepulveda, CA 91343, USA
e-mail: felix.leung@va.gov

F. W. Leung
David Geffen School of Medicine at UCLA, Los Angeles, CA, USA

F. W. Leung
VA Sepulveda Ambulatory Care Center, VAGLAHS, North Hills, CA, USA

O. M. E. Abdel-Salam (ed.), *Capsaicin as a Therapeutic Molecule*, Progress in Drug Research 68, DOI: 10.1007/978-3-0348-0828-6_7, © Springer Basel 2014

consumption of foods containing capsaicin is associated with a lower prevalence of obesity. Clinical evidence supports a role of capsaicin as an anti-obesity agent. Both oral and gastrointestinal exposure to capsaicin increase satiety and reduce energy and fat intake; the stronger reduction with oral exposure suggests a sensory effect of capsaicin. Bioactive components containing capsaicin may support weight maintenance after a hypocaloric diet. Capsaicin consumption 1 h before low intensity exercise is a valuable supplement for the treatment of individuals with hyperlipidemia and/or obesity because it improves lipolysis. Capsinoid ingestion increases energy expenditure through the activation of brown adipose tissue in humans. Capsinoid ingestion is associated with an increase in fat oxidation that is nearly significant; and two common genetic variants may be predictors of response. Further clinical research to develop convenient approaches for obese individuals to take advantage of this common dietary ingredient to prevent the onset or curtail the progression of obesity will be instructive and clinically relevant.

7.1 Introduction

Laboratory and clinical studies support a role of capsaicin as an anti-obesity agent. This chapter reviews recent developments in this field. Systemic treatment with capsaicin, the active ingredient of hot pepper, or its analog is an accepted experimental method to induce functional ablation of the capsaicin-sensitive afferent nerves (Holzer 1991). Such functional impairment retarded body weight gain (Leung et al. 2007) and reduced total body fat (Melnyk and Himms-Hagen 1995) in rats. The capsaicin (vanilloid) receptor agonist (resiniferatoxin) (Gram et al. 2005; Moesgaard et al. 2005) reduced body fat and body weight and improved glucose tolerance in obese rats (Gram et al. 2005; Moesgaard et al. 2005). In experimental studies, when oral capsaicin was provided to rodents as 0.014 % of the diet (Kawada et al. 1986; Ohnuki et al. 2001), a dose equivalent to that ingested by rural Thai people (Interdepartment Committee on Nutrition for National Defense 1962), there was a significant 24 % (Kawada et al. 1986) and 29 % (Ohnuki et al. 2001) reduction in the weight of visceral (peri-renal) fat, but no effect on total caloric intake. These studies suggested the possibility that oral capsaicin treatment might regulate visceral adipose tissue metabolism.

Capsaicin absorbed from the gut lumen was almost completely metabolized before reaching the general circulation (Donnerer et al. 1990). A direct effect (Do et al. 2004; Hsu and Yen 2007a; Kang et al. 2003; Zhang et al. 2007) of oral capsaicin on adipose tissue at remote sites was unlikely. In support of this was also the fact that repeated administration of oral capsaicin (Leung et al. 2007) functionally desensitized the intestinal mucosal but not the corneal afferent nerves. The wiping reflex of the front paw of the eye exposed briefly to dilute capsaicin irritation was preserved in these rats treated with oral capsaicin for 14 days. Thus, if oral capsaicin could regulate adipose tissue distribution, the process might involve the intestinal mucosal afferent nerves.

The development of visceral obesity may be the result of the normal pattern of postprandial blood flow distributing absorbed fat nutrients preferentially to the adipose tissue at visceral sites. Ingested fat must pass through the intestinal lumen to be digested prior to absorption and distribution to various adipose tissue sites. Fat stored at any site must be delivered there by the systemic circulation. The intestinal mucosa is well-endowed with afferent nerve terminals (sensors), which mediate postprandial changes in intestinal and visceral adipose tissue blood flow. Their usual function may play a role in the accumulation of fat at visceral sites and impairment of their usual function may result in the accumulation of adipose tissue in nonvisceral sites. The results of a series of experiments (Leung et al. 2007; Leung et al. 2001; Leung et al. 2008) summarized in one review (Leung 2008) showed that attenuation of intestinal mucosal afferent nerve function may be a plausible approach to the treatment of visceral obesity. Stimulation of the intestinal mucosal capsaicin-sensitive afferent nerves by capsaicin produced a significant vasoconstriction in adipose tissue (Leung et al. 2001). Functional ablation of the intestinal mucosal capsaicin-sensitive afferent nerves led to loss of this vasoconstriction in the visceral but not subcutaneous adipose tissue (Leung et al. 2007). Further studies showed that the intestinal mucosal capsaicin-sensitive afferent nerves elicit events mediated by angiotensin II in adipose tissue (vasoconstriction) when nutrients were present in the intestinal lumen. When the intestinal mucosal capsaicin-sensitive afferent nerves were functionally ablated by repeated intragastric capsaicin treatment (Leung et al. 2007), the angiotensin II-mediated events were abolished in the visceral, but partially retained in the subcutaneous adipose tissue. The net effect was an angiotensin II-mediated and blood flow (vasoconstriction)-dependent distribution of absorbed fat nutrient(s) preferentially to the subcutaneous rather than the visceral adipose tissue. These studies provide the evidence to implicate the intestinal mucosal afferent nerves in the regulation of adipose tissue distribution.

7.2 Laboratory Studies

Long-term feeding experiments were undertaken in wild-type mice and transient receptor potential channel vanilloid type 1 (TRPV1) knockout mice. Compared with lean counterparts, in the visceral adipose tissue from obese db/db and ob/ob mice, and from obese human male subjects, there was a reduced expression of TRVP1. The oral administration of capsaicin for 120 days prevented the development of obesity in male wild-type mice but not in TRPV1 knockout mice assigned to high-fat diet. This activation of TRPV1 channels by capsaicin prevented adipogenesis and obesity (Zhang et al. 2007).

On a 4.5 % fat diet, wild-type and TRPV1-null mice gained equivalent body mass. On a 11 % fat diet, however, TRPV1-null mice gained significantly less mass and adiposity; at 44 weeks the mean body weights of wild-type and TRPV1-null mice were approximately 51 and 34 gm, respectively. Both groups of mice consumed equivalent energy and absorbed similar amounts of lipids. TRPV1-null mice, however, exhibited a significantly greater thermogenic capacity. Furthermore, 3T3-L1 preadipocytes expressed functional calcitonin gene-related peptide receptors. A potential neurogenic mechanism by which TRPV1-sensitive sensory nerves may regulate energy and fat metabolism (Motter and Ahern 2008).

Intragastric administration of capsiate resulted in a time- and dose-dependent increase in integrated brown adipose tissue sympathetic nerve activity over 180 min. This increase in brown adipose tissue sympathetic nerve activity was abolished by blockade of TRP channels as well as of sympathetic ganglionic transmission and was inhibited by ablation of the gastrointestinal vagus nerve. The activation of sympathetic nerve activity was delimited to brown adipose tissue and did not occur in the heart or pancreas. A neural pathway enables the selective activation of the central network regulating the brown adipose tissue sympathetic nerve activity in response to a specific stimulation of gastrointestinal TRP channels (Ono et al. 2011).

Based on the premise that metabolic dysregulation (hyperglycemia, hyperinsulinemia, hyperlipidemia) is a hallmark of obesity-related diseases such as insulin resistance, type 2 diabetes, and fatty liver disease, investigators assessed whether dietary capsaicin attenuated the metabolic dysregulation in genetically obese diabetic KKAy mice, which have severe diabetic phenotypes. Male KKAy mice fed a high-fat diet for 2 weeks received a 0.015 % capsaicin supplement for a further 3 weeks and were compared with nonsupplemented controls. Dietary capsaicin markedly decreased fasting glucose/insulin and triglyceride levels in the plasma and/or liver, as well as expression of inflammatory adipocytokine genes (e.g., monocyte chemoattractant protein-1 and interleukin-6) and macrophage infiltration. Expression of the adiponectin gene/protein and its receptor, AdipoR2, increased in adipose tissue and/or plasma, was accompanied by increased activation of hepatic adenosine monophosphate (AMP)-activated protein kinase, a marker of fatty acid oxidation. Dietary capsaicin reduces metabolic dysregulation in obese/diabetic KKAy mice by enhancing expression of adiponectin and its receptor (Kang et al. 2011).

Whether dietary capsaicin can reduce obesity-induced inflammation and metabolic disorders such as insulin resistance and hepatic steatosis was assessed in male C57BL/6 obese mice fed a high-fat diet for 10 weeks. They received a supplement of 0.015 % capsaicin for a further 10 weeks and were compared with unsupplemented controls. Dietary capsaicin lowered fasting glucose, insulin, leptin levels, and markedly reduced the impairment of glucose tolerance in obese mice. Levels of tumor necrosis factor-alpha (TNFα), monocyte chemoattractant protein-1 (MCP-1), and interleukin (IL)-6 mRNAs and proteins in adipose tissue and liver decreased markedly, as did macrophage infiltration, hepatic triglycerides, and TRPV-1 expression in adipose tissue. The messenger ribonucleic acid/protein of adiponectin in the adipose tissue and peroxisome proliferator-activated receptor alpha/peroxisome proliferator-activated receptor-γ coactivator 1 alpha messenger ribonucleic acid in the liver increased. Luciferase assays revealed that capsaicin is capable of binding peroxisome proliferator-activated receptor alpha. Dietary capsaicin may reduce obesity-induced glucose intolerance by not only suppressing inflammatory responses but also enhancing fatty acid oxidation in adipose tissue and/or liver, both of which are important peripheral tissues affecting insulin resistance. The effects of capsaicin in adipose tissue and liver are related to its dual action on peroxisome proliferator-activated receptor alpha and TRPV-1 expression/activation (Kang et al. 2010).

Intraperitoneal capsaicin (5 mg/kg) desensitizes the local afferent vagal nerve endings for approximately 3 weeks. Following such desensitization, male Wistar rats deprived of food for 120 h lost significantly (18.9 ± 0.4 % vs. 15.8 ± 1.0 %), i.e., 20 % more weight than the controls, suggesting defective hypometabolic adaptation in desensitized animals. Upon re-feeding following a period of fasting, in the first 0.5–3 h the food intake was significantly greater in capsaicin pretreated compared to the control group, demonstrating blockade of satiety as a sign of desensitization. The delayed gastrointestinal passage supported that vagal afferent nerve endings were in a desensitized state in these rats. Local desensitization of the abdominal capsaicin-sensitive fibers attenuates the hypometabolic adaptation to food deprivation (Garami et al. 2010).

The impact of disrupting vagal signaling by total vagotomy or selective vagal de-afferentation on weight gain and fat content in diet-induced obese rats was assessed. Male Sprague–Dawley rats (n = 5–8) underwent truncal vagotomy, selective vagal de-afferentation with capsaicin, or sham procedure. Animals were maintained for 11 months on a high-caloric diet. At 11-months, vagotomized rats weighed 19 % less ($P = 0.003$) and de-afferented rats 7 % less ($P = 0.19$) than shams. Vagotomized and de-afferented animals had 52 % ($P < 0.0001$) and 18 % reduction ($P = 0.039$) in visceral abdominal fat, respectively. There were no changes in blood glucose or glycemic indexes. Jejunal sodium-glucose linked transporter 1 messenger ribonucleic acid, protein and function were unchanged across all cohorts at 11-months postoperatively. Truncal vagotomy led to significant reductions in both diet-induced weight gain and visceral abdominal fat deposition; and vagal de-afferentation led to a more modest, but clinically and statistically significant, reduction in visceral abdominal fat (Stearns et al. 2012).

The anti-obesity effect of capsaicin was examined in rats (5-week old) treated with capsaicin (10 mg/kg) along with a high-fat diet. In comparison with saline-treated rats, body weight of those in the capsaicin-treated group decreased by 8 %. Protein mapping of white adipose tissue homogenates revealed significant alterations to a number of proteins. Significant down-regulation of heat shock protein 27 (Hsp27) and Steap3 protein, as well as upregulation of olfactory receptor (Olr1434) in obese white adipose tissue was documented. Most of the identified proteins are associated with lipid metabolism and redox regulation. Thermogenesis and lipid metabolism-related proteins were markedly altered upon capsaicin treatment in white adipose tissue (Joo et al. 2010).

The effects of capsaicin on the induction of apoptosis and inhibition of lipid accumulation in 3T3-L1 preadipocytes and adipocytes were investigated. Capsaicin decreased cell population growth of 3T3-L1 preadipocytes. 3T3-L1 preadipocytes exposed to capsaicin showed that apoptotic cells increased in a time- and dose-dependent manner. Treatment with capsaicin decreased the number of normal cells and increased the number of early apoptotic and late apoptotic cells in a dose-dependent manner. The treatment of cells with capsaicin caused the loss of mitochondrial membrane potential. The induction of apoptosis in 3T3-L1 preadipocytes by capsaicin was mediated through the activation of caspase-3, Bax, and Bak, and then through the cleavage of poly ADP ribose polymerase (PARP) and the down-regulation of Bcl-2. Capsaicin significantly decreased the amount of intracellular triglycerides and glycerol-3-phosphate dehydrogenase (GPDH) activity in 3T3-L1 adipocytes. Capsaicin also inhibited the expression of peroxisome proliferator-activated receptors gamma (PPARγ), CCAAT-enhancer-binding protein alpha (C/EBPα), and leptin, but induced upregulation of adiponectin at the protein level. Capsaicin efficiently induces apoptosis and inhibits adipogenesis in 3T3-L1 preadipocytes and adipocytes (Hsu and Yen 2007b).

7.3 Clinical Studies

Early epidemiological data revealed that the consumption of foods containing capsaicin was associated with a lower prevalence of obesity (Wahlqvist and Wattanapenpaiboon 2001). Clinical studies in recent years support a role of capsaicin in the treatment of obesity. For 24 subjects, 16 h food intake was assessed four times during 2 consecutive days by offering macronutrient-specific buffets and boxes with snacks. At 30 min before each meal, 0.9 gm red pepper (0.25 % capsaicin; 80,000 Scoville Thermal Units) or a placebo was offered in either tomato juice or in two capsules that were swallowed with tomato juice. Hunger and satiety were recorded using Visual Analogue Scales. Only in the oral exposure condition was the reduction in energy intake and the increase in satiety related to perceived spiciness. Both oral and gastrointestinal exposure to capsaicin increased satiety and reduced energy and fat intake; the stronger reduction with oral exposure suggests a sensory effect of capsaicin (Westerterp-Plantenga et al. 2005).

The acute and subchronic effect of a supplement containing tyrosine, capsaicin, catechines, and caffeine or placebo on thermogenesis, body fat loss and fecal fat excretion was assessed. Eighty overweight-obese subjects ((body mass index) 31.2 ± 2.5 kg/m^2, mean $\pm$ SD) underwent an initial 4-week hypocaloric diet (3.4 MJ/day). Those who lost >4 % body weight were instructed to consume a hypocaloric diet (-1.3 MJ/day) and were randomized to receive either placebo ($n = 23$) or bioactive supplement ($n = 57$) in a double-blind, 8-week intervention. Weight loss during the induction phase was 6.8 ± 1.9 kg. At the first exposure the thermogenic effect of the bioactive supplement exceeded that of placebo by 87.3 kJ/4 h (95 % CI: 50.9; 123.7, $P = 0.005$) and after 8 weeks this effect was sustained (85.5 kJ/4 h (47.6; 123.4), $P = 0.03$). Body fat mass decreased more in the supplement group by 0.9 kg (0.5; 1.3) compared to placebo ($P < 0.05$). The bioactive supplement had no effect on fecal fat excretion, blood pressure, or heart rate. Bioactive supplement increased 4-hours thermogenesis by 90 kJ more than placebo, and the effect was maintained after 8 weeks and accompanied by a slight reduction in fat mass. Bioactive components containing capsaicin may support weight maintenance after a hypocaloric diet (Belza et al. 2007).

Capsaicin significantly induced a lower respiratory gas exchange ratio (0.92 (0.02) vs. 0.94 (0.02), means (SE), $P < 0.05$) and higher fat oxidation (0.17 (0.04) vs. 0.12 (0.04) gm/min, means (SE), $P < 0.05$) during exercise. Other measured effects were not significant. Capsaicin consumption 1 h before low intensity exercise (50 % VT(max)) is a valuable supplement for the treatment of individuals with hyperlipidemia and/or obesity because it improves lipolysis (Shin and Moritani 2007).

The acute effect of nonpungent capsaicin analogs (capsinoids) on energy expenditure in brown adipose tissue in humans was studied. Eighteen healthy men aged 20–32 years underwent fludeoxyglucose positron emission tomography (FDG-PET) after 2 h of cold exposure (19 °C) while wearing light clothing. Whole-body energy expenditure and skin temperature, after oral ingestion of capsinoids (9 mg), were measured for 2 h under warm conditions (27 °C) in a single-blind, randomized, placebo-controlled, crossover design. When exposed to cold, 10 subjects showed marked fludeoxyglucose uptake into adipose tissue of the supraclavicular and paraspinal regions (brown adipose tissue-positive group), whereas the remaining 8 subjects (brown adipose tissue-negative group) showed no detectable uptake. Under warm conditions (27 °C), the mean (±SEM) resting energy expenditure was 6114 ± 226 kJ/day in the brown adipose tissue-positive group and 6307 ± 156 kJ/day in the brown adipose tissue-negative group (NS). Energy expenditure increased by 15.2 ± 2.6 kJ/hour in 1 h in the brown adipose tissue-positive group and by 1.7 ± 3.8 kJ/hour in the brown adipose tissue-negative group after oral ingestion of capsinoids ($P < 0.01$). Placebo ingestion produced no significant change in either group. Neither capsinoids nor placebo changed the skin temperature in various regions, including regions close to brown adipose tissue deposits. Capsinoid ingestion increases energy expenditure through the activation of brown adipose tissue in humans (Yoneshiro et al. 2012).

In a 12-week, placebo-controlled, double-blind, randomized study, the safety and efficacy of capsinoids taken orally (6 mg/day) on weight loss, fat loss, change in metabolism, and candidate genes as predictors of capsinoid response were evaluated. Forty women and 40 men with a mean (±SD) age of 42 ± 8 years and body mass index of 30.4 ± 2.4 were randomly assigned to a capsinoid or placebo group. Capsinoids were well tolerated. Mean (±SD) weight change was 0.9 ± 3.1 and 0.5 ± 2.4 kg in the capsinoid and placebo groups, respectively ($P = 0.86$). There was no significant group difference in total change in adiposity, but abdominal adiposity decreased more ($P = 0.049$) in the capsinoid group (−1.11 ± 1.83 %) than in the placebo group (−0.18 ± 1.94 %), and this change correlated with the change in body weight ($r = 0.46$, $P < 0.0001$). Changes in resting energy expenditure did not differ significantly between groups, but fat oxidation was higher at the end of the study in the capsinoid group. Of 13 genetic variants tested, TRPV1 Val585Ile and mitochondrial uncoupling protein 2 (UCP2) −866 G/A correlated significantly with change in abdominal adiposity. Capsinoid ingestion was associated with an increase in fat oxidation that was nearly significant. Two common genetic variants may be predictors of therapeutic response (Snitker et al. 2009).

7.4 Conclusion

The hypothesis that capsaicin and TRVP1 play a role in regulating adipose tissue is supported by laboratory and clinical evidence. Further clinical research to develop convenient approaches for obese individuals to take advantage of this common dietary ingredient to prevent the onset or curtail the progression of obesity will be instructive and clinically relevant.

Acknowledgments Supported in part by Veterans Affairs Medical Research Funds.

References

Belza A, Frandsen E, Kondrup J (2007) Body fat loss achieved by stimulation of thermogenesis by a combination of bioactive food ingredients: a placebo-controlled, double-blind 8-week intervention in obese subjects. Int J Obes (Lond) 31:121–130

Do MS, Hong SE, Jung-Heun Ha JH, Sun-Mi Choi SM, Ahn IS, Yoon JY, Park KY (2004) Increased lipolytic activity by high-pungency red pepper extract (var. Chungyang) in rat adipocytes in vitro. J Food Sci Nutr 9:34–38

Donnerer J, Amann R, Schuligoi R, Lembeck F (1990) Absorption and metabolism of capsaicinoids following intragastric administration in rats. Naunyn-Schmiedebergs Arch Pharmacol 342:357–361

Garami A, Balaskó M, Székely M, Solymár M, Pétervári E (2010) Fasting hypometabolism and refeeding hyperphagia in rats: effects of capsaicin desensitization of the abdominal vagus. Eur J Pharmacol 644:61–66

Gram DX, Hansen AJ, Deacon CF, Brand CL, Ribel U, Wilken M, Carr RD, Svendsen O, Ahren B (2005) Sensory nerve desensitization by resiniferatoxin improves glucose tolerance and increases insulin secretion in Zucker Diabetic Fatty rats and is associated with reduced plasma activity of dipeptidyl peptidase IV. Eur J Pharmacol 509:211–217

Holzer P (1991) Capsaicin: cellular targets, mechanisms of action, and selectivity for thin sensory neurons. Pharmacol Rev 43:143–201

Hsu CL, Yen GC (2007a) Effects of capsaicin on induction of apoptosis and inhibition of adipogenesis in 3T3-L1 cells. J Agric Food Chem 55:1730–1736

Hsu CL, Yen GC (2007b) Effects of capsaicin on induction of apoptosis and inhibition of adipogenesis in 3T3-L1 cells. J Agric Food Chem 7(55):1730–1736

Interdepartment Committee on Nutrition for National Defense (1962) Nutrition survey—the kingdom of Thailand. US Government Priniting Office, Washington, pp 57–59

Joo JI, Kim DH, Choi JW, Yun JW (2010) Proteomic analysis for antiobesity potential of capsaicin on white adipose tissue in rats fed with a high fat diet. J Proteome Res 9:2977–2987

Kang J, Kim C, Han I, Kawada T, Yu R (2003) Capsaicin, a spicy component of hot peppers, modulates adipokine gene expression and protein release from obese-mouse adipose tissues and isolated adipocytes, and suppresses the inflammatory responses of adipose tissue macrophages. FEBS Lett 581:4389–4396

Kang JH, Goto T, Han IS, Kawada T, Kim YM, Yu R (2010) Dietary capsaicin reduces obesity-induced insulin resistance and hepatic steatosis in obese mice fed a high-fat diet. Obesity (Silver Spring). 18:780–787

Kang JH, Tsuyoshi G, Le Ngoc H, Kim HM, Tu TH, Noh HJ, Kim CS, Choe SY, Kawada T, Yoo H, Yu R (2011) Dietary capsaicin attenuates metabolic dysregulation in genetically obese diabetic mice. J Med Food 14:310–315

Kawada T, Hagihara K, Iwai K (1986) Effects of capsaicin on lipid metabolism in rats fed a high fat diet. J Nutr 116:1272–1278

Leung FW (2008) Capsaicin-sensitive intestinal mucosal afferent mechanism and body fat distribution. Life Sci 83:1–5

Leung FW, Golub M, Tuck M, Yip I, Go VLW (2001) Stimulation of intestinal mucosal afferent nerves increases superior mesenteric artery and decreases mesenteric adipose tissue blood flow. Dig Dis Sci 46:1217–1222

Leung FW, Go VLW, Scremin OU, Obenaus A, Tuck ML, Golub MS, Eggena P, Leung JW (2007) Pilot studies to demonstrate intestinal mucosal afferent nerves are functionally linked to visceral adipose tissue. Dig Dis Sci 52:2695–2702

Leung FW, Murray E, Murray S, Go VLW (2008) Determination of body fat distribution by dual excitation X-ray absorptiometry and attenuation of visceral fat vasoconstriction by enalapril. Dig Dis Sci 53:1084–1087

Melnyk A, Himms-Hagen J (1995) Resistance to aging-associated obesity in capsaicin-desensitized rats one year after treatment. Obesity Res 3:337–344

Moesgaard SG, Brand CL, Sturis J, Ahren B, Wilken M, Fleckner J, Carr RD, Svendsen O, Hansen AJ, Gram DX (2005) Sensory nerve inactivation by resiniferatoxin improves insulin sensitivity in male obese Zucker rats. Am J Physiol Endocrinol Metab 288:E1137–E1145

Motter AL, Ahern GP (2008) TRPV1-null mice are protected from diet-induced obesity. FEBS Lett 582:2257–2262

Ohnuki K, Haramizu S, Oki K, Watanabe T, Yazawa S, Fushiki T (2001) Administration of capsiate, a non-pungent capsaicin analog, promotes energy metabolism and suppresses body fat accumulation in mice. Biosci Biotechnol Biochem 65:2735–2740

Ono K, Tsukamoto-Yasui M, Hara-Kimura Y, Inoue N, Nogusa Y, Okabe Y, Nagashima K, Kato F (2011) Intragastric administration of capsiate, a transient receptor potential channel agonist, triggers thermogenic sympathetic responses. J Appl Physiol 110:789–798

Shin KO, Moritani T (2007) Alterations of autonomic nervous activity and energy metabolism by capsaicin ingestion during aerobic exercise in healthy men. J Nutr Sci Vitaminol 53:124–132

Snitker S, Fujishima Y, Shen H, Ott S, Pi-Sunyer X, Furuhata Y, Sato H, Takahashi M (2009) Effects of novel capsinoid treatment on fatness and energy metabolism in humans: possible pharmacogenetic implications. Am J Clin Nutr 89:45–50

Stearns AT, Balakrishnan A, Radmanesh A, Ashley SW, Rhoads DB, Tavakkolizadeh A (2012) Relative contributions of afferent vagal fibers to resistance to diet-induced obesity. Dig Dis Sci 57:1281–1290

Wahlqvist ML, Wattanapenpaiboon N (2001) Hot foods–unexpected help with energy balance? Lancet 358(9279):348–349

Westerterp-Plantenga MS, Smeets A, Lejeune MP (2005) Sensory and gastrointestinal satiety effects of capsaicin on food intake. Int J Obes (Lond) 29:682–688

Yoneshiro T, Aita S, Kawai Y, Iwanaga T, Saito M (2012) Nonpungent capsaicin analogs (capsinoids) increase energy expenditure through the activation of brown adipose tissue in humans. Am J Clin Nutr 95:845–850

Zhang LL, Liu DY, Ma LQ, Luo ZD, Cao TB, Zhong J, Yan ZC et al (2007) Activation of transient receptor potential vanilloid type-1 channel prevents adipogenesis and obesity. Cir Res 100:1063–1070

Chapter 8
The Potential Antitumor Effects of Capsaicin

Inés Díaz-Laviada and Nieves Rodríguez-Henche

Abstract Capsaicin, one of the major pungent ingredients found in red peppers, has been recently demonstrated to induce apoptosis in many types of malignant cell lines including colon adenocarcinoma, pancreatic cancer, hepatocellular carcinoma, prostate cancer, breast cancer, and many others. The mechanism whereby capsaicin induces apoptosis in cancer cells is not completely elucidated but involves intracellular calcium increase, reactive oxygen species generation, disruption of mitochondrial membrane transition potential, and activation of transcription factors such as NFκB and STATS. Recently, a role for the AMP-dependent kinase (AMPK) and autophagy pathways in capsaicin-triggered cell death has been proposed. In addition, capsaicin shows antitumor activity in vivo by reducing the growth of many tumors induced in mice. In this chapter, we report the last advances performed in the antitumor activity of capsaicin and review the main signaling pathways involved.

8.1 Capsaicin

Capsaicin (8-methyl-*N*-vanillyl-6-noneamide) is the major constituent of the peppers belonging to the genus *Capsicum* and responsible for their spicy flavor and burning sensation, also known as pungency. Besides capsaicin, a family of related compounds are present in *Capsicum sp.* plants, all referred as capsaicinoids. These compounds are capsaicin, dihydrocapsaicin, nordihydrocapsaicin, and homocapsaicin. Capsaicin

---

Conflict of Interest. Authors declare that there is no conflict of interest.

I. Díaz-Laviada (✉) · N. Rodríguez-Henche
Biochemistry and Molecular Biology Unit, Department of System Biology,
University of Alcala, 28871 Madrid, Spain
e-mail: ines.diazlaviada@uah.es

N. Rodríguez-Henche
e-mail: nieves.rhenche@uah.es

O. M. E. Abdel-Salam (ed.), *Capsaicin as a Therapeutic Molecule*, Progress in Drug Research 68, DOI: 10.1007/978-3-0348-0828-6_8, © Springer Basel 2014

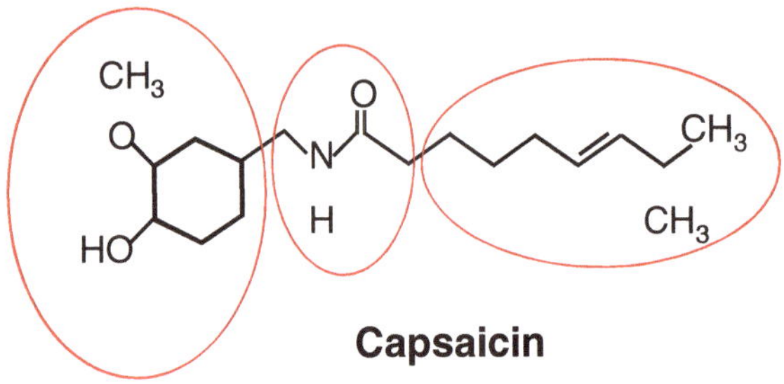

Fig. 8.1 Structure of capsaicin. Capsaicin has three main moieties: vannillyl (methylcatechol group), amide bond, and an alkyl side chain

and dihydrocapsaicin are the two major capsaicinoids found in hot peppers (more than 90 % of the total capsaicinoids) (Wahyuni et al. 2013).

The naturally occurring content of capsaicinoids in spices have been determined by use of liquid chromatography and ranges typically from 0.1 mg/g in chili pepper to 2.5 mg/g in red pepper and 60 mg/g in oleoresin red pepper (Alothman et al. 2012). Pungency is measured by the Scoville scale that considers the times a sample must be diluted to make the pungency imperceptible. By definition, one part per million (ppm) of capsaicin has a pungency of 15 Scoville Heat units (SHU) (Wahyuni et al. 2013).

Capsaicin consists of three functional moieties: vanillyl (methylcatechol group), amide bond, and alkyl side chain (Fig. 8.1). Analyses of the structure–activity relationship of numerous capsaicin analogs suggest that the vanillyl motif and amide bond regions are essential for pharmacological activity at TRPV1 and thus maintaining the excitation of sensory neurons, which could be alternatively expressed as maintaining pungency (Walpole et al. 1996). In contrast, the aliphatic chain in the C region is presumed to be essential for maximal potency (Walpole et al. 1993). Recently, a capsaicin analog was synthesized by a ring closure of the methylcatechol, a replacement of amide bond by a bioisosteric sulfonamide group, and a modification of the alkyl chain to incorporate a rigid ring. This compound was named RPF 101 and exhibited much higher potency against breast tumor cell growth than capsaicin (de-Sa-Junior et al. 2013).

Capsaicin is absorbed very rapidly by a nonactive process from the stomach and whole intestine with a maximum blood concentration observed at 1 h after administration (Suresh and Srinivasan 2010). Capsaicin is mainly metabolized in the liver through cytochrome P450-dependent reactions and peroxydase enzymes, producing three major metabolites, 16-hydroxycapsaicin, 17-hydroxycapsaicin, and 16, 17-hydroxycapsaicin, and is scarcely excreted in the urine (Suresh and Srinivasan 2010). Although many enzymes may play some role in hepatic drug metabolism, cytochrome P450 enzymes are quantitatively the most important, and it has been proposed that many drug–drug interactions result from the alteration (increase or decrease) in the activities of these enzymes (Zhang et al. 2012; Zhai et al. 2013). However, Babbar et al. demonstrated that at concentrations occurring after ingestion of chili peppers or topical administration of a high-concentration patch, capsaicin did not cause direct inhibition of any CYP enzyme (Babbar et al. 2010). Capsaicin toxicity is minimal at low doses. Previous research on the metabolism of capsaicin has proposed the formation of potentially deleterious reactive intermediates. It has been suggested that capsaicin is converted into a mutagenic or carcinogenic form through metabolism, such as an electrophilic epoxide or quinone derivatives (Surh and Lee 1995). However, research by Reilly et al. (2003) support the hypothesis that P450-mediated metabolism of capsaicin represents a detoxification mechanism by decreasing its pharmacological and/or toxicological activity and may serve to ameliorate the effects of capsaicin by preventing key biochemical interactions with molecular determinants of toxicity (Reilly et al. 2003). It must be taken into account that the metabolism of capsaicin by different P450 enzymes expressed in different tissues may yield different reactive intermediates in different cell types, which may partially explain conflicting reports related to the cytotoxic, procarcinogenic, and chemoprotective effects of capsaicinoids in different cells and/or organ systems (Reilly et al. 2013).

8.2 TRPV1 Receptor

It has been well documented that capsaicin targets the receptor TRPV1, first cloned from rat (Caterina et al. 1997) (see Chap. 2 of this book). TRPV1 is a cation channel belonging to the superfamily of transient potential receptors (TRPs) which are subdivided into seven subfamilies based on their amino acid sequence homology: TRPC (canonical), TRPV (vanilloid), TRPA1 (the only member of the subfamily ankyrin), TRPM (melastatin or long TRPs), TRPP (polycystin), TRPN (nonmechanoreceptor potential C), and TRPML (mucolipin). The vanilloid TRP subfamily comprises six members (TRPV1-6). Based on sequence homology and functional similarity, the six TRPV channels are divided into nonselective cation channels group 1 (TRPV1, TRPV2, TRPV3, and TRPV4), and selective Ca^{2+} channels group 2 (TRPV5 and TRPV6). TRPV1 is a nonselective cation channel but prefers Ca^{2+} over Na^{+}. Until now, capsaicin has been identified uniquely as an agonist at TRPV1.

Structurally, a functional TRPV1 channel is a tetrameric membrane protein with four identical subunits assembled around a central aqueous pore which forms the cation channel. Each subunit harbors six membrane-spanning domains with a short, pore-forming hydrophobic loop between the fifth and sixth transmembrane domains, an N-terminal domain with six ankyrin repeats (ARD), and a C-terminal domain residue within the cytoplasm (Fig. 8.2). Capsaicin binds to the TRPV1 protein channel in the intracellular S2–S4 region with high affinity mediated by interactions between the vanilloid group of capsaicin and the benzene ring of aromatic residues (Jordt and Julius 2002). The ARD of the N-terminal region contains an ATP-binding as well as a Ca-calmodulin binding site (Lishko et al. 2007). Phosphatidylinositol-4,5-bisphosphate (PIP2) binds to the C-terminus of the receptor and inhibits channel gating (Prescott and Julius 2003). Either ATP or PIP2 prevent desensitization to repeated applications of capsaicin whereas calmodulin has the opposite effect (Lishko et al. 2007).

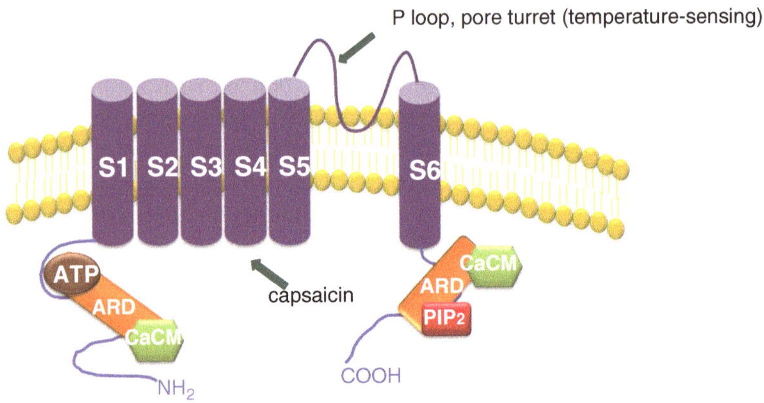

Fig. 8.2 The TRPV1 receptor. TRPV1 channel is a tetrameric membrane protein with four identical subunits. Each subunit harbors six membrane-spanning domains with a short, pore-forming hydrophobic loop between the fifth and sixth transmembrane domains, an N-terminal domain with six ankyrin repeats (ARD), and a C-terminal domain residue within the cytoplasm. The ARD of the N-terminal region contains an ATP-binding as well as a Ca-calmodulin binding site

Besides by capsaicin, TRPV1 receptor is activated by heat, low pH, and other ligands, leading to a burning pain sensation. Recent findings suggest that heat and capsaicin activate TRPV1 at different sites and they may act synergistically to stimulate channel gating (Cui et al. 2012).

The expression of TRPV1 has been demonstrated in most of the tumor cells analyzed. TRPV1 is expressed in human breast cancer MCF-7 and BT-20 cells (Chang et al. 2011; Vercelli et al. 2013) as well as in canine mammary cancer cells (Vercelli et al. 2013). Prostate cancer derived LNCaP and PC-3 cells as well as Benign Prostate Hyperplasia (BPH) tissue expresses TRPV1 (Sanchez et al. 2005). In those cells, capsaicin evokes an increase in the intracellular calcium concentration which is blocked by the TRPV1 antagonist capsazepine, implying a functional receptor (Sanchez et al. 2005). TRPV1 ion channels are expressed in glioma cell lines and in glioma tissues as well as in several tumor cells of astrocytic origin, and in normal human astrocytes (Biggs et al. 2007).

Changes in the expression of TRPV1 are often associated with changes in tumor progression and prognosis. Clinical investigation found a remarkably elevated TRPV1 expression in the epithelial cells of prostate cancer samples when compared to either the healthy or the BPH sections (Czifra et al. 2009). The expression of TRPV1 increased in parallel and gradually with the Gleason grade (Czifra et al. 2009). High TRPV1 expression in tumorigenic cell lines may play roles in the development and progression of hepatocellular carcinoma and metastatic liver cancers (Rychkov and Barritt 2011). By contrary, a decrease of TRPV1 expression can occur during the development of human urothelial cell carcinoma (UCC). Levels of TRPV1 are strongly reduced in high-grade and stage invasive of transitional cell carcinoma of human bladder and low TRPV1 expression is related with poor prognosis (Santoni et al. 2012). In line with this, it has been proposed that chronic blockade of TRPV1 might increase the risk of tumor development. Topical administration of a TRPV1 antagonist in mice promoted mouse skin tumorigenesis (Li et al. 2011). Likewise, capsaicin treatment induced a more aggressive gene phenotype and invasiveness in null-TRPV1 urothelial cancer cells (Caprodossi et al. 2011).

However, as described below, in most studies performed, capsaicin-induced tumor cell growth inhibition and apoptosis is independent of its stimulatory effects on the TRPV1 receptor, because co-treatment with competitive vanilloid receptor inhibitors like capsazepin did not protect the cells from capsaicin-induced death (Kim et al. 2004; Athanasiou et al. 2007; Zhang et al. 2008); moreover, it increases the cytotoxic effect of capsaicin (Sanchez et al. 2006; Sung et al. 2012).

8.3 Antitumor Properties of Capsaicin in Different Cancer Cells

Cancer is caused by defects in the mechanisms underlying cell proliferation and cell death. The development of tumors results from excessive cell proliferation combined with inhibition of cell apoptosis, which eventually leads to imbalances in tissue homeostasis and uncontrolled proliferation. Hence, targeting cell proliferation or induction of cancer cell apoptosis is one of the major challenges in cancer research. Capsaicin has been shown to inhibit cell proliferation, to induce cell cycle arrest and to trigger apoptosis in many cancer cell types (summarized in Table 8.1).

8.3.1 Colorectal Cancer

Colorectal cancer (CRC) is one of the most lethal cancers worldwide and the third leading cause of cancer-related death in the United States (Siegel et al. 2012; Quaglia et al. 2013). It is estimated that there are nearly 1.2 million men and women living in the United States with a previous diagnosis of colorectal cancer, and an additional ~150,000 will be diagnosed each year (Siegel et al. 2012). The poor prognostic outcome of colorectal cancer is due to its resistance to current therapies. Although about half of individuals with CRC could be cured by surgery, radiation therapy, and/or chemotherapy treatment before tumor cell dissemination, 40–50 % of patients had metastatic diseases and prognosis is poor with a 5-year survival <10 % (Quaglia et al. 2013).

Recent findings suggest that deregulation of the mucosal immune system predisposes to inflammatory bowel disease (IBD) and CRC. The role of inflammation in carcinogenesis was first proposed by R. Wirchow in the nineteenth century after observations in tumor samples which were infiltrated by high numbers of leukocytes (Bochalli 1952). A tumorigenic niche, composed of inflammatory

Table 8.1 Cancer cell lines sensitive to capsaicin-induced cell death

	Effective doses (μM)	IC50 (μM)	References
Colorectal cancer			
LoVo	100–200	100	Lee et al. (2012)
HCT-116	50–250	250, 25	Chueh et al. (2004), Oh et al. (2008), Yang et al. (2013)
SW480			
COLO 205	25–500	150	Lu et al. (2010)
Prostate cancer			
PC-3	5–50	20	Mori et al. (2006), Sanchez et al. (2006, 2007)
DU-145	0.01–500	10	Mori et al. (2006)
LNCaP	0.01–500	200	Mori et al. (2006)
Breast cancer			
MCF-7, SKBR-3, T47D, BT-474	1–200	50, 200, 300	Oh et al. (2008), Chou et al. (2009), Thoennissen et al. (2010), Chang et al. (2011), Dou et al. (2011), de-Sa-Junior et al. (2013)
MDA-MB-231		200, 22	Thoennissen et al. (2010), de-Sa-Junior et al. (2013)
Urinary bladder			
T24	50–200	150	Yang et al. (2010)
Myeloid leukemia			
NB4, Kasumi-1	10–200	50	Ito et al. (2004)
UF-1, HL60	50–1,000	80, 150	Ito et al. (2004), Tsou et al. (2006), Moon et al. (2012)
U937	50–250	500, 200	Moon et al. (2012)
HPB-ATL-T, HPB-CTL-I, HUT-102	50–200		Zhang et al. (2003)
HPB-ALL, Jurkat T		100	
Gastric carcinoma			
SCM1	0.1–200	200	Wang et al. (2008)
Hepatocellular carcinoma			
HepG2	10–200	75, 200, >200	Huang et al. (2009), Popovich et al. (2010), Moon et al. (2012)
Pancreatic cáncer			
PANC-1	50–300	200	Zhang et al. (2013)
AsPC-1 and BxPC-3	25–250	150	Zhang et al. (2008)
Cutaneous squamous cell carcinoma			
COLO 16	25–200	100	Hail and Lotan (2002)
Melanoma			
A375			Kim (2012)

(continued)

Table 8.1 (continued)

	Effective doses (μM)	IC50 (μM)	References
Nasopharyngeal carcinoma			
NPC, NPC-TW 039	200–400	250	Ip et al. (2012)
Small cell lung cancer			
H69	1–100	50	Brown et al. (2010)
Others			
KB cells	50–250	150	Lin et al. (2013)

cells, myofibroblasts, other cell types, and extracellular components, is essential for the maintenance of malignancies and facilitates tumor initiation, progression, and survival. Indeed, human colon cancer tissues are infiltrated by inflammatory cells and plasma levels of cytokines are often raised in CRC patients (Vaiopoulos et al. 2013). Regulation of the inflammatory response is very complicated but many signaling pathways involve the transcription factor NFκB. Capsaicin down-regulates NFκB (see below) behaving as a very potent inhibitor of inflammation (revised in this book) and hence may contribute to prevent CRC. Besides this, capsaicin functions as an antitumoral drug as it inhibits the growth and proliferation of different CRC cell lines. High-concentration capsaicin (≥200 μM for SW480 and CT-26 cell lines; ≥25 μM for HCT116 cell line) showed antiproliferative activity in CRC cells in a dose-dependent manner (Yang et al. 2013). In another study, an inhibition of cell growth and transcriptional activity was observed at 100 μM (Lee et al. 2012) (Table 8.1).

8.3.2 Pancreatic Cancer

Pancreatic cancer, one of the most fatal types of solid malignancy, is the fourth leading cause of cancer-related mortality in the USA and other industrialized countries. Despite efforts over the past three decades to improve diagnosis and treatment, the prognosis for patients with pancreatic cancer is extremely poor with or without treatment, and incidence rates are virtually identical to mortality rates (Tamburrino et al. 2013). Srivastava et al. demonstrated that capsaicin-triggered apoptosis in human pancreatic cancer cells, which represent one of the most difficult types of cancer to treat. Capsaicin increased the number of apoptotic proteins and increased cytochrome c levels in the cytosol in pancreatic AsPC-1 and BxPC-3 cells. Capsaicin-induced apoptosis in pancreatic cancer cells was associated with the generation of reactive oxygen species (ROS) and persistent disruption of mitochondrial transmembrane potential without affecting the normal cells (Zhang et al. 2008; Pramanik et al. 2011). Likewise, in pancreatic cancer PANC-1 cells, capsaicin dose-dependently induced apoptosis, via downregulation of the PI3 K/Akt pathway (Zhang et al. 2013).

8.3.3 Hepatocellular Carcinoma

Hepatocellular carcinoma is the most common form of liver cancer, and its incidence has been increasing worldwide, representing 70–85 % of primary hepatic malignancies in adults. Liver transplant is the first choice of treatment because it eliminates malignant cells and restores liver function. However, unfortunately 20 % of patients suffer tumor recurrence and in spite of intense research on HCC treatment, no relevant improvement in the survival of patients with HCC has been achieved so far (Llovet and Bruix 2008). Therefore it is urgent to identify novel therapeutic strategies for the management of HCC.

Capsaicin induced apoptosis in the hepatocellular carcinoma cell line HepG2 with the involvement of intracellular Ca^{2+}, ROS, Bcl-2 family, cytochrome *c* protein expression, and caspase-3 activity (Huang et al. 2009). In the same cells, capsaicin increased ROS production and induced expression of heme oxygenase-1 (HO-1) (Lee et al. 2004; Joung et al. 2007). Likewise, capsaicin sensitized hepatocellular carcinoma cells as well as breast cancer cells and leukemia cells to apoptosis induced by tumor necrosis factor-related, apoptosis-inducing ligand (TRAIL) (Moon et al. 2012). Co-treatment with capsaicin and TRAIL potentiated the caspase 3, 8, and 9 activation, the release of cytochrome C, and the disruption of mitochondrial transmembrane potential.

8.3.4 Prostate Cancer

Prostate cancer is one of the most prevalent forms of cancer in men worldwide. It is estimated that there are nearly 2.8 million men living with a history of prostate cancer in the United States, and an additional 241,740 cases have been diagnosed in 2012. Although prostate-specific antigen (PSA)-based screening has substantially reduced the incidence of mortality from prostate cancer (Carter et al. 2013; Vickers et al. 2013), it has increased the number of new cases diagnosed. Therefore, the increasing prevalence and the complexity of cancer treatment techniques require a great effort to avoid negative treatment effectiveness. Treatment options vary depending on the stage and grade of the cancer, as well as patient comorbidity, age, and personal preferences. More than one-half (57 %) of men aged younger than 65 years are treated with radical prostatectomy. Those aged 65–74 years commonly undergo radiation therapy (42 %), although radical prostatectomy (33 %) is also often used. Androgen deprivation therapy, chemotherapy, bone-directed therapy (such as zoledronic acid or denosumab), radiation therapy, or a combination of these treatments are used to treat more advanced disease. Unfortunately, too often the appearance of hormone refractory cancer cells leads eventually to the recurrence of cancer which turns to a hormone-independent state for which there is not treatment. The development of such lethal, castration-resistant prostate cancer (CRPC) is associated with adaptive changes to the androgen receptor (AR), including the emergence of mutant receptors and truncated, constitutively active AR variants.

Scientific progress in prostate cancer treatment has often been based on the use of established cell lines which mimics different prostate cancer stages. The LNCaP cell line is derived from a biopsy of a lymph node of a 50-year-old Caucasian male with confirmed diagnosis of metastatic prostate carcinoma (Horoszewicz et al. 1983). These cells are responsive to classic AR agonists and therefore are used as a model for androgen-sensitive prostate cancer. It has been shown that in the LNCaP cells high doses of capsaicin downregulates the expression of the AR (Mori et al. 2006). AR regulates the transcription of the PSA gene, as the 5′ upstream promoter and enhancer region of the PSA gene has several androgen response elements (ARE). Capsaicin at high doses inhibits the ability of dihydrotestosterone to activate the PSA promoter/enhancer even in the presence of exogenous AR which suggests that capsaicin inhibits the transcription of PSA not only via downregulation of expression of AR, but also by a direct inhibitory effect on PSA transcription (Mori et al. 2006). Those effects are TRPV1 receptor independent since the antagonists, capsazepine and ruthenium red, do not have any effect (Mori et al. 2006). Moreover, doses used to induce apoptosis on LNCaP prostate cells are very high (200 μM) and far away from the Kd of the receptor. However, capsaicin at lower doses (10–20 μM) induces upregulation of androgen receptor expression in LNCaP cells which is prevented by the TRPV1 antagonist capsazepine (Malagarie-Cazenave et al. 2009).

PC-3 cell line was originally derived from advanced (grade IV) androgen-independent prostate adenocarcinoma metastasized to bone (Iype et al. 1998). They are tumorigenic and have been widely used as a model for androgen-resistant prostate cancer. DU-145 cells were derived from a human prostate adenocarcinoma metastatic to the brain and are also used to study the androgen-resistant prostate cancer (Stone et al. 1978). In this androgen-independent cell lines, capsaicin dose-dependently induces cell cycle arrest and apoptosis (Mori et al. 2006; Sanchez et al. 2006, 2007, 2008). The mechanisms underlying vanilloid-induced apoptosis seem to occur independently of the TRPV1 receptor. In fact the apoptotic effect elicited by capsaicin in PC-3 cells cannot be reversed by the TRPV1 antagonist capsazepine, which in turn exerts cytotoxic effect on prostate cells (Mori et al. 2006; Sanchez et al. 2006). The androgen-resistant cell lines are more sensitive to capsaicin-induced cell death as doses of capsaicin required to induce cell death are lower than that required in the LNCaP cells (Table 8.1).

8.3.5 Breast Cancer

Breast cancer is the second leading cause of cancer death in women, exceeded only by lung cancer. It is estimated that 1 out of 10 women will develop breast cancer during her life and that there are nearly 3 million women living in the United States with a history of invasive breast cancer (Siegel et al. 2012). Although significant advances have been made in the treatment of this cancer, only less than half of the patients treated for localized breast cancer benefit from adjuvant chemotherapy; and most patients with metastatic cancer eventually develop disease that is resistant to therapy. In addition to stage, factors that influence survival include tumor grade, hormone receptor status, and human epidermal growth factor receptor 2 (HER2) status.

Several reports indicate that capsaicin inhibits the growth of breast cancer cell lines. Inhibition of growth is associated with cell cycle arrest in the S-phase and increased levels of apoptosis both in caspase-3-deficient MCF-7 cells and in non-caspase-3-deficient BT-20 cells suggesting that apoptosis induction is caspase-3 independent (Chou et al. 2009; Thoennissen et al. 2010; Chang et al. 2011).

Notably, in breast cancer cell lines, capsaicin was able to decrease the protein levels of both HER-2 and EGFR (Thoennissen et al. 2010). In HER-2 overexpressing BT-474 and SKBR-3 cell lines, which only have low to moderate levels of EGFR, capsaicin was able to clearly reduce expression levels of both types of receptors. In contrast, the drug showed less activity in the MDA-MB231 cell line, which is known to overexpress HER-2 as well as EGFR. However, capsaicin did not alter the mRNA levels of EGFR and HER-2 in all three breast cancer cell lines, suggesting that capsaicin decreases the two receptors by affecting their protein stability (Thoennissen et al. 2010).

In another study performed by Yoon et al. capsaicin treatment of MCF-7 cells induced S-phase arrest and the accumulation of p53 in the nucleus and cytosol. Capsaicin also induced autophagy through the AMPKα-mTOR signaling pathway which was further confirmed by Atg5 induction, LC3 conversion, and decreased p62 in a dose-dependent manner (Yoon et al. 2012).

Likewise, Dou et al. showed that whole pepper extracts were effective in inhibiting cell growth and inducing apoptosis in breast cancer cell lines MDA-MB-231 and MCF-7 and in Jurkat T leukemia cells. The peppers used in this study ranged in capsaicin levels from the bell pepper (0 Scoville heat units) to the habanero chili (100,000–350,000 Scoville heat units) and they were compared with purified capsaicin (16,000,000 units) (Dou et al. 2011). The effectiveness of the pepper extracts was correlated with the levels of capsaicin present according to the Scoville scale. Both pepper extracts and purified capsaicin induced apoptosis and decreased VEGF secretion in breast cancer cells whereas has minimal effect in breast normal cells (Dou et al. 2011). The mechanism whereby the extracts and capsaicin induced apoptosis was not related to the presence/absence of estrogen receptors since both cell lines differ in the ER expression (MCF-7 are estrogen receptor-positive and MDA-MB-231 are estrogen receptor-negative) (Thoennissen et al. 2010). However, it was reduced by the hydroxyl radical scavenger thiourea, suggesting the involvement of reactive oxygen species in the apoptotic effect.

8.3.6 Leukemic Cells

Capsaicin suppressed the growth of leukemic cells, but not normal bone marrow mononuclear cells, via induction of G_0–G_1 phase cell cycle arrest and apoptosis. Capsaicin-induced apoptosis was in association with the elevation of intracellular reactive oxygen species and Ca^{2+} production accompanying a downregulation of mitochondrial membrane potential ($\Delta\psi_m$) (Ito et al. 2004; Tsou et al. 2006). Interestingly, capsaicin-sensitive leukemic cells were possessed of wild-type p53, resulting in the phosphorylation of p53 at the Ser-15 residue by the treatment of capsaicin which was abrogated by pre-treatment with the antioxidant NAC (Ito et al. 2004). In human myeloid leukemia cells capsaicin binds to prohibitin (PHB) 2, which is normally localized to the inner mitochondrial membrane, and induces its translocation to the nucleus thereby causing apoptosis. In human acute monocytic leukemia cells THP-1, capsaicin increases the gene expression of carnitine palmitoyltransferase 1 (CPT-1) and the oxidation rate of palmitate. This data suggests that capsaicin-induced attenuation of palmitate-induced inflammatory gene expression is associated with reduced activation of JNK, c-Jun, and p38 and improved β-oxidation (Choi et al. 2011).

The approach of treating cancer with combinations of standard chemotherapeutic drugs has become increasingly common. In line with this, studies performed by Schwartz et el. demonstrated that the addition of capsaicin to a combination of molecules targeting the cancer metabolism markedly decreased lung or bladder carcinoma and melanoma tumor cell growth in mice (Schwartz et al. 2013).

8.3.7 *Lung and Bronchus*

Lung cancer is a major cause of morbidity and mortality worldwide in both men and women, accounting for 29 % of all cancers. The median age at diagnosis for lung cancer is 70 years for males and 71 years for females. The majority of lung cancers (56 %) are diagnosed at a distant stage because early disease is typically asymptomatic; only 15 % of cases are diagnosed at a local stage (Matsuda and Machii 2013). Lung cancer is classified as small cell (14 % of cases) or non-small cell (85 % of cases) for the purposes of treatment. Radiation therapy alone (for limited disease) or combined with chemotherapy (for extensive disease) is the standard treatment for small cell lung cancer. Although it has been reported the chemopreventive effect of capsaicin in experimental models of lung carcinogenesis, there are few studies showing the antitumor activity in lung cancer. In four human small cell lung cancer (SCLC) cells, capsaicin displays potent antiproliferative activity with the contribution of the E2F family of transcription factors which mediate cell cycle arrest (Brown et al. 2010).

8.4 Capsaicin Cancer-Promoter Activity

Despite our increasing understanding of the anticancer effects of capsaicin on the above-mentioned cancer cell lines, conflicting data from animal models and basic research suggest that in some circumstances capsaicin may promote tumor growth.

Low doses of capsaicin may exert protumorigenic effects in several cancer cell lines. Human colorectal carcinoma cell line SW480 and HCT116, and murine colorectal carcinoma CT-26 cell line revealed a 4-fold elevation in cell motility upon treatment with 12.5 μM capsaicin, which had no impact on cell proliferation (Yang et al. 2013). Likewise, HCT116 human colon carcinoma cells treatment with low concentrations of capsaicin (≤10 μM) enhanced cell proliferation and migration in association with upregulation of ENOX2 (tumor-associated NADH oxidase) expression (Liu et al. 2012). The same group has demonstrated that higher doses of capsaicin (250 μM) inhibit HCT116 cell proliferation and downregulate ENOX2 (Mao et al. 2008). In human keratinocytes from perilesional vitiligo skin, capsaicin used at a concentration of 10 μM, induced an increase in mitochondrial activity and reduced ROS accumulation and NFκB and p53 activation (Becatti et al. 2010).

In the same line, the group of Yang et al. demonstrated that low doses of capsaicin (12.5 μM) enhanced both migratory and invasive capability of HCT116 cell line whereas higher doses (200 μM) induced cell cycle arrest and inhibit cell proliferation (Yang et al. 2013). Furthermore, 100 μM capsaicin induced epithelial-to-mesenchymal transition, upregulated expression of MMP-2 and MMP-9, and activated Akt/mTOR and STAT-3 pathways in colorectal cancer cells (Yang et al. 2013). We have observed that capsaicin at lower doses (10–20 μM) induces cell proliferation and upregulation of the androgen receptor expression in prostate cancer LNCaP cells (Malagarie-Cazenave et al. 2009). Interestingly, this effect was TRPV1 receptor-dependent since it was prevented by the TRPV1 receptor antagonist capsazepine (Malagarie-Cazenave et al. 2009).

The biphasic effect of capsaicin observed in many tumor cells might be due to the activation of TRPV1. As stated above, most tumor cell lines expressed TRPV1 which has an affinity for capsaicin of Kd = 710 nM. Low doses of capsaicin (≤20 μM) were effective in inducing calcium entry through TRPV1 receptor in cultured cells (Vriens et al. 2004; Sanchez et al. 2005). In line with this, it has been observed that Ca^{2+} entry via a capsaicin-sensitive membrane channel may play a role in stimulating hepatocellular carcinoma HepG2 cells cell migration (Vriens et al. 2004). Therefore at low doses capsaicin presumably activates TRPV1 which could influence intracellular calcium levels affecting cancer cell aggressiveness. However, the capsaicin-induced apoptotic effect at high doses is a receptor-independent mechanism, as observed in most cancer cell lines. In addition, recent findings demonstrate that in TRPV1 null cells, capsaicin exhibits a more aggressive antiproliferative effect than in TRPV1 expressing cells (Caprodossi et al. 2011).

8.5 Mechanisms Underlying the Capsaicin Antitumor Activity

In spite of the well-known antiproliferative effect of capsaicin in tumor cell lines, the mechanism underlying the intracellular signaling pathways are poorly understood. In this section, we will summarize the best established intracellular phenomena as well as recent pathways involving AMP-dependent kinase (AMPK) and autophagy.

8.5.1 Intracellular Calcium

The calcium dependence of apoptosis has been well defined and comprises a sustained elevation of intracellular calcium as well as a decrease in endoplasmic reticulum calcium. Sustained elevation in intracellular calcium concentration activates various secondary mechanisms that induce the increased production of reactive oxygen and nitrogen species and ultimately the programmed cell death. Several studies showed that capsaicin-induced apoptosis via increased Ca^{2+} levels in different carcinoma cells models (Chou et al. 2009; Huang et al. 2009; Lu et al. 2010), although the molecular mechanisms of the Ca^{2+} signaling pathways leading to capsaicin-induced cell death are still misunderstood. The release of intracellular Ca^{2+} may be an important regulatory factor on early apoptosis induced by capsaicin as calcium chelators prevent capsaicin-induced cell death (Lee et al. 2009). In most cancer cell types other than neuroblastoma or glioma cells, the increase in intracellular calcium is secondary to ER stress-dependent responses rather than a massive calcium entry by a calcium-permeable channel (Huang et al. 2009; Lee et al. 2009; Ip et al. 2012).

8.5.2 Reactive Oxygen Species

Reactive oxygen species (ROS), including superoxide (O_2^-), hydroxyl radical (HO^-), and hydrogen peroxide (H_2O_2), have a dual role in cellular environments. Whereas low ROS levels are involved in normal cell events, excess ROS cause cellular damage and ultimately lead to cell death (Sinha et al. 2013). The involvement of ROS in vanilloid-induced apoptosis has been demonstrated in most of the cell lines analyzed (Sanchez et al. 2007; Huang et al. 2009; Lu et al. 2010) and revised by Surh (Surh 2002; Lu et al. 2010). In recent years, a number of studies have shown that oxidative stress could cause cellular apoptosis via both the mitochondria dependent and mitochondria-independent pathways (Sinha et al. 2013).

The plasma membrane of cells contains an electron transport chain (tPMET), cyanide-insensitive, comprised by two cytoplasmic NADH-coenzyme Q reductases, one NADH cytochrome b reductase, the lipophilic electron carrier coenzyme Q (CoQ), and a terminal coenzyme Q oxidase located on the external plasma membrane surface (Fig. 8.3). The last one oxidizes externally supplied NADH and hence they are NADH oxidases (NOX). Since they are located on the outside cell surface, they are referred to as ECTO-NOX or ENOX proteins (Crane and Low 2008; Jiang et al. 2008). The tPMET reduces extracellular oxidants by using the reducing power of intracellular antioxidants, making the cell

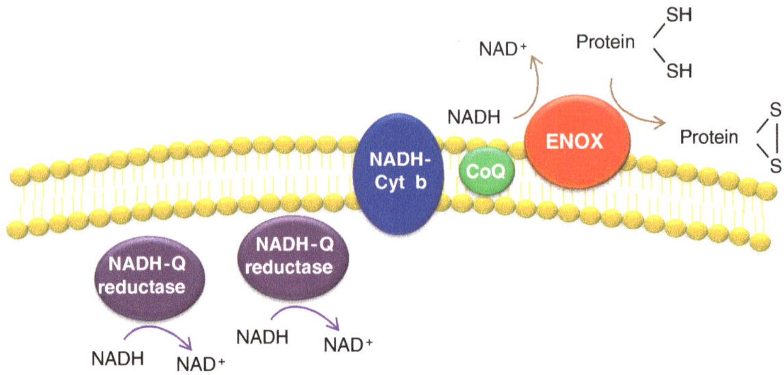

Fig. 8.3 Trans-Plasma membrane electron transport chain (tPMET). It is comprised by two cytoplasmic NADH-coenzyme Q reductases, one NADH cytochrome b reductase, the lipophilic electron carrier coenzyme Q, and a terminal coenzyme Q oxidase located on the external plasma membrane surface

metabolism respond to changes in the local redox environment. They also exhibit protein disulfide-thiol interchange activities (Bosneaga et al. 2008). In tumor cells, this plasma membrane NADH oxidase is upregulated (Morre et al. 1995). It seems that at least one function of this redox system is to regenerate NADP from NADH accumulated in the glycolytic production of ATP, increased in tumor cells. CoQ blockage inhibits the plasma membrane NADH-oxidoreductase electron transport chain and promotes reactive oxygen species production that may result in apoptosis.

The group of Morré has demonstrated that cancer cells contains a specific isoform of ENOX only expressed in tumor cells designated ENOX2 (former tNOX) that is inhibited by several quinone site inhibitors with anticancer activity, all of which result in cell cycle arrest and induce apoptosis. ENOX2 is expressed only in tumoral cells and not in normal cells. In line with this, ENOX2 overexpression in noncancerous MCF-10A cells results in the acquisition of invasivity, an aggressive characteristic of cancer (Chueh et al. 2004). The role of ENOX2 in tumor formation is evidenced by the fact that ENOX2 knockdown suppresses the growth of HCT116 xenografts in vivo and metastatic potential following colon cancer cells tail-vein injections in mice (Liu et al. 2012). This activity has been also detected in the sera of prostate cancer patients (Morre et al. 1997) whereas it is absent in serum from healthy volunteers or patients of other conditions (Morre et al. 2008). Different ENOX2 isoforms are specifically expressed in cancers of different tissue origins providing a very useful tool for diagnosis and management (Morre et al. 2008). It is relevant to note that this enzyme is completely inhibited by capsaicin, since capsaicin can behave like a quinone analog (Morre et al. 1995, 1996; Macho et al. 1999), which has no activity in constitutive ENOX (Jiang et al. 2008). Likewise, preincubation of cancer cells with coenzyme Q prevents capsaicin-induced apoptosis (Wolvetang et al. 1996), suggesting that capsaicin induces apoptosis by competing with coenzyme Q in the plasma membrane redox system. Inhibition of ENOX2 can affect the redox balance with an overall shift toward a pro-oxidative status which results in the redirection of the normal electron flow in the plasma membrane complex, favoring the one electron processes that generates superoxides and other aggressive oxidants (Hail 2003; Macho et al. 2003). Capsaicin also decreases the half-life of ENOX2 in human gastric carcinoma cells concurrently with apoptosis (Wang et al. 2008).

By other hand, research performed by Srivastava et al. has demonstrated the involvement of thioredoxine (Trx) in capsaicin-induced apoptosis in pancreatic cancer cells. Intracellular antioxidant thioredoxin (Trx) negatively regulates apoptosis signal-regulating kinase 1 (ASK1,) a member of mitogen-activated protein kinase kinase kinase family, which is involved in apoptosis induction. Authors demonstrated that the expression of Trx was significantly reduced by capsaicin, resulting in the activation of ASK1 mainly by phosphorylation at Thr845. Capsaicin-mediated ROS generation was involved in the inhibition of Trx and activation of the ASK-1 cascade, leading to apoptosis in pancreatic cancer cells (Pramanik and Srivastava 2012) (Fig. 8.4).

However, one cannot exclude the possibility that some of the ROS generation promoted by vanilloid treatment is attributable to a disruption of the mitochondrial respiratory system since capsaicin can also inhibit the NADH:coenzyme Q oxidoreductase (i.e., complex I) activity of the mitochondrial electron transport system. Hail and Lotan have demonstrated that in skin squamous cell carcinoma capsaicin induces the inhibition of mitochondrial respiration (Hail and Lotan 2002). The induction of apoptosis was associated with the mitochondrial permeability transition (i.e., an increase in the permeability of the inner mitochondrial membrane associated with the opening of a nonspecific pore) concomitant with a rapid increase in hydroperoxide generation and a decrease in oxygen consumption. This may be due to an inhibition of mitochondrial electron transport by capsaicin, presumably at complex I, which may promote the production of ROS. In human pancreatic cancer cells capsaicin causes ROS (superoxide radical and hydrogen peroxide) generation by inhibiting mitochondrial complex I and complex III activity and drastically disrupts mitochondrial functions decreasing ATP levels. However, normal pancreatic epithelial cells were resistant to the effects of capsaicin (Pramanik et al. 2011). Therefore, capsaicin targets both mitochondrial and plasma membrane electron transport systems, thereby generating ROS that can mediate apoptosis (Surh 2002). In line with this notion we have observed that capsaicin treatment of prostate cancer PC-3 cells induces an increase in ROS in a biphasic manner with an acute peak after a 15-min treatment and a second peak after 10 h (Sanchez et al. 2006). Whereas the second peak is inhibited by mitochondrial electron chain inhibitors, as rotenone and cyanide, the first peak seems not to have a mitochondrial origin (Sanchez et al. 2006). Macho et al. demonstrated that in transformed cells capsaicin and capsaicinoids selectively induced a rapid increase of ROS followed by a subsequent disruption of the mitochondrial transmembrane potential and had no effect in normal cells (Macho et al. 1999). Similar results were observed in prostate PC-3 cells (Sanchez et al. 2006). Therefore, it appeared that capsaicin exposure of tumor cells initiates ROS production at the plasma membrane tPMET resulting in oxidative stress, which triggered mitochondrial-induced apoptosis (Fig. 8.3).

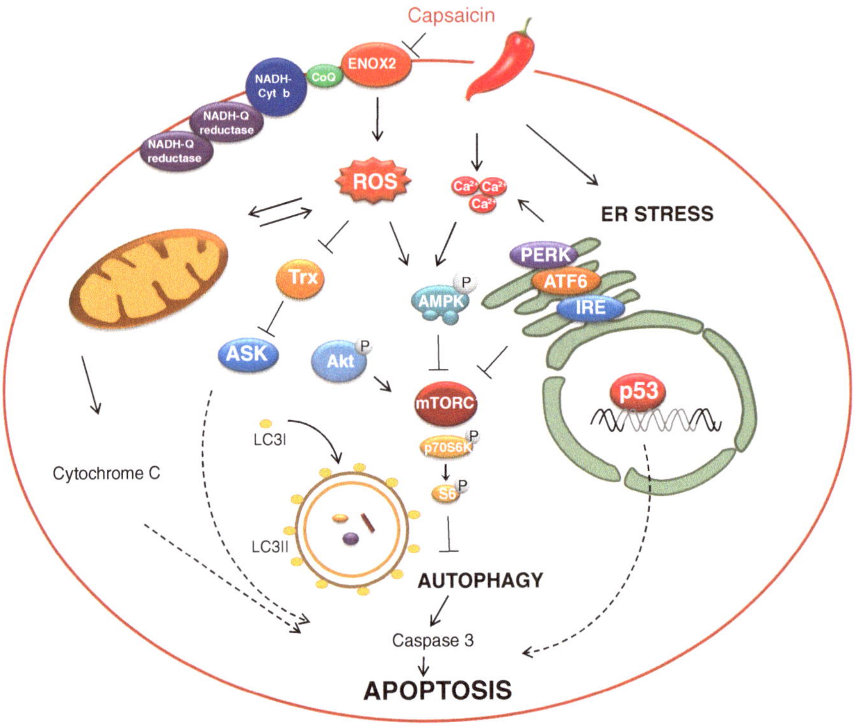

Fig. 8.4 Scheme of the main signaling pathways activated by capsaicin in tumoral cells. Capsaicin induces apoptosis by several mechanisms. Capsaicin impacts the NADH-oxidoreductase electron transport chain present in cancer cells and inhibits its activity. Deregulation of plasma membrane electron transport chain produces accumulation of ROS which inactivates thioredoxin (Trx) activating the apoptosis signal-regulated kinase ASK1. Excess of ROS may also activate mitochondrial-dependent apoptosis. In most cell lines, capsaicin increases intracellular calcium concentration secondary to ER stress. ER stress responses may induce autophagy. Activation of AMPK may occur by ROS or by a calcium-dependent pathway. AMPK inhibits the mTOR7S6 pathway and activates autophagy (see text for explanation)

8.5.3 AMPK and Autophagy

Cancer cells can reprogram their metabolism, and thus their energy production, to support the anabolic requirements associated with cell growth and proliferation, by limiting their energy metabolism largely to glycolysis, leading to a state that has been termed "aerobic glycolysis" (Schulze and Harris 2012; Ward and Thompson 2012). Those changes constitute a fundamental adaptation of tumor cells to a relatively hostile environment, and support the evolution of aggressive and metastatic phenotypes. The importance of metabolic reprogramming in cancer is being increasingly recognized and represents one of the major fields of research in this area.

The AMP-dependent protein kinase (AMPK) is considered the principal metabolic gatekeeper of the cell. It is activated by metabolic stresses that increase cellular ADP/ATP and/or AMP/ATP ratios (Hardie et al. 2012; Hardie and Alessi 2013). Upon energetic imbalance, intracellular concentrations of AMP increase, thus promoting AMPK activation. Activated AMPK stimulates catabolic pathways (e.g. glycolysis and fatty acid oxidation) and, concomitantly, inhibits the rate of anabolic reactions (protein, cholesterol, triglyceride and fatty acid synthesis) to restore the correct adenylate energy charge. Capsaicin treatment of colon cancer HT29 cells induced AMPK activation and inhibition of ACC, a well-known AMPK substrate, suggesting that capsaicin is inhibiting lipid biosynthesis. Both phenomena were involved in capsaicin-induced apoptosis (Kim et al. 2007). We have also observed that capsaicin at 40 μM induces activation of AMPK in prostate PC-3 cells through a mechanism independent of TRPV1 receptor (data not shown). In line with this, capsaicin was shown to inhibit adipogenesis in 3T3-L1 preadipocytes cells through direct activation of caspase-3 (Hsu and Yen 2007). The mechanism whereby capsaicin could activate AMPK is not clear but recent research indicates that pro-oxidant conditions or the selective inhibition of the mitochondrial electron transport chain, also plays a pivotal role in the stimulation of AMPK activity (Cardaci et al. 2012). As capsaicin increases intracellular ROS and impairs mitochondrial transmembrane potential, this could be a sufficient signal to trigger AMPK activation (Fig. 8.3).

AMPK is not only an energy-responsive enzyme but has been identified as a regulator of autophagy. Autophagy is a cellular self-digestive process whereby bulk cytoplasmic components and intracellular organelles are sequestered into double membrane vesicles named autophagosomes and delivered for degradation fusing with lysosomes to form single-membrane autophagolysosomes. The contents of the autophagolysosomes are ultimately degraded by lysosomal hydrolase (Caffarel et al. 2006; Eisenberg-Lerner and Kimchi 2009; Dikic et al. 2010; Glick et al. 2010). Accumulating data have demonstrated that autophagy is involved in cell death, referred to as type II programmed cell death. Stimulation of autophagy in many cellular settings relies on the inhibition of the mTORC1 complex, which plays a central role in the control of protein synthesis, cell growth and cell proliferation through the regulation of several downstream targets. As a result of its central position in the control of cellular homeostasis, mTORC1 integrates signals from different inputs. One of the most important upstream regulators of mTORC1 is the pro-survival kinase Akt, which phosphorylates and inactivates TSC2 (an inhibitor of the mTORC1 activator Rheb) and PRAS-40. Thus, Akt activation stimulates mTORC1 and inhibits autophagy. On the other hand, AMPK has also been shown to negatively regulate mTORC1 via TSC2 activation, which also leads to autophagy stimulation (Alers et al. 2012; Cardaci et al. 2012). The autophagic pathway has been extensively investigated in yeast and mammalian cells. During autophagy, microtubule-associated protein 1 light chain 3 (LC3) is cleaved at its C-terminal arginine residue to form LC3-I. LC3-I is easily activated and conjugated to phosphatidylethanolamine (PE) and bound to the autophagosome membrane to form LC3-II. LC3-II localized to the autophagosome has been used as an autophagosome marker. Capsaicin-induced autophagy has been demonstrated in various cancer cell types. In HCT116 and MCF-7 cells, dihydrocapsaicin (DHC) and capsaicin induce autophagy that may contribute to cell death (Oh et al. 2008). The effect of capsaicin and DHC was abrogated by the catalase inhibitor 3-amino-1,2,4-triazole (3AT) and catalase genetic knockdown, indicating that DHC-induced autophagy was regulated by catalase activity (Oh et al. 2008).

The endoplasmic reticulum (ER) performs several functions, which include protein-folding, trafficking, and intracellular calcium concentration regulation. When ER functions are disrupted causing an imbalance between protein-folding capacity and protein load ER triggers a series of signaling and transcriptional events known as the unfolded protein response (UPR). The UPR attempts to restore homeostasis in the ER but if unsuccessful can trigger apoptosis in the stressed cells and local inflammation (Wang et al. 2010). Three pathways may be activated during the ER stress response: the inositol-requiring enzyme-1 (IRE-1) pathway, the PERK pathway and the ATF6 pathway. In prostate PC-3 cells, capsaicin treatment induced an upregulation of CHOP protein which was detected by microarray studies, RT-PCR and western blot (Sanchez et al. 2008). The increase in CHOP protein expression was preceded by an increase in ATF4 expression and in an enhancement of eIF2α phosphorylation, which indicates that the PERK ER stress pathway is activated by capsaicin in prostate cells (Sanchez et al. 2008). In human breast cancer cells, capsaicin treatment triggered ER stress by increasing levels of IRE1, CHOP, GRP78/Bip, and activated caspase-4. It led to an increase in cytosolic Ca^{2+}, calpain activation, loss of the mitochondrial transmembrane potential, release of mitochondrial cytochrome c, and caspase-9 and -7 activation (Lee et al. 2009). In line with these results, Choi et al. demonstrated that in breast cancer cells capsaicin induced ER stress by upregulation of IRE-1 and CHOP. Moreover, capsaicin treatment caused an increase in the conversion of LC3I into LC3II which was reduced by transfection of MCF-7 cells with p38 siRNA. IRE1 knockdown with selective siRNA was found to reduce the phosphorylations of p38 and Akt and eventually to reduce LC3II conversion. Authors demonstrate that p38 MAPK is required for capsaicin-induced autophagy at the sequestration step of autophagosome formation (Choi et al. 2010a). This observation link capsaicin-induced ER stress with autophagy as is schematized in Fig. 8.4.

In a recent study, Choi et al. demonstrated that the capsaicin analog, dihydrocapsaicin (DHC) induced autophagy through catalase activation, although it might be involved in cell protection against apoptotic and necrotic cell death rather than in apoptosis induction (Choi et al. 2010b).

8.5.4 Peroxisome Proliferator-Activated Receptors

Peroxisome Proliferator-Activated Receptors (PPAR) are ligand-activated transcription factors which belong to the nuclear receptor superfamily and mediate several physiological functions, among which the best characterized are lipid metabolism, energy balance and anti-inflammation (Youssef and Badr 2011). There are three PPAR subtypes alpha, delta (also known as beta), and gamma, all of which have long been known to be expressed in most tissues although at different levels (Yessoufou and Wahli 2010). PPARγ exists in two major isoforms (γ_1 and γ_2) which arise by differential transcription start sites and alternative splicing (Zhu et al. 1995) although PPARγ_1 expression is very low in most tissues.

Recent research has shown that capsaicin activates PPARα in vitro with an EC_{50} of 50 μM (Mueller et al. 2011). In addition, dietary capsaicin enhances fatty acid oxidation in adipose tissue through PPARα activation (Kang et al. 2010). Moreover, dietary capsaicin lowered fasting glucose, insulin, leptin levels, and markedly reduced the impairment of glucose tolerance in obese mice pointing to a beneficial effect of capsaicin in metabolic-related diseases. In line with this observation, topical application of capsaicin cream in male mice lowered serum levels of fasting glucose, total cholesterol, and triglycerides and increased expression of PPARα and PPARγ (Lee et al. 2013). The involvement of PPAR receptors in the capsaicin antitumor activity has been demonstrated by several groups. In HT-29 human colon cancer cells treatment with capsaicin or the PPARγ ligand troglitazone-induced apoptotic cell death in a dose-dependent manner (Kim et al. 2004). Capsaicin-induced cell death was completely blocked by a specific PPARγ antagonist and was independent of the TRPV1 receptor as capsazepine did not have any effect (Kim et al. 2004).

8.5.5 P53

The tumor suppressor protein p53 regulates the cellular response to DNA damage by mediating cell cycle arrest, DNA repair, and cell death. Activation of p53 induces apoptosis typically through the mitochondrial pathway, although p53 can also modulate cell death through death receptors although the mechanisms involved in p53-mediated cell death remain controversial. In response to stress signals, the levels of p53 protein are rapidly increased, and activity is enhanced after phosphorylation at the Ser-15 residue, resulting in the upregulation of various proapoptotic genes, including the cyclin-dependent kinase inhibitor *p21*WAF1/CIP1 and those encoding members of the Bcl-2 family as the proapoptotic protein Bax. In turn, increased levels of Bax induce mitochondrial depolarization, release of cytochrome *c*, and activation of caspase cascade, leading to apoptosis.

Following capsaicin treatment an increase in p53 and phosphorylated p53 has been observed in several cancer cell lines (Huang et al. 2009; Kim et al. 2009; Maity et al. 2010; Kim 2012; Yoon et al. 2012) (reviewed in (Rajput and Mandal 2012)). Several studies have demonstrated that ROS generation plays a significant role in phosphorylation of p53 at the Ser-15 residue.

However, the role of p53 in the mechanism of capsaicin-induced cell death is not critical since in cells lacking p53 as PC-3 cells or null capsaicin also triggers apoptosis and cell death. It has been suggested that in the absence of p53, programmed cell death proceeds and is partly mediated by the "tumor suppressor lipid", ceramide (Hage-Sleiman et al. 2013). Ceramide either de novo synthetized or produced by sphingomyelin hydrolysis, can induce cell death through both caspase-dependent and caspase-independent mechanisms. As ceramide accumulation has been observed in capsaicin-treated p53 null cells (Sanchez et al. 2007), this could explain the p53-independent apoptosis induction triggered by capsaicin.

8.5.6 Transcription factors: NFκB and STATs

NF-κB is a family of transcription factors ubiquitously expressed and well-known for their central role in immunity, inflammation. However, NF-κB also plays a major role in development and progression of cancer because it regulates a number of genes involved in inflammation, cell survival, cell proliferation, invasion, angiogenesis, and metastasis. Capsaicin is a potent inhibitor of NFκB and blocks NFκB activation induced by proinflammatory stimuli (Singh et al. 1996). The group of Mori described that the activity of NF-κB was dramatically inhibited by capsaicin in PC-3 cells (Mori et al. 2006). NFκB proteins are maintained in the cytoplasm by their binding with inhibitory proteins (IKBs). The degradation of IKB allows NFκB to translocate to the nucleus and bind cognate DNA-binding sites to regulate the transcription of a large number of genes, including inflammatory cytokines. Capsaicin treatment of human myeloid ML-1a cells blocked the degradation of I kappa B alpha, and thus the nuclear translocation of the p65 subunit of NF-kappa B, which is essential for NF-kappa B activation (Singh et al. 1996). Mori et al. also observed that capsaicin inhibited the TNF-α-induced IκBα degradation in the cytoplasm, thus preventing the TNF-α-dependent translocation of NF-κB to the nucleus. Moreover, IκBα protein levels increased in PC-3 cells cultured with capsaicin for 2 h compared with the levels in untreated cells (Mori et al. 2006). In line with this, in adult T cell leukemia cells, capsaicin treatment induced the decrease in phosphorylated Iκ-Bα accompanied by a decrease in the NF-κB binding activity of p65, but not p50, indicating selective inhibition of p65 subunit by capsaicin. Decrease in the NF-κB activity, at least in part, may be responsible for induction of apoptosis in these cells (Zhang et al. 2003).

8.6 In Vivo Antitumoral Action of Capsaicin

Given the large number of publications that have described the antiproliferative effect of capsaicin in vitro it is somewhat surprising that there are relatively few studies that have investigated the in vivo antitumoral action of capsaicin. However, although they differ in the cell type used, the inoculation site and the administration route of capsaicin (Table 8.2), all show a substantial reduction of tumor growth in xenograft and orthotopic mouse models.

Table 8.2 In vivo antitumor activity of capsaicin

	Tumor site	Cells injected	Dose (mg/kg)	Administration route	References
Colon cancer	Subcutaneous	COLO 250	1 and 3	Injection	Lu et al. (2010)
Pancreatic cancer	Subcutaneous	PANC-1	5 (3 times per week)	Oral gavage	Zhang et al. (2013)
		AsPC-1	2.5 (5 days a week)	Oral gavage	Pramanik et al. (2011)
	Orthotopic	PANC-1	5	Oral gavage	Pramanik and Srivastava (2012)
Prostate cancer	Subcutaneous	PC-3	5	Injection	Sanchez et al. (2006)
	Subcutaneous	PC-3	5 (3 times per week)	Oral gavage	Mori et al. (2006)
Breast cancer	Orthotopic	MDAMB231	5 (3 times per week)	Oral gavage	Thoennissen et al. (2010)
Urinary bladder cancer	Subcutaneous	T24	5	Injection	Yang et al. (2010)
Leukemia	Subcutaneous	NB4	50	Injection	Ito et al. (2004)
Small cell carcinoma	Subcutaneous	H69	10	Injection	Brown et al. (2010)

In vivo studies in immunodeficient nu/nu mice bearing colo 205 tumor xenografts showed that capsaicin at 1 and 3 mg/Kg injected each 3 days effectively inhibited tumor growth (Table 8.2) (Lu et al. 2010). Interestingly, dietary exposure of capsaicin during the initiation phase was found to significantly reduce the incidence of colonic adenocarcinoma in a model of azoxymethane-induced colon tumorigenesis (Yoshitani et al. 2001).

Capsaicin at 5 mg/kg administered by oral gavage 3 days a week reduced 30 % the volume and weight of pancreatic tumors (Pramanik and Srivastava 2012; Zhang et al. 2013) and urinary bladder tumors (Yang et al. 2010). Capsaicin was an extremely effective inhibitor of the cancer process, inducing apoptosis in cancer cells.

The in vivo activity of capsaicin against prostate cancer has only been studied in the PC-3 cell line because it is the best tumorigenic. Xenograft PC-3 tumors were induced intradermically in mice and a significant reduction of tumor growth was observed in the mice treated during 14 days with capsaicin when injected near the tumor. Biochemical parameters revealed that the treatments did not affect liver or kidney. Tunnel labeling showed that capsaicin was able to induce apoptosis of PC-3 cells also in vivo (Sanchez et al. 2006). Moreover, capsaicin exhibit a protective anticarcinogenic activity in mice injected s.c. with PC-3 cells. PC-3 cells were injected into the flanks, and from the next day, capsaicin was given by gavage 3 days per week. Tumor volumes were measured weekly and all mice were killed at the end of the 4th week when tumors were dissected and weighted. Tumors in capsaicin-treated mice compared with those in vehicle-treated mice were statistically significantly smaller (Mori et al. 2006). Those results indicate that capsaicin is a promising new chemotherapeutic agent that exerts effects in preventing and in reducing tumor growth.

In addition, the aggressive EGFR-positive MDAMB231 breast cancer cells were grown orthotopically in the breast tissue of female mice following oral capsaicin administration 3 days a week. Capsaicin treatment caused a reduction of 70 % in the weight of breast cancer tumors compared to controls (Thoennissen et al. 2010). Concordantly with the in vitro studies, breast tumors of mice treated with capsaicin had lower levels of activated ERK, as well as HER-2 and cyclin D1, whereas caspase-3, -7, -9 activity along with PARP cleavage products was increased compared to the tumors from the control mice (Thoennissen et al. 2010).

In a model of mice with subcutaneous leukemic tumors, treatment of animals with capsaicin (50 mg/kg) in 5 % ethanol as an emulsion fluid injected daily for 6 days significantly decreased tumor weight and increased apoptosis (Ito et al. 2004).

To the best of our knowledge, no human clinical trials on capsaicin efficacy against cancer have been carried out. However, it has recently been reported a case of a patient with recurrent adenocarcinoma of the prostate with Gleason grade 7, who experienced a slowing of his prostate-specific antigen doubling time while taking capsaicin (Jankovic et al. 2010).

8.7 Conclusions and Future Perspectives

Despite our improved understanding of cancer biology and ability to perform more complex therapeutic strategies that produce better short-term outcomes, major progress toward increasing survival times has been exhaustively slow. It is, therefore, of particular interest to impose new therapeutic strategies of this fatal disease. The development of preventive approaches using specific natural or synthetic compounds, or both, requires a depth of understanding of the cross-talk between cancer signaling pathways and networks to retain or enhance chemopreventive activity while reducing known toxic effects. Capsaicin has shown to have antitumoral properties both in vitro and in vivo against many cancer cell types. Although the in vitro doses required to trigger apoptosis are very high, in the in vivo studies no toxic side effects have been observed suggesting that capsaicin-based chemotherapy could be a safety treatment. In fact, antitumoral capsaicin effective doses used in the in vivo studies (range between 1 and 50 mg/kg, Table 8.2) suggest that therapeutic doses could be achievable without toxic side effects. Considering that red peppers have a capsaicin content ranging from 0.1 to 60 mg/g, to reach a therapeutically effective dose, a person of about 70 kg should take daily 3 kg of the soft pepper or 6 g of the most hot pepper during the treatment. Although this is not a daily consuming quantity, could be used in case of chemotherapy. Global differences in the daily consumption of capsicum spices vary from 2.5 g/person in India, 5 g/person in Thailand, 15 g/person in Saudi Arabia, or 20 g/person (one chili pepper) in Mexico (O'Neill et al. 2012). This suggests that at least 20 g pepper/person can be consumed daily without side toxic effects. Overall, these findings show that capsaicinoids could be considered as a useful cancer therapeutic approach.

Acknowledgments This work has been supported by Spanish Minneco (grant BFU2012-31444), Comunidad de Madrid (Grant S2010/BMD-2308), and Fundación Tatiana Pérez de Guzmán.

References

Alers S, Loffler AS, Wesselborg S, Stork B (2012) Role of AMPK-mTOR-Ulk1/2 in the regulation of autophagy: cross talk, shortcuts, and feedbacks. Mol Cell Biol 32:2–11

Alothman ZA, Wabaidur SM, Khan MR, Abdel Ghafar A, Habila MA, Ahmed YB (2012) Determination of capsaicinoids in Capsicum species using ultra performance liquid chromatography-mass spectrometry. J Sep Sci 35:2892–2896

Athanasiou A, Smith PA, Vakilpour S, Kumaran NM, Turner AE, Bagiokou D et al (2007) Vanilloid receptor agonists and antagonists are mitochondrial inhibitors: how vanilloids cause non-vanilloid receptor mediated cell death. Biochem Biophys Res Commun 354:50–55

Babbar S, Chanda S, Bley K (2010) Inhibition and induction of human cytochrome P450 enzymes in vitro by capsaicin. Xenobiotica 40:807–816

Becatti M, Prignano F, Fiorillo C, Pescitelli L, Nassi P, Lotti T et al (2010) The involvement of Smac/DIABLO, p53, NF-kB, and MAPK pathways in apoptosis of keratinocytes from perilesional vitiligo skin: protective effects of curcumin and capsaicin. Antioxid Redox Signal 13:1309–1321

Biggs JE, Yates JM, Loescher AR, Clayton NM, Boissonade FM, Robinson PP (2007) Vanilloid receptor 1 (TRPV1) expression in lingual nerve neuromas from patients with or without symptoms of burning pain. Brain Res 1127:59–65

Bochalli R (1952) To the 50th anniversary of death of Rudolf Wirchow. Hippokrates 23:647–649

Bosneaga E, Kim C, Shen B, Watanabe T, Morre DM, Morre DJ (2008) ECTO-NOX (ENOX) proteins of the cell surface lack thioredoxin reductase activity. BioFactors 34:245–251

Brown KC, Witte TR, Hardman WE, Luo H, Chen YC, Carpenter AB et al (2010) Capsaicin displays anti-proliferative activity against human small cell lung cancer in cell culture and nude mice models via the E2F pathway. PLoS ONE 5:e10243

Caffarel MM, Sarrio D, Palacios J, Guzman M, Sanchez C (2006) Delta9-tetrahydrocannabinol inhibits cell cycle progression in human breast cancer cells through Cdc2 regulation. Cancer Res 66:6615–6621

Caprodossi S, Amantini C, Nabissi M, Morelli MB, Farfariello V, Santoni M et al (2011) Capsaicin promotes a more aggressive gene expression phenotype and invasiveness in null-TRPV1 urothelial cancer cells. Carcinogenesis 32:686–694

Cardaci S, Filomeni G, Ciriolo MR (2012) Redox implications of AMPK-mediated signal transduction beyond energetic clues. J Cell Sci 125:2115–2125

Carter HB, Albertsen PC, Barry MJ, Etzioni R, Freedland SJ, Greene KL et al (2013) Early detection of prostate cancer: AUA guideline. J Urol 190:419–426

Caterina MJ, Schumacher MA, Tominaga M, Rosen TA, Levine JD, Julius D (1997) The capsaicin receptor: a heat-activated ion channel in the pain pathway. Nature 389:816–824

Crane FL, Low H (2008) Reactive oxygen species generation at the plasma membrane for antibody control. Autoimmun Rev 7:518–522

Cui Y, Yang F, Cao X, Yarov-Yarovoy V, Wang K, Zheng J (2012) Selective disruption of high sensitivity heat activation but not capsaicin activation of TRPV1 channels by pore turret mutations. J Gen Physiol 139:273–283

Czifra G, Varga A, Nyeste K, Marincsak R, Toth BI, Kovacs I et al (2009) Increased expressions of cannabinoid receptor-1 and transient receptor potential vanilloid-1 in human prostate carcinoma. J Cancer Res Clin Oncol 135:507–514

Chang HC, Chen ST, Chien SY, Kuo SJ, Tsai HT, Chen DR (2011) Capsaicin may induce breast cancer cell death through apoptosis-inducing factor involving mitochondrial dysfunction. Hum Exp Toxicol 30:1657–1665

Choi CH, Jung YK, Oh SH (2010a) Autophagy induction by capsaicin in malignant human breast cells is modulated by p38 and extracellular signal-regulated mitogen-activated protein kinases and retards cell death by suppressing endoplasmic reticulum stress-mediated apoptosis. Mol Pharmacol 78:114–125

Choi CH, Jung YK, Oh SH (2010b) Selective induction of catalase-mediated autophagy by dihydrocapsaicin in lung cell lines. Free Radic Biol Med 49:245–257

Choi SE, Kim TH, Yi SA, Hwang YC, Hwang WS, Choe SJ et al (2011) Capsaicin attenuates palmitate-induced expression of macrophage inflammatory protein 1 and interleukin 8 by increasing palmitate oxidation and reducing c-Jun activation in THP-1 (human acute monocytic leukemia cell) cells. Nutr Res 31:468–478

Chou CC, Wu YC, Wang YF, Chou MJ, Kuo SJ, Chen DR (2009) Capsaicin-induced apoptosis in human breast cancer MCF-7 cells through caspase-independent pathway. Oncol Rep 21:665–671

Chueh PJ, Wu LY, Morre DM, Morre DJ (2004) tNOX is both necessary and sufficient as a cellular target for the anticancer actions of capsaicin and the green tea catechin (-)-epigallocatechin-3-gallate. BioFactors 20:235–249

de Sa Junior PL, Pasqualoto KF, Ferreira AK, Tavares MT, Damiao MC, de Azevedo RA et al (2013) RPF101, a new capsaicin-like analogue, disrupts the microtubule network accompanied by arrest in the G2/M phase, inducing apoptosis and mitotic catastrophe in the MCF-7 breast cancer cells. Toxicol Appl Pharmacol 266:385–398

Dikic I, Johansen T, Kirkin V (2010) Selective autophagy in cancer development and therapy. Cancer Res 70:3431–3434

Dou D, Ahmad A, Yang H, Sarkar FH (2011) Tumor cell growth inhibition is correlated with levels of capsaicin present in hot peppers. Nutr Cancer 63:272–281

Eisenberg-Lerner A, Kimchi A (2009) The paradox of autophagy and its implication in cancer etiology and therapy. Apoptosis 14:376–391

Glick D, Barth S, Macleod KF (2010) Autophagy: cellular and molecular mechanisms. J Pathol 221:3–12

Hage-Sleiman R, Esmerian MO, Kobeissy H, Dbaibo G (2013) p53 and ceramide as collaborators in the stress response. Int J Mol Sci 14:4982–5012

Hail N Jr (2003) Mechanisms of vanilloid-induced apoptosis. Apoptosis 8:251–262

Hail N Jr, Lotan R (2002) Examining the role of mitochondrial respiration in vanilloid-induced apoptosis. J Natl Cancer Inst 94:1281–1292

Hardie DG, Alessi DR (2013) LKB1 and AMPK and the cancer-metabolism link-ten years after. BMC Biol 11:36

Hardie DG, Ross FA, Hawley SA (2012) AMP-activated protein kinase: a target for drugs both ancient and modern. Chem Biol 19:1222–1236

Horoszewicz JS, Leong SS, Kawinski E, Karr JP, Rosenthal H, Chu TM et al (1983) LNCaP model of human prostatic carcinoma. Cancer Res 43:1809–1818

Hsu CL, Yen GC (2007) Effects of capsaicin on induction of apoptosis and inhibition of adipogenesis in 3T3-L1 cells. J Agric Food Chem 55:1730–1736

Huang SP, Chen JC, Wu CC, Chen CT, Tang NY, Ho YT et al (2009) Capsaicin-induced apoptosis in human hepatoma HepG2 cells. Anticancer Res 29:165–174

Ip SW, Lan SH, Lu HF, Huang AC, Yang JS, Lin JP et al (2012) Capsaicin mediates apoptosis in human nasopharyngeal carcinoma NPC-TW 039 cells through mitochondrial depolarization and endoplasmic reticulum stress. Hum Exp Toxicol 31:539–549

Ito K, Nakazato T, Yamato K, Miyakawa Y, Yamada T, Hozumi N et al (2004) Induction of apoptosis in leukemic cells by homovanillic acid derivative, capsaicin, through oxidative stress: implication of phosphorylation of p53 at Ser-15 residue by reactive oxygen species. Cancer Res 64:1071–1078

Iype PT, Iype LE, Verma M, Kaighn ME (1998) Establishment and characterization of immortalized human cell lines from prostatic carcinoma and benign prostatic hyperplasia. Int J Oncol 12:257–263

Jankovic B, Loblaw DA, Nam R (2010) Capsaicin may slow PSA doubling time: case report and literature review. Can Urol Assoc J 4:E9–E11

Jiang Z, Gorenstein NM, Morre DM, Morre DJ (2008) Molecular cloning and characterization of a candidate human growth-related and time-keeping constitutive cell surface hydroquinone (NADH) oxidase. Biochemistry 47:14028–14038

Jordt SE, Julius D (2002) Molecular basis for species-specific sensitivity to "hot" chili peppers. Cell 108:421–430

Joung EJ, Li MH, Lee HG, Somparn N, Jung YS, Na HK et al (2007) Capsaicin induces heme oxygenase-1 expression in HepG2 cells via activation of PI3 K-Nrf2 signaling: NAD(P) H:quinone oxidoreductase as a potential target. Antioxid Redox Signal 9:2087–2098

Kang JH, Goto T, Han IS, Kawada T, Kim YM, Yu R (2010) Dietary capsaicin reduces obesity-induced insulin resistance and hepatic steatosis in obese mice fed a high-fat diet. Obesity (Silver Spring) 18:780–787

Kim CS, Park WH, Park JY, Kang JH, Kim MO, Kawada T et al (2004) Capsaicin, a spicy component of hot pepper, induces apoptosis by activation of the peroxisome proliferator-activated receptor gamma in HT-29 human colon cancer cells. J Med Food 7:267–273

Kim MY (2012) Nitric oxide triggers apoptosis in A375 human melanoma cells treated with capsaicin and resveratrol. Mol Med Rep 5:585–591

Kim MY, Trudel LJ, Wogan GN (2009) Apoptosis induced by capsaicin and resveratrol in colon carcinoma cells requires nitric oxide production and caspase activation. Anticancer Res 29:3733–3740

Kim YM, Hwang JT, Kwak DW, Lee YK, Park OJ (2007) Involvement of AMPK signaling cascade in capsaicin-induced apoptosis of HT-29 colon cancer cells. Ann N Y Acad Sci 1095:496–503

Lee GR, Shin MK, Yoon DJ, Kim AR, Yu R, Park NH et al (2013) Topical application of capsaicin reduces visceral adipose fat by affecting adipokine levels in high-fat diet-induced obese mice. Obesity (Silver Spring) 21:115–122

Lee MJ, Kee KH, Suh CH, Lim SC, Oh SH (2009) Capsaicin-induced apoptosis is regulated by endoplasmic reticulum stress- and calpain-mediated mitochondrial cell death pathways. Toxicology 264:205–214

Lee SH, Richardson RL, Dashwood RH, Baek SJ (2012) Capsaicin represses transcriptional activity of beta-catenin in human colorectal cancer cells. J Nutr Biochem 23:646–655

Lee YS, Kang YS, Lee JS, Nicolova S, Kim JA (2004) Involvement of NADPH oxidase-mediated generation of reactive oxygen species in the apototic cell death by capsaicin in HepG2 human hepatoma cells. Free Radic Res 38:405–412

Li S, Bode AM, Zhu F, Liu K, Zhang J, Kim MO et al (2011) TRPV1-antagonist AMG9810 promotes mouse skin tumorigenesis through EGFR/Akt signaling. Carcinogenesis 32:779–785

Lin CH, Lu WC, Wang CW, Chan YC, Chen MK (2013) Capsaicin induces cell cycle arrest and apoptosis in human KB cancer cells. BMC Complement Altern Med 13:46

Lishko PV, Procko E, Jin X, Phelps CB, Gaudet R (2007) The ankyrin repeats of TRPV1 bind multiple ligands and modulate channel sensitivity. Neuron 54:905–918

Liu NC, Hsieh PF, Hsieh MK, Zeng ZM, Cheng HL, Liao JW et al (2012) Capsaicin-mediated tNOX (ENOX2) up-regulation enhances cell proliferation and migration in vitro and in vivo. J Agric Food Chem 60:2758–2765

Lu HF, Chen YL, Yang JS, Yang YY, Liu JY, Hsu SC et al (2010) Antitumor activity of capsaicin on human colon cancer cells in vitro and colo 205 tumor xenografts in vivo. J Agric Food Chem 58:12999–13005

Llovet JM, Bruix J (2008) Molecular targeted therapies in hepatocellular carcinoma. Hepatology 48:1312–1327

Macho A, Calzado MA, Munoz-Blanco J, Gomez-Diaz C, Gajate C, Mollinedo F et al (1999) Selective induction of apoptosis by capsaicin in transformed cells: the role of reactive oxygen species and calcium. Cell Death Differ 6:155–165

Macho A, Sancho R, Minassi A, Appendino G, Lawen A, Munoz E (2003) Involvement of reactive oxygen species in capsaicinoid-induced apoptosis in transformed cells. Free Radic Res 37:611–619

Maity R, Sharma J, Jana NR (2010) Capsaicin induces apoptosis through ubiquitin-proteasome system dysfunction. J Cell Biochem 109:933–942

Malagarie-Cazenave S, Olea-Herrero N, Vara D, Diaz-Laviada I (2009) Capsaicin, a component of red peppers, induces expression of androgen receptor via PI3 K and MAPK pathways in prostate LNCaP cells. FEBS Lett 583:141–147

Mao LC, Wang HM, Lin YY, Chang TK, Hsin YH, Chueh PJ (2008) Stress-induced down-regulation of tumor-associated NADH oxidase during apoptosis in transformed cells. FEBS Lett 582:3445–3450

Matsuda A, Machii R (2013) Worldwide relative burden of cancer death in 2008 extrapolated from the WHO mortality database. Jpn J Clin Oncol 43:102

Moon DO, Kang CH, Kang SH, Choi YH, Hyun JW, Chang WY et al (2012) Capsaicin sensitizes TRAIL-induced apoptosis through Sp1-mediated DR5 up-regulation: involvement of Ca(2+) influx. Toxicol Appl Pharmacol 259:87–95

Mori A, Lehmann S, O'Kelly J, Kumagai T, Desmond JC, Pervan M et al (2006) Capsaicin, a component of red peppers, inhibits the growth of androgen-independent, p53 mutant prostate cancer cells. Cancer Res 66:3222–3229

Morre DJ, Caldwell S, Mayorga A, Wu LY, Morre DM (1997) NADH oxidase activity from sera altered by capsaicin is widely distributed among cancer patients. Arch Biochem Biophys 342:224–230

Morre DJ, Chueh PJ, Morre DM (1995) Capsaicin inhibits preferentially the NADH oxidase and growth of transformed cells in culture. Proc Natl Acad Sci U S A 92:1831–1835

Morre DJ, Hostetler B, Weston N, Kim C, Morre DM (2008) Cancer type-specific tNOX isoforms: a putative family of redox protein splice variants with cancer diagnostic and prognostic potential. BioFactors 34:201–207

Morre DJ, Sun E, Geilen C, Wu LY, de Cabo R, Krasagakis K et al (1996) Capsaicin inhibits plasma membrane NADH oxidase and growth of human and mouse melanoma lines. Eur J Cancer 32A:1995–2003

Mueller M, Beck V, Jungbauer A (2011) PPAR alpha activation by culinary herbs and spices. Planta Med 77:497–504

O'Neill J, Brock C, Olesen AE, Andresen T, Nilsson M, Dickenson AH (2012) Unravelling the mystery of capsaicin: a tool to understand and treat pain. Pharmacol Rev 64:939–971

Oh SH, Kim YS, Lim SC, Hou YF, Chang IY, You HJ (2008) Dihydrocapsaicin (DHC), a saturated structural analog of capsaicin, induces autophagy in human cancer cells in a catalase-regulated manner. Autophagy 4:1009–1019

Popovich DG, Tiaras F, Yeo CR, Zhang W (2010) Lovastatin interacts with natural products to influence cultured hepatocarcinoma cell (hep-g2) growth. J Am Coll Nutr 29:204–210

Pramanik KC, Boreddy SR, Srivastava SK (2011) Role of mitochondrial electron transport chain complexes in capsaicin mediated oxidative stress leading to apoptosis in pancreatic cancer cells. PLoS ONE 6:e20151

Pramanik KC, Srivastava SK (2012) Apoptosis signal-regulating kinase 1-thioredoxin complex dissociation by capsaicin causes pancreatic tumor growth suppression by inducing apoptosis. Antioxid Redox Signal 17:1417–1432

Prescott ED, Julius D (2003) A modular PIP2 binding site as a determinant of capsaicin receptor sensitivity. Science 300:1284–1288

Quaglia A, Lillini R, Crocetti E, Buzzoni C, and Vercelli M (2013) Incidence and mortality trends for four major cancers in the elderly and middle-aged adults: an international comparison. Surg Oncol 22(2):e31–e38

Rajput S, Mandal M (2012) Antitumor promoting potential of selected phytochemicals derived from spices: a review. Eur J Cancer Prev 21:205–215

Reilly CA, Ehlhardt WJ, Jackson DA, Kulanthaivel P, Mutlib AE, Espina RJ et al (2003) Metabolism of capsaicin by cytochrome P450 produces novel dehydrogenated metabolites and decreases cytotoxicity to lung and liver cells. Chem Res Toxicol 16:336–349

Reilly CA, Henion F, Bugni TS, Ethirajan M, Stockmann C, Pramanik KC et al (2013) Reactive intermediates produced from the metabolism of the vanilloid ring of capsaicinoids by P450 enzymes. Chem Res Toxicol 26(1):55–66

Rychkov GY, Barritt GJ (2011) Expression and function of TRP channels in liver cells. Adv Exp Med Biol 704:667–686

Sanchez AM, Malagarie-Cazenave S, Olea N, Vara D, Chiloeches A, Diaz-Laviada I (2007) Apoptosis induced by capsaicin in prostate PC-3 cells involves ceramide accumulation, neutral sphingomyelinase, and JNK activation. Apoptosis 12:2013–2024

Sanchez AM, Martinez-Botas J, Malagarie-Cazenave S, Olea N, Vara D, Lasuncion MA et al (2008) Induction of the endoplasmic reticulum stress protein GADD153/CHOP by capsaicin in prostate PC-3 cells: a microarray study. Biochem Biophys Res Commun 372:785–791

Sanchez AM, Sanchez MG, Malagarie-Cazenave S, Olea N, Diaz-Laviada I (2006) Induction of apoptosis in prostate tumor PC-3 cells and inhibition of xenograft prostate tumor growth by the vanilloid capsaicin. Apoptosis 11:89–99

Sanchez MG, Sanchez AM, Collado B, Malagarie-Cazenave S, Olea N, Carmena MJ et al (2005) Expression of the transient receptor potential vanilloid 1 (TRPV1) in LNCaP and PC-3 prostate cancer cells and in human prostate tissue. Eur J Pharmacol 515:20–27

Santoni G, Caprodossi S, Farfariello V, Liberati S, Gismondi A, Amantini C (2012) Antioncogenic effects of transient receptor potential vanilloid 1 in the progression of transitional urothelial cancer of human bladder. ISRN Urol 2012:458238

Schulze A, Harris AL (2012) How cancer metabolism is tuned for proliferation and vulnerable to disruption. Nature 491:364–373

Schwartz L, Guais A, Israel M, Junod B, Steyaert JM, Crespi E et al (2013) Tumor regression with a combination of drugs interfering with the tumor metabolism: efficacy of hydroxycitrate, lipoic acid and capsaicin. Invest New Drugs 31:256–264

Siegel R, DeSantis C, Virgo K, Stein K, Mariotto A, Smith T et al (2012) Cancer treatment and survivorship statistics, 2012. CA Cancer J Clin 62:220–241

Singh S, Natarajan K, Aggarwal BB (1996) Capsaicin (8-methyl-N-vanillyl-6-nonenamide) is a potent inhibitor of nuclear transcription factor-kappa B activation by diverse agents. J Immunol 157:4412–4420

Sinha K, Das J, Pal PB, Sil PC (2013) Oxidative stress: the mitochondria-dependent and mitochondria-independent pathways of apoptosis. Arch Toxicol 87(7):1157–1180

Stone KR, Mickey DD, Wunderli H, Mickey GH, Paulson DF (1978) Isolation of a human prostate carcinoma cell line (DU 145). Int J Cancer 21:274–281

Sung B, Prasad S, Ravindran J, Yadav VR, Aggarwal BB (2012) Capsazepine, a TRPV1 antagonist, sensitizes colorectal cancer cells to apoptosis by TRAIL through ROS-JNK-CHOP-mediated upregulation of death receptors. Free Radic Biol Med 53:1977–1987

Suresh D, Srinivasan K (2010) Tissue distribution & elimination of capsaicin, piperine & curcumin following oral intake in rats. Indian J Med Res 131:682–691

Surh YJ (2002) More than spice: capsaicin in hot chili peppers makes tumor cells commit suicide. J Natl Cancer Inst 94:1263–1265

Surh YJ, Lee SS (1995) Capsaicin, a double-edged sword: toxicity, metabolism, and chemopreventive potential. Life Sci 56:1845–1855

Tamburrino A, Piro G, Carbone C, Tortora G, Melisi D (2013) Mechanisms of resistance to chemotherapeutic and anti-angiogenic drugs as novel targets for pancreatic cancer therapy. Front Pharmacol 4:56

Thoennissen NH, O'Kelly J, Lu D, Iwanski GB, La DT, Abbassi S et al (2010) Capsaicin causes cell-cycle arrest and apoptosis in ER-positive and -negative breast cancer cells by modulating the EGFR/HER-2 pathway. Oncogene 29:285–296

Tsou MF, Lu HF, Chen SC, Wu LT, Chen YS, Kuo HM et al (2006) Involvement of Bax, Bcl-2, Ca^{2+} and caspase-3 in capsaicin-induced apoptosis of human leukemia HL-60 cells. Anticancer Res 26:1965–1971

Vaiopoulos AG, Athanasoula KC, Papavassiliou AG (2013) NF-kappaB in colorectal cancer. J Mol Med (Berl) 91(9):1029–1037

Vercelli C, Barbero R, Cuniberti B, Odore R, Re G (2013) Expression and functionality of TRPV1 receptor in human MCF-7 and canine CF.41 cells. Vet Comp Oncol. doi:10.1111/vco.12028 [Epub ahead of print]

Vickers AJ, Ulmert D, Sjoberg DD, Bennette CJ, Bjork T, Gerdtsson A et al (2013) Strategy for detection of prostate cancer based on relation between prostate specific antigen at age 40–55 and long term risk of metastasis: case-control study. BMJ 346:f2023

Vriens J, Janssens A, Prenen J, Nilius B, Wondergem R (2004) TRPV channels and modulation by hepatocyte growth factor/scatter factor in human hepatoblastoma (HepG2) cells. Cell Calcium 36:19–28

Wahyuni Y, Ballester AR, Sudarmonowati E, Bino RJ, Bovy AG (2013) Secondary metabolites of capsicum species and their importance in the human diet. J Nat Prod 76(4):783–793

Walpole CS, Bevan S, Bloomfield G, Breckenridge R, James IF, Ritchie T et al (1996) Similarities and differences in the structure-activity relationships of capsaicin and resiniferatoxin analogues. J Med Chem 39:2939–2952

Walpole CS, Wrigglesworth R, Bevan S, Campbell EA, Dray A, James IF et al (1993) Analogues of capsaicin with agonist activity as novel analgesic agents; structure-activity studies. 3. The hydrophobic side-chain "C-region". J Med Chem 36:2381–2389

Wang G, Yang ZQ, Zhang K (2010) Endoplasmic reticulum stress response in cancer: molecular mechanism and therapeutic potential. Am J Transl Res 2:65–74

Wang HM, Chueh PJ, Chang SP, Yang CL, Shao KN (2008) Effect of Ccapsaicin on tNOX (ENOX2) protein expression in stomach cancer cells. BioFactors 34:209–217

Ward PS, Thompson CB (2012) Metabolic reprogramming: a cancer hallmark even Warburg did not anticipate. Cancer Cell 21:297–308

Wolvetang EJ, Larm JA, Moutsoulas P, Lawen A (1996) Apoptosis induced by inhibitors of the plasma membrane NADH-oxidase involves Bcl-2 and calcineurin. Cell Growth Differ 7:1315–1325

Yang J, Luo B, Xu G, Li T, Chen Y, Zhang T (2013) Low-concentration capsaicin promotes colorectal cancer metastasis by triggering ROS production and modulating Akt/mTOR and STAT-3 pathways. Neoplasma 60(4):364–372

Yang ZH, Wang XH, Wang HP, Hu LQ, Zheng XM, Li SW (2010) Capsaicin mediates cell death in bladder cancer T24 cells through reactive oxygen species production and mitochondrial depolarization. Urology 75:735–741

Yessoufou A, Wahli W (2010) Multifaceted roles of peroxisome proliferator-activated receptors (PPARs) at the cellular and whole organism levels. Swiss Med Wkly 140:w13071

Yoon JH, Ahn SG, Lee BH, Jung SH, Oh SH (2012) Role of autophagy in chemoresistance: regulation of the ATM-mediated DNA-damage signaling pathway through activation of DNA-PKcs and PARP-1. Biochem Pharmacol 83:747–757

Yoshitani SI, Tanaka T, Kohno H, Takashima S (2001) Chemoprevention of azoxymethane-induced rat colon carcinogenesis by dietary capsaicin and rotenone. Int J Oncol 19:929–939

Youssef J, Badr M (2011) Peroxisome proliferator-activated receptors and cancer challenges and opportunities. Br J Pharmacol 164(1):68–82

Zhai XJ, Chen JG, Liu JM, Shi F, Lu YN (2013) Food-drug interactions: effect of capsaicin on the pharmacokinetics of simvastatin and its active metabolite in rats. Food Chem Toxicol 53:168–173

Zhang J, Nagasaki M, Tanaka Y, Morikawa S (2003) Capsaicin inhibits growth of adult T-cell leukemia cells. Leuk Res 27:275–283

Zhang JH, Lai FJ, Chen H, Luo J, Zhang RY, Bu HQ et al (2013) Involvement of the phosphoinositide 3-kinase/Akt pathway in apoptosis induced by capsaicin in the human pancreatic cancer cell line PANC-1. Oncol Lett 5:43–48

Zhang QH, Hu JP, Wang BL, Li Y (2012) Effects of capsaicin and dihydrocapsaicin on human and rat liver microsomal CYP450 enzyme activities in vitro and in vivo. J Asian Nat Prod Res 14:382–395

Zhang R, Humphreys I, Sahu RP, Shi Y, Srivastava SK (2008) In vitro and in vivo induction of apoptosis by capsaicin in pancreatic cancer cells is mediated through ROS generation and mitochondrial death pathway. Apoptosis 13:1465–1478

Zhu Y, Qi C, Korenberg JR, Chen XN, Noya D, Rao MS et al (1995) Structural organization of mouse peroxisome proliferator-activated receptor gamma (mPPAR gamma) gene: alternative promoter use and different splicing yield two mPPAR gamma isoforms. Proc Natl Acad Sci U S A 92:7921–7925

Chapter 9
Capsaicin as New Orally Applicable Gastroprotective and Therapeutic Drug Alone or in Combination with Nonsteroidal Anti-Inflammatory Drugs in Healthy Human Subjects and in Patients

Gyula Mózsik

Abstract Background: Capsaicin is a specific compound acting on capsaicin-sensitive afferent nerves. Aim: Capsaicin was used to study the different events of human gastrointestinal physiology, pathology, and clinical pharmacology, and possible therapeutic approaches to enhance gastrointestinal mucosal defense in healthy human subjects and in patients with various different gastrointestinal disorders as well as its use with nonsteroidal anti-inflammatory drugs (NSAIDs) in healthy subjects and in patients. Materials and Methods: The observations were carried out in 198 healthy human subjects and in 178 patients with different gastrointestinal (GI) diseases (gastritis, erosions, ulcer, polyps, cancer, inflammatory bowel diseases, colorectal polyps, cancers), and in 69 patients with chronic (Helicobacter pylori positive and negative) gastritis (before and after eradication treatment). The gastric secretory responses and their chemical composition, gastric emptying, sugar loading test, gastric transmucosal potential difference (GTPD) with application of capsaicin alone, after ethanol alone and with capsaicin, indomethacin-induced gastric mucosal microbleeding without and with capsaicin were studied. The immunohistochemical examinations of the capsaicin receptor (TRVP1), calcitonin gene- related peptide (CGRP), and substance P (SP) were carried out in gastrointestinal tract, and especially in patients with chronic gastritis (with and without Helicobacter infection, before and after classical eradication treatment). Classical molecular pharmacological methods were applied to study the drugs inhibiting the gastric basal acid output. Results: Capsaicin decreased the gastric basal output, enhanced the "non-parietal" (buffering) component of gastric secretory responses, and gastric emptying, and the release of glucagon. Capsaicin

G. Mózsik (✉)
First Department of Medicine Medical and Health Centre, University of Pécs, Pécs H-7643, Hungary
e-mail: gyula.mozsik@aok.pte.hu; gyula.mozsik@gmail.com

O. M. E. Abdel-Salam (ed.), *Capsaicin as a Therapeutic Molecule*, Progress in Drug Research 68, DOI: 10.1007/978-3-0348-0828-6_9, © Springer Basel 2014

prevented the indomethacin- and ethanol-induced gastric mucosal damage; meanwhile capsaicin itself enhanced (GTPD). Capsaicin prevented the indomethacin-induced gastric mucosal microbleeding. The expression of TRVP1 and CGRP increased in the gastric mucosa of patients with chronic gastritis (independently of the presence of Helicobacter pylori infection), and the successfully carried out eradication treatment. The human first phase examinations (the application of acetylsalicylic acid (ASA), diclofenac, and naproxen together with capcaicinoids) (given in doses that stimulate capsaicin-sensitive afferent vagal nerves) showed no change in the pharmacokinetic parameters of ASA and diclofenac and the ASA and diclofenac-induced platelet aggregation. Conclusions: Capsaicin represents a new orally applicable gastroprotective agent in healthy human subjects and in patients with different chemical and Helicobacter pylori-induced mucosal damage and in many other diseases requiring treatment with NSAIDs.

9.1 Introduction

Capsaicin is an active ingredient of red pepper and paprika. These plants are well known and used in every day of the culinary practice for about 7500 years.

It was an important discovery that capsaicin (capsaicin, dihydrocapsaicin, nordihydrocapsaicin, and other capsaicinoids) specifically modify the function of capsaicin-sensitive afferent nerves (Jancsó et al. 1967, 1968, 1970).

Capsaicin activates the capsaicin (vanilloid) receptor expressed in a subgroup of primary afferent nociceptive neurons (Szolcsányi 2004). The capsaicin receptor has been cloned (Caterina et al. 1997) and turned out to be a cation channel. It is gated besides capsaicin and other capsaicinoids (some vanilloids) by low pH, noxious heat, and various pain-producing endogenous and exogenous chemicals. Thus, these sensory nerve endings equipped with these ion channels are prone to be stimulated in gastric mucosa.

The action of capsaicin on capsaicin-sensitive afferent nerves is a dose-dependent (Szolcsányi and Barthó 1981; Szolcsányi 1984, 1997, 2004; Abdel-Salam et al. 1999, 2001; Mózsik et al. 2001). Szolcsányi indicated four different stages of capsaicin action (depending on the dose and duration of the exposure to the compound): (a) Excitation (stage 1); (b) Sensory blocking effect (stage 2); (c) Long-term selective neurotoxin impairment (stage 3), and (d) Irreversible cell destruction (stage 4) (Szolcsányi 1984). The stages 1 and 2 are reversible, while the stages 3 and 4 are irreversible compound-induced actions on capsaicin sensitive afferent nerves. These stages of capsaicin actions can be detected in the gastrointestinal tract (Mózsik et al. 2001) in animal experiments.

The vagal nerve has a key role in the development of gastrointestinal mucosal damage and prevention (Mózsik et al. 1982). The key role of vagal nerve has been emphasized dominantly in the aggressive processes to gastrointestinal (GI) mucosa (such as peptic ulcer disease, gastric mucosal damage, etc.) in both animal models and as well as in human clinical practice. The "chemical" and "surgical" vagotomy were widely used in the treatment of patients with peptic ulcer disease in the years up to middle of 1970 (Karádi and Mózsik 2000). By other words, the primary aim of this therapy was to decrease the activity of vagal nerve at the level of efferent nerve.

The application of capsaicin in the animals experiments was used as a specific tool to approach the group of primary afferent nociceptive neurons (Szolcsányi 2004; Buck and Burks 1986; Holzer 1988, 1991, 2013; Szállasi and Blumberg 1999) involved in the different physiological, pathological processes, and medical therapy in healthy human subjects, and in patients with different GI disorders as well as those treated with NSAIDs.

Szolcsányi and Barthó (1981) were the first who clearly indicated the beneficial and harmful effect of capsaicin in the peptic ulcer disease in rats that depended on the applied doses of capsaicin. Later, Holzer started a very extensive research work with capsaicin in the field of gastroenterology (Holzer 1998, 1999, 2013; Buck and Burks 1986; Szállasi and Blumberg 1999; Holzer and Sametz 1986; Holzer and Lippe 1988). Our group also participated in the GI capsaicin research in animal experiments beginning from 1980 (Mózsik et al. 1997).

Even the new drug "Lafutidine" a Histamin-2-receptor (H_2R) blocking compound, that was developed in the medical treatment of GI mucosal damage and marketed in Japan (Ajioka et al. 2000, 2002; Onodera et al. 1999; Takeuchi 2006) showed typical capsaicin actions at the target organ.

The new and interesting results obtained with capsaicin application in animal experiments offered excellent tools to approach the different events of human gastrointestinal physiology, pathology, and pharmacology, and to produce new drug or new drug combinations in healthy human subjects and patients with different GI and other diseases (myocardial infarction, thrombophilia, rheumatoid arthritis, chronic pain killer use).

We started with clinical studies with capsaicin from 1997 (Debreceni et al. 1999; Mózsik et al. 1999, 2004a, b, 2005) and these studies incorporated the different regulatory mechanisms of capsaicin in the human stomach, gastric mucosal preventive effects of capsaicin(noids) on the NSAIDs-induced gastric mucosal damage, chronic gastritis with Helicobacter pylori (H. pylori) positive and negative gastritis (with and without eradication treatment). We performed immunohistochemical examinations of capsaicin receptor (TRVP1), Calcitonin Gene-Related Peptide (CGRP), SP in the human gastrointestinal mucosa of patients with different GI disorders, took significant steps for the development of a capsaicin containing drug (alone) and in combination with NSAIDs (capsaicin plus aspirin, diclofenac, naproxen), including the preparation of protocols for human phase I examinations (and to carry out these examinations after the receiving permission from the National Institute of Pharmacy (Budapest, Hungary) and National Clinical Pharmacological and Ethical Committee of Hungary).

These studies were carried out in prospective, randomized, and multiclinical studies of healthy human subjects, patients with various gastrointestinal disorders including gastric mucosal damage produced by application of NSAIDs or H. pylori infection.

The aims of this review are: (1) to give a short summary on the actions of capsaicin on the human gastrointestinal tract (dominantly on the stomach); (2) to indicate some details of gastroprotective actions of capsaicin in healthy human subjects; (3) to demonstrate the capsaicin-induced gastric protective actions against the NSAIDs-(COX-1 and COX-2 inhibitor or a nonselective COX inhibitor) drug-induced gastric microbleedings in healthy human subjects; (4) to prove the independency the expression of TRPV1 and CGRP expression from the presence of the Helicobacter pylori positive or Helicobacter pylori −ve chronic gastritis, the efficacy of successfully carried out eradication treatment in patients with Helicobacter pylori positive gastritis in patients; (5) to indicate the clinical pharmacological problems of plant origin capsaicin in humans (in term of drug processing); (6) to draw attention to capsaicin actions (given orally in stimulatory doses) on capsaicin-sensitive afferent nerves); (7) to illustrate these gastroprotective effects of capsaicin in healthy human subjects in the treatment of those who have been under chronic NSAID use (like patients with myocardial infarction, stroke, thrombophilia, rheumatic diseases, etc.).

In terms of classical pharmacology, we would like to demonstrate clearly that the applied doses of capsaicin in the human observations stimulates capsaicin-sensitive afferent nerve with a clear-cut exclusion of capsaicin desensitization.

On the other hand, our research activity clearly demonstrates the different difficulties of capsaicin(oids) application as new gastroprotective drug for healthy subjects and patients with different GI disorders and NSAIDs used in regards to toxicology plant cultivation, storage, chemical detection and standardization questions as well as permission request from authorities needed prior the launch of industrial processing of plant-derived, orally applicable drug or drug combinations.

Our attention was focused toward the effects of capsaicin on the human gastrointestinal tract in healthy conditions and in various gastrointestinal disorders, and the development of a new capsaicin containing drug (alone) or in different combinations (NSAIDs plus capsaicin: aspirin, diclofenac, naproxen) together with nationally and internationally accepted by the responsible authorities working in this field.

9.2 Materials and Methods

9.2.1 Subjects

The observations were carried out in 198 healthy human subjects aged 25–65 years (40 ± 10 years) and in 178 patients with various gastrointestinal disorders (gastritis, erosion, ulcer, polyps, cancer, and chronic inflammatory bowel diseases, polyps, precancerous states, colorectal cancer) aged 25–75 years (45 ± 10) as well as on 69 patients with chronic gastritis aged 39–68 years (mean: 56.4 years) (altogether 445 healthy persons and GI patients).

The observations were carried out at First Department of Medicine and Institute of Cardiology, Medical and Health Centre of Pécs, Hungary, Department of Gastroenterology of Petz Aladár Teaching Hospital, Győr, Hungary, Department of Gastroenterology of Markusovszky Hospital, Szombathely, Hungary (and their relevant Departments of Pathology), Department of Pharmacology and Pharmacotherapy and Institute of Pharmaceutical Chemistry, Medical and Health Centre, University of Pécs, Hungary, Histopathology Ltd., Pécs, Hungary and our industrial research partner (PannonPharma Ltd., Pécsvárad, Hungary).

The healthy human subjects and patients were included into the groups of different randomized, prospective studies (see later).

The classical human phase I examinations were carried out in 15 healthy males in each protocol (additionally up today, 30 healthy human subjects for human phase I examinations for aspirin plus capsaicin and diclofenac plus capsaicin).

The physical, laboratory, and iconographic examinations were normal in the healthy human subjects, in patients with various gastrointestinal disorders.

The healthy persons were randomized into different groups of prospective, randomized, and prospective studies for evaluation of the effects of capsaicin on:

1. Basal gastric acid secretion (Mózsik et al. 1999);
2. Changes in cations, anions, albumin concentration (and outputs) of gastric secretory responses (Mózsik et al. 2004a, 2005);
3. Gastric emptying (Debreceni et al. 1999);
4. Sugar (glucose) loading test (75 g given orally) (Dömötör et al. 2006b);
5. Gastric transmucosal potential difference (GTPD) alone (Mózsik et al. 2005);
6. GTPD measurement after intragastric administration of ethanol and capsaicin application (Mózsik et al. 2005);
7. Indomethacin-induced gastric microbleedings without and with capsaicin (Fisher and Hunt 1976).

The different doses of capsaicin (1–8 μg/100 mL in saline solution) were intragastrically given to identify the ED_{50} values on the gastric basal acid secretion. These doses of capsaicin were used to determine direct action of capsaicin on the GTPD (without and with intragastric administration of ethanol) and indomethacin-induced gastric microbleedings.

All of the healthy volunteers received capsaicin in doses in random allocation. In the observations to study the gastric emptying, sugar loading test, the effect of the ED_{50} value (400 μg intragastrically given) of capsaicin was tested.

The 178 patients with different gastrointestinal disorders were studied by immunohistochemical examinations of biopsy samples. The histological diagnosis was established based on the opinion of independent pathologist. The immunohistochemical examinations for TRVP1, CGRP, and SP were carried out on the same paraffin-embedded tissue samples from which the classical histological diagnosis was established by the independent pathologist.

The patients with chronic gastritis (69 patients) were divided into Helicobacter positive and negative groups. Smaller group of patients with Helicobacter pylori infection were further studied after classical eradication treatment had been performed.

The observations were carried out according to the method of Good Clinical Practice (GCP). The studies were carried out from 1997 up to now and which were permitted by the Regional Ethical Committee of Pécs University, Hungary. Written informed consent was obtained from all participants.

The human phase I examinations were permitted by the National Institute of Pharmacy (Budapest, Hungary) and National Clinical Pharmacological and Ethical Committee (Budapest, Hungary). These studies were performed in years of 2011–2012.

The following main methods were used in the human observations:

9.2.2 Determination of Gastric Basal Acid Out

Determination of Gastric Basal Acid Out (BAO) in healthy human subjects. After an overnight fasting, a nasogastric tube was introduced at 8.00 a.m., and the total gastric content was suctioned. Then the newly secreted gastric juice was suctioned every 15 min for 1 h (BAO). The healthy subjects received intragastrically capsaicin (100, 200, 400 and 800 μg ig.), atropine (0.1–1.0 mg sc.), Pirenzepine 25–50 mg, famotidine (20–40 mg orally), ranitidine (150–300 mg orally), cimetidine (100–1000 mg orally), Omeprazole (20–40 mg iv.), and Esomeprazole (20–40 mg orally) given for determination of their dose responses curves (Mózsik et al. 2005, 2007; Szabó et al. 2013).

Gastric acid secretion was measured by titration of gastric juice with 0.1 N NaOH to pH 7.0 (pH titrimeter, Radelkis, Budapest). The gastric acid outputs were expressed as mmol/h (mean ± SEM).

9.2.3 Determination of Affinity and Intrinsic Activity Curves

Determination of affinity and intrinsic activity curves for drugs inhibiting BAO in healthy human subjects. The applied doses of drugs were expressed in molar values, which were used to determine the affinity and intrinsic activity curves of the different drugs by the method of Csáky (1969). For drawing the affinity and intrinsic activity curves the doses of various drugs were expressed in (−) molar values, which offered to analyze the drug actions on the BAO according to the classical molecular pharmacological methods. We identified the pD_2 values (necessary doses of drugs to produce 50 % inhibition on BAO values). The effect of atropine ($\alpha_{atropine} = 1.00$) in case of identification of intrinsic activity curves for other drugs and capsaicin (Mózsik 2006).

9.2.4 Chemical Composition of Gastric Juice Without and with Capsaicin Application

These observations were carried out in the same healthy human subjects. The concentrations of Na^+, K^+, and calcium^{2+} in the gastric juice were measured flame photometrically. The concentration of Mg^{2+} was measured by atomic absorption spectrophotometrically, the chloride concentration by colorimetric method, the protein content by the method of biuret reaction. The 400 μg of capsaicin (as ED_{50} value) was used in these studies.

9.2.5 *Calculation of "Parietal" and "Non-Parietal" Components of Gastric Secretory Responses Without and with Capsaicin*

The chloride linked to H^+ and sodium was calculated for the determination of "parietal" (chloride linked to H^+) and "non-parietal" (linked to sodium) components of gastric BAO (Hollander 1934).

9.2.6 *Measurement of Gastric Transmucosal Potential Difference*

Gastric Transmucosal Potential Difference (GTPD) was measured during endoscopy. The exploring mucosal electrode was passed through the biopsy channel of gastroscope and the reference electrode was placed on the volar surface of the left forearm. The electrodes were connected to a digital voltmeter (Radelkis, Budapest, Hungary, OP 211/1). GTPD measurements were done at the greater curvature of the gastric body and the results were expressed in –mV (without and with intragastrically administration of different doses of capsaicin) (Hossennbocus et al. 1975; Mózsik et al. 2005). Five mL capsaicin (300 mL/L, diluted in saline) was intragastrically applied and only saline solution was given to identify the baseline in GTPD. The Δ GTPD values were expressed in –mV, ΔGTPD max was calculated at 5 min after intragastric application of capsaicin.

9.2.7 *Effect of Capsaicin on Ethanol-Induced Changes GTPD Changes*

The GTPD baseline was identified. Then ethanol (5 mL, 300 mL/L) was intragastrically given. The GTPD change was determined after the ethanol had been passed through the biopsy channel of gastroscope without and with capsaicin administration (given in different doses in the same pathway after 1 min of ethanol administration).

9.2.8 Gastric Microbleeding Measurements Produced by Application of Indomethacin Produced by Acute Administration of Indomethacin (Without with Capsaicin Administration) in Healthy Human Subjects

Indomethacin (IND) (as one of the non- selective COX-inhibitors) produces gastric microbleeding. The extent of indomethacin-induced gastric microbleeding was measured in healthy human subjects by the method of hemoglobin concentration in the gastric juice respecting the value of gastric emptying rate (Fisher and Hunt 1976). The details of this method were described earlier (Mózsik et al. 2005).

9.2.8.1 Indomethacin (IND)-Induced Gastric Mucosal Microbleedings in Acute Observations in Healthy Human Subjects

The baseline of gastric microbleeding was measured in the gastric juice without application of any drug and/or capsaicin.

The hemoglobin concentration was determined. The extent of gastric emptying was measured with application of phenol red into the stomach (by the method of Fisher and Hunt 1976; Nagy et al. 1984). The extent of gastric microbleeding was expressed in mL/day (mean $\pm$ SEM), and this value was taken as baseline (used as control for other observations).

9.2.8.2 Capsaicin-Induced Acute Mucosal Protection on the IND-Induced Acute Gastric Microbleeding in Healthy Human Subjects

The healthy human subjects received IND (3×25 mg given orally for a day), and the forthcoming day the gastric microbleeding was measured on forthcoming day, when these healthy human subjects also received 25 mg IND orally. The extent of gastric microbleeding was measured as mentioned above, and its value was expressed as mL/day (mean $\pm$ SEM).

9.2.9 Measurement of Gastric Emptying by Stable Isotope Method (Infrared Spectroscopy, IRIS, Izinta, Budapest, Hungary)

The gastric emptying measurements were performed on two consecutive days by the same protocol, without capsaicin on first day and with capsaicin on second day. The measurement procedure was the following. The healthy human subjects went on an overnight starvation and the observations were started at 8.00 a.m. In total, 100 mL of ^{13}C-octanoid acid (Izinta, Budapest, Hungary) was given for the gastric emptying measurements. This material was given in 200 mL physiological saline and 75 g glucose was added to the solution. The volunteers exhaled into a plastic bag with a volume of 0.5 L. The first air sample was considered as reference. Then, the volunteers swallowed the test solution and gave air samples in every 15 min. The IRIS performed the infrared spectroscopy (IRIS, Izinta, Budapest, Hungary) measurements and calculated the delta over base (DOB) values. This value was directly proportional to the ratio $^{13}CO_2$ and $^{12}CO_2$ (DOB is about $^{13}CO_2/^{12}CO_2$) in the air sample. When we respected the DOB values against the time in the graph, we obtained a curve (gastric emptying curve). On this curve, we could consider the following four parameters to characterize gastric emptying rate: (1) maximal value of DOB (DOB_{max} unit) (U); (2) the time at DOB_{max} (U/min); (3) the slope of the rising part of the curve (U/min), and (4) time at 50 % of area under curve ($AUC_{50\ \%}$, min). The DOB_{max} and slope are direct, meanwhile the time at DOB_{max} and the tome at $AUC_{50\ \%}$ are inversely proportional to gastric emptying (Debreceni et al. 1999; Mózsik et al. 2004a).

9.2.10 *Sugar Loading Test in Healthy Human Subjects (75 g Glucose Given Orally)*

The glucose (75 g) was orally given in 100 mL water. The plasma level of glucose was measured enzymatically (Boehringer, Germany). The plasma levels of insulin (μIU/mL) (Biochem Immunsystem), C-peptide and glucagon (pg/mL) (Byk-Sangtect Diagnostic GmbH) were measured by RIA. All measurements were carried out before and after administration repeatedly every 15 min for 4 h period (Dömötör et al. 2006b).

9.2.11 *Immunohistochemical Examinations in the Gastric and Large Bowel Mucosa in Patients with Various Disorders*

The classical histopathological examinations were carried out by an independent pathologist for giving the histopathological diagnosis of patients (besides the classical laboratory, iconographic examinations).

The specific immunohistochemical examinations were used for the same biopsy specimens used for pathological examination. Specific immune antisera were used for detection of vanilloid (TRVP1) receptor (polyclonal anti-TRVP1, Abcam, Cambridge, UK), CGRP (polyclonal anti-CGRP, Abcam, Cambridge, UK), and substance P (monoclonal anti SP, Abcam, Cambridge, UK).

The TRVP1 and CGRP positivity and/or negativity was detected, meanwhile SP staining was evaluated by a semiquantitative scale (Dömötör et al. 2005).

9.2.12 Detection of Helicobacter Pylori in Patients with Chronic Gastritis

The presence of Helicobacter pylori was detected by ^{13}C-urea breath test (Izinta, Hungary) and with specific histological staining of biopsy specimens. The diagnosis of chronic gastritis was based on the classical pathological histology. The results of observations were expressed as mean $\pm$ SEM. The unpaired and paired Student's t tests were used for the calculation of results between the identical observations. *P* value ≤ 0.05 was considered statistically significant.

9.2.13 Evaluation of Capsaicin-Stimulated Gastric Mucosal Protection on IND-Induced Gastric Microbleeding and Capsaicin-Produced Gastric Mucosal Protection on the IND-Induced Gastric Microbleeding Before and After 2 Weeks Capsaicin Treatment (Based on Randomized, Prospective and Multiclinical Study in Healthy Subjects) (Mózsik et al. 2004a, 2005, 2007)

9.2.13.1 Measurement of Gastric Microbleeding Before and After 2 Weeks Capsaicin Treatment

The baseline in gastric microbleeding was measured and carried out as those under the point of Sect. 9.2.8.1. The gastric microbleeding was expressed in mL/day (mean $\pm$ SEM).

9.2.13.2 Measurement of IND-Induced Acute Gastric Microbleeding Before and After 2 Week Capsaicin Treatment

These measurements were carried out in healthy human subjects as those written under Sect. 9.2.8.2. These healthy subjects received 3×25 mg IND for 1 day and 25 mg IND on the next day before the measurement of the extent of gastric microbleeding. The gastric microbleeding was expressed in mL/day (mean $\pm$ SEM).

9.2.13.3 Measurement of Capsaicin-Induced Acute Gastric Mucosal Protection Against the IND-Induced Acute Gastric Microbleeding Before and After 2 Week Capsaicin Treatment

The observations were carried out under the observational circumstances mentioned in 12.2, however, different doses of capsaicin (200 and 400 μg given orally) were used. 200 and 400 μg capsaicin were applied given orally before the measurement of IND-induced acute gastric microbleeding before and after 2 week capsaicin treatment.

9.2.14 Evaluation of Capsaicin's Effect by Randomized, Prospective, Multiclinical Studies in Patients with Chronic Helicobacter Pylori Positive Gastritis Before and After Eradication Treatment to Capsaicin Effect Due to Stimulation of Capsaicin-Sensitive Neural Afferentation (Lakner et al. 2011)

These studies were carried out in 38 persons (including 20 healthy persons and 18 patients with H. pylori positive gastritis). The histologically normal controls were 41–67 years, mean: 52.1 years, meanwhile the ages of patients with chronic Helicobacter pylori infection were 39–68 years, mean: 56.4 years (Lakner et al. 2011).

The presence of H. pylori was determined by the methods mentioned above.

The eradication therapy involved a 7 days treatment with double dose proton pump inhibitor consisting of pantoprazole (2 × 40 mg/day), amoxicillin (1000 mg twice daily), and clarithromycin (500 mg twice daily) according to European guidelines (Malfertheiner et al. 2007). Following this 1 week of eradication period, the patients were further treated with normal dose of pantoprazole for another week.

The gastroscopies, gastric biopsies, general, and special immunohistochemical examinations were carried out at the time of entry of patients into the eradication treatment and after the eradication treatment (Lakner et al. 2011).

9.2.15 Animal Toxicological Examinations Required by Hungarian Authorities to Receiving Permission for Human Phase I. Examinations

The National Institute of Pharmacy (Budapest, Hungary) and National Clinical Pharmacological and Ethical Committee (Budapest, Hungary) requested additional geno- and other toxicological examinations with natural capsaicin (Capsaicin Natural USP 27), since limited knowledge were known about the circumstances of its cultivation, collection, storage, stability, preparation, and chemical composition. Few literature data suggested genotoxicity in certain preparation. Further research suggested that to be dependent on environmental factors, since these tested were negative for synthetic capsaicin.

These required studies with natural capsaicin from India were: (1) testing of natural capsaicin with bacterial reverse mutation assay; (2) testing of mutagenic effect of test item natural capsaicin by mouse micronucleus test; (3) 14 day oral average dose 120 mg/kg body weight given orally for 14 days; (4) determination of natural capsaicin's toxic oral dose in Beagle dogs (placebo, 0.3–0.6–0.9 mg/kg body weight given orally for 14 days); (5) 28 day oral toxicology study of natural capsaicin in rats (used placebo treatment, 5, 15, and 30 mg/kg body weight); (6) 28 day oral toxicology and kinetic study in Beagle dogs (placebo, 0.1, 0.3, and 0.9 mg/kg body weight/day orally given for 28 days) (Mózsik et al. 2010).

9.2.16 Human Phase I. Clinical Pharmacological Studies

The National Institute of Pharmacy (Budapest, Hungary) permitted to carry out three human phase I. examinations. The aims of these studies were: (1) The safety of capsaicin containing drug combinations (capsaicin plus aspirin, capsaicin plus diclofenac, and capsaicin plus naproxen); (2) The measurements of different pharmacokinetic parameters (capsaicin and NSAIDs); (3) The measurements of different orally given capsaicin on the pharmacokinetic parameters of NSAIDs; (4) Testing the effects of NAIDs or capsaicin (given alone and co-administrations) on the platelet aggregations.

These observations were carried out in healthy males (15 healthy persons participated in each protocol study) (for further details, see below).

9.2.17 Used Drugs and Compounds

Anticholinergic (atropine, Egis, Budapest, Hungary), antimuscarinic (Pirenzepine, Boehringer, Ingelheim, Germany) agents; (histamine H_2-receptor antagonists (Cimetidine, PannonPharma, Hungary), ranitidine (Biogal-Teva, Hungary), famotidine (Richter Gedeon, Hungary), proton pump inhibitors (PPI) (Omeprazole, Astra-Zeneca, Sweden), Esomeprazole (Astra-Zeneca, Sweden)); indomethacin (Chinoin, Budapest, Hungary).

Capsaicin was applied in these studies was obtained from Asian Herbex Ltd (Capsaicin USP as manufactured in Andhra Pradesh, India). The Drug Master File (DMF) is signed in the documentation of Drug and Food Administration (FDA) in the United States as only one capsaicin preparation for orally applicable preparation (17856 A II 26.10.2004 Asian Herbex Ltd.: Capsaicin USP as manufactured in Andhra Pradesh, India) (for further details, see Mózsik et al. 2009a, b).

9.2.18 Statistical Evaluation of the Results

The results were expressed as mean ± SEM. The paired, unpaired Student's t test, and ANOVA test were used for the statistical analysis of the results. The results were taken to be significant if the $P \leq 0.05$. Special mathematical programs were applied for the evaluation of results of human phase I. examinations.

9.3 Results

9.3.1 Capsaicin-Induced Gastric BAO in Healthy Human Subjects

Capsaicin (given in doses of 100, 200, 400, and 800 μg orally) dose-dependently inhibited the gastric acid output ($Y = -0.13X + 1.164$; $r = 0.97$; $n = 16$; $P < 0.001$)

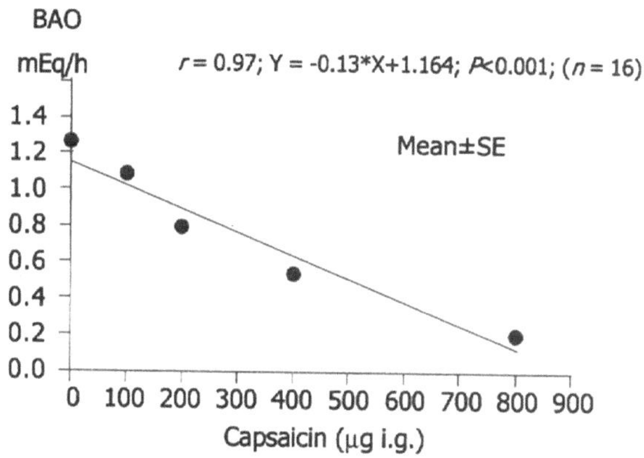

Fig. 9.1 Inhibition of gastric acid basal output (BAO) by capsaicin in 16 healthy human subjects. (After Mózsik et al. 2005)

(Mózsik et al. 1999, 2005). The ED_{50} value of capsaicin was obtained as 400 μg/person on the gastric BAO (in case of administration of capsaicin in doses which stimulates capsaicin-sensitive afferent nerves) (Fig. 9.1) (Mózsik et al. 2005).

9.3.2 *Affinity and Intrinsic Affinity Curves for the Capsaicin, Muscarinic (Atropine, Pirenzepine), H2-Receptor Antagonists (Cimetidine, Ranitidine, Famotidine), and Proton Pump Inhibitors (Omeprazole and Esomeprazole) on the Gastric BAO in Healthy Human Subjects*

The action of the compounds inhibiting the gastric basal acid secretion is shown in Fig. 9.2. The curve indicates that no competitive actions of these drugs exist on the gastric basal acid output. The pD_2 values were calculated from the affinity curves obtained in the molecular pharmacological studies.

The intrinsic activity curves for the drugs inhibiting the gastric basal acid outputs in healthy human subjects were calculated. The intrinsic activity ($\alpha_{atropine} = 1.00$) was taken to be equal to 1.00, and the values for other drugs were expressed to action of atropine (Fig. 9.3). The pA_2 values (50 % inhibition of intrinsic activity in (−) molar values) were calculated from the intrinsic activity curves.

For the molecular pharmacological understanding the background of the action of drugs, action the molecular weights, pD_2 values, of the intrinsic activity (in comparison to atropine action) and pA_2 values were calculated and shown in Table 9.1.

The Figs. 9.2 and 9.3, Table 9.1 clearly indicate that capsaicin acts in the smaller doses as those drugs acting on the muscarinic (atropine, Pirenzepine), H_2R (cimetidine, ranitidine, famotidine, nizatidine) receptors and proton pump inhibitors (omeprazole, esomeprazole).

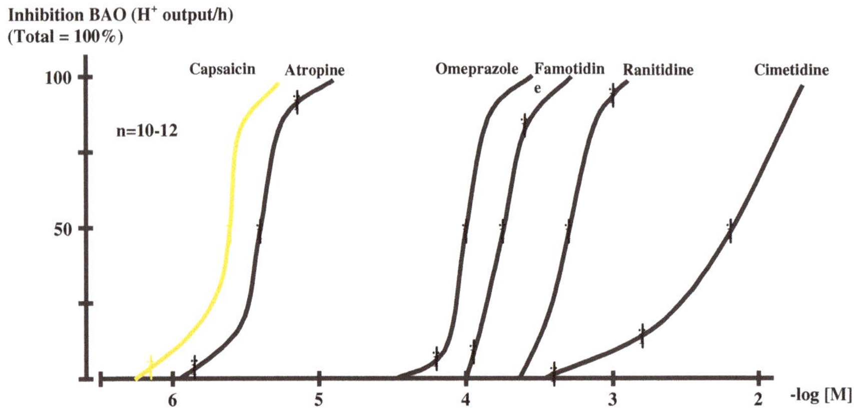

Fig. 9.2 Affinity curves for drugs inhibitory actions of different antisecretory drugs on the BAO in healthy human subjects. The absolute values were calculated as H^+ output/h, the presentations of curves expressed in percent value (total = 100 %) (mean ± SEM). (After Mózsik et al. 2007)

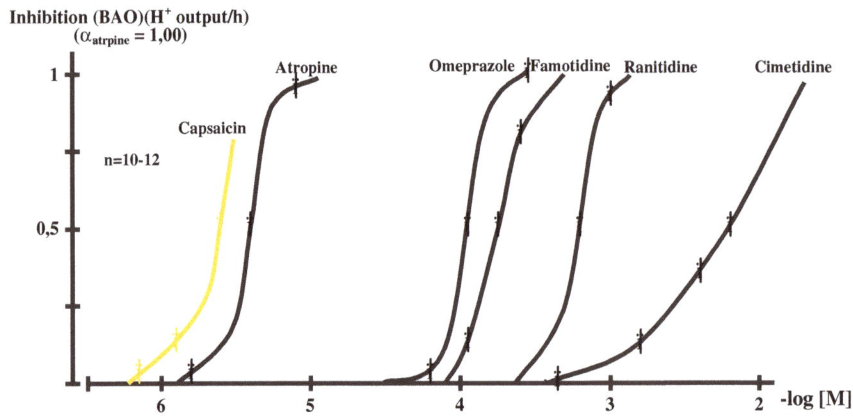

Fig. 9.3 Intrinsic activity curves for the inhibitory drugs of different antisecretory drugs and capsaicin (given in stimulatory doses of capsaicin-sensitive afferent nerves) on the BAO in healthy human subjects, which were expressed to action of atropine (1.00) (α atropine) (mean ± SEM). (After Mózsik et al. 2007)

9.3.3 Changes in the "Parietal" and "Non-Parietal" Components of Gastric Secretory Responses in Healthy Human Subjects

The measurements of cations (H^+, sodium, potassium, calcium, magnesium) and of chloride$^-$ offered the possibility to identify the "parietal" and "non-parietal"

Table 9.1 Summary of the affinity (pD_2) and intrinsic activity (expressed in value of $\alpha_{atropine} = 1.00$) (pA_2) values of capsaicin, atropine, Pirenzepine, cimetidine, ranitidine, famotidine, Omeprazole, and Esomeprazole on the gastric basal acid output (BAO) in healthy human subjects. (After Mózsik et al. 2007)

Compounds	M.W.	pD_2	Intrinsic activity	pA_2
Capsaicin	305.4	5.88	0.76	5.87
Atropine	289.38	5.40	1.00	5.40
Pirenzepine	424.34	3.93	0.89	3.93
Cimetidine	252.34	2.23	1.00	2.23
Ranitidine	314.41	3.33	1.00	3.33
Famotidine	337.43	3.77	1.00	3.77
Nizatidine	331.47	3.34	1.00	3.34
Omeprazole	345.42	3.97	1.00	3.97
Esomeprazole	345.42	3.97	1.00	3.97

components of gastric secretion in humans without and with administration of different drugs (or compounds) (Hollander 1934).

Using the Hollander's method for the calculation and evaluation of measurements of cations, chloride in the gastric juice indicated clearly the significant decrease of "parietal component" ($\Delta - 18 \pm 2$ mmol/L, $P < 0.001$) in association with significant increase of " non-parietal component" ($\Delta + 19 \pm 2$ mmol/L, $P < 0.001$) component of the gastric secretion after application of 400 μg (given orally) of capsaicin ($n = 10$) (Mózsik et al. 2005) (Table 9.2).

9.3.4 Changes in Albumin Level in the Gastric Juice After Capsaicin Administration in Healthy Human Subjects

The albumin concentration increased from 1.24 ± 0.001 g/L versus 1.63 ± 0.02 g/L ($P < 0.001$; $n = 10$) after 400 μg capsaicin (i.g. given) application (Mózsik et al. 2005).

9.3.5 Action of Capsaicin on the GTPD in the Healthy Human Subjects

Capsaicin (given ig. in doses of 100, 200, 400, and 800 μg) dose-dependently increased the GTPD alone (Δ value from to baseline 10 (−mV)) (Mózsik et al. 2005).

When we applied capsaicin in double dose (800 μg, intragastrically) then we received the same increase in GTPP and in the same time period (Hossenbocus et al. 1975; Mózsik et al. 2005) (Fig. 9.4).

Table 9.2 Chemical composition of gastric juice without (A) and with (B) application of capsaicin ($ED_{50} = 400\ \mu g$) in healthy human subjects

H^+		Na^+		K^+		Ca^{2+}		Mg^{2+}	
A	B	A	B	A	B	A	B	A	B
43 ± 3	25 ± 1	73 ± 4	89 ± 2	13 ± 1	8 ± 0.6	0.98 ± 0.02	0.88 ± 0.01	0.49 ± 0.01	0.38 ± 0.01
$P < 0.001$		$P < 0.001$		$P < 0.001$		$P < 0.001$		$P < 0.001$	
100 ± 7	58 ± 2	100 ± 5	122 ± 3	100 ± 8	62 ± 5	100 ± 2	90 ± 1	100 ± 2	78 ± 2

"Parietal" component		"Non-parietal" component		Albumin (g/L)	
A	B	A	B	A	B
43 ± 3	25 ± 2	126 ± 4	145 ± 4	1.24 ± 0.001	1,630,002
$P < 0.001$		$P < 0.001$		$P < 0.001$	
100 ± 7	58 ± 5	100 ± 3	115 ± 3	100 ± 1	131 ± 2

The results are given as mmol/L or % (mean ± SEM) ($n = 10$). (After Mózsik et al. 2005)

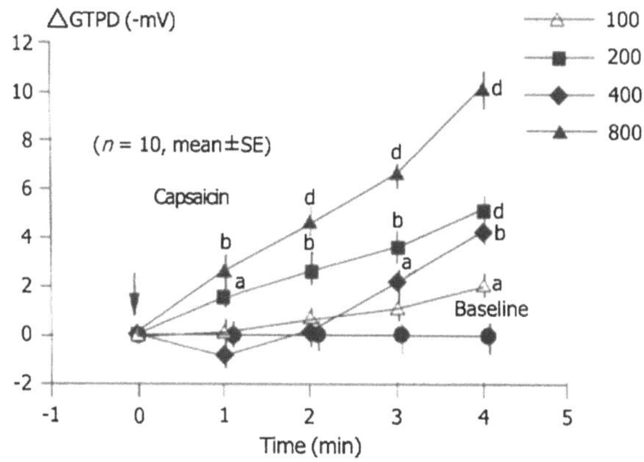

Fig. 9.4 Capsaicin dose-dependent gastric mucosal protective effect of capsaicin on GTPD in 10 healthy subjects. (After Mózsik et al. 2005)

9.3.6 Action of Ethanol on GTPD in Healthy Human Subjects

The intragastrically applied ethanol immediately and significantly decreased the GTPD (Δ 25 (−mV)) (Mózsik et al. 2005).

9.3.7 Preventive Action of Capsaicin on the Ethanol-Induced Decrease of GTPD in Healthy Human Subjects

The intragastrically applied capsaicin (given in doses of 100, 200, 400, and 800 μg) dose-dependently prevented the ethanol-induced decrease of GTPD in healthy human subjects (Mózsik et al. 2003, 2005). 800 μg capsaicin was intragastrically given after each other with 5 min interval (Fig. 9.5).

9.3.8 Indomethacin-Induced Acute Gastric Microbleeding and the Acute Gastric Mucosal Preventive Effect of Capsaicin on the Indomethacin-Induced Acute Gastric Mucosal Damage in Healthy Human Subjects (Based on the Results of Prospective, Randomized and Multiclinical Study)

9.3.8.1 Extent of Indomethacin-Induced Acute Gastric Mucosal Damage in Healthy Human Subjects

The baseline of blood losing was 2.0 ± 0.2 mL/day ($n = 14$) without application of IND, which was increased to 8.1 ± 0.2 mL/day ($n = 14$; $P < 0.001$).

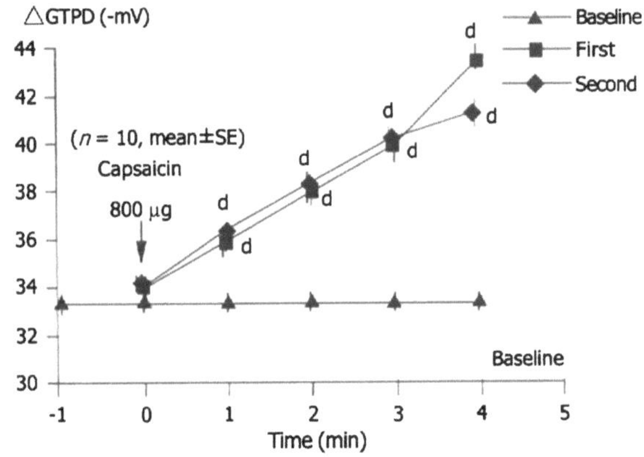

Fig. 9.5 Dose-dependent gastric mucosal protective effect of capsaicin is repeated (800 μg) on the GTPD with 5 min time interval ($n = 10$, mean ± SEM) in healthy human subjects (after Mózsik et al. 2005; with permission)

9.3.8.2 Gastric Mucosal Preventive Effect of Capsaicin on the Indomethacin-Induced Acute Gastric Microbleeding in Healthy Human Subjects

Capsaicin was given in doses of 200, 400, and 800 μg orally before the administration of indomethacin. The acutely applied capsaicin prevented by dose-dependent manner of indomethacin-induced gastric microbleeding in healthy human subjects ($Y = -0.0071*X + 7.78$; $r = -0.98$, $n = 14$; $P < 0.001$) (Mózsik et al. 2005; Sarlós et al. 2003) (Fig. 9.6).

9.3.9 Effect of Capsaicin on the Gastric Emptying in Healthy Human Subjects

Capsaicin was intragastrically given in dose of ED_{50}, which increased significantly the gastric acid emptying: (1) Capsaicin (400 μg, ig = ED_{50})-induced changes in the maximal values of Delta Over Base (DOB $_{max}$) decreased from 18 ± 1 to 14 ± 1 U ($P < 0.01$); (2) the time to reach the DOB $_{max}$ decreased from 148 ± 13 to 70 ± 12 min ($P < 0.01$); (3) the slope (in U/min) increased from 0.11 ± 0.01 to 14 ± 0.001 ($P < 0.001$); (4) the time to reach the AUC_{50} decreased from 115 ± 10 to 80 ± 8 (min) ($n = 10$; $P < 0.01$) (Debreceni et al. 1999).

9.3.10 Increased Glucose Absorption from Small Intestine and of Glucagon Release by capsaicin During the Glucose Loading Test in Healthy Human Subjects

During glucose loading test we measured the glucose absorption in the proximal part of the small intestine, insulin, C peptide, glycagon using the plasma level of glucose as markers substance (Dömötör et al. 2006a, b) (Figs. 9.7, 9.8).

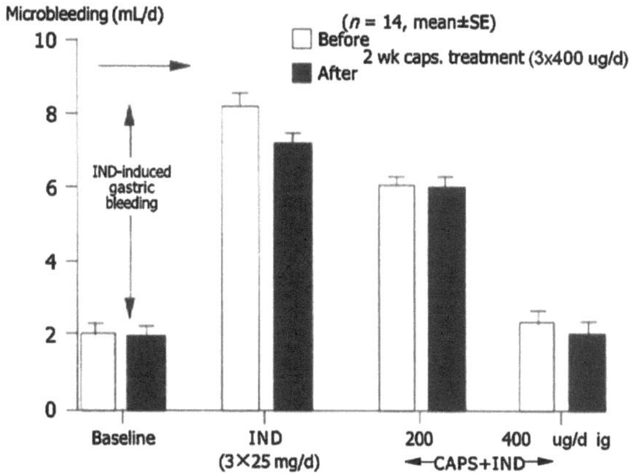

Fig. 9.6 Gastric mucosal protection demonstrated by reduced microbleeding before and after two weeks capsaicin treatment of indomethacin (IND)-induced mucosal damage. (After Mózsik et al. 2005)

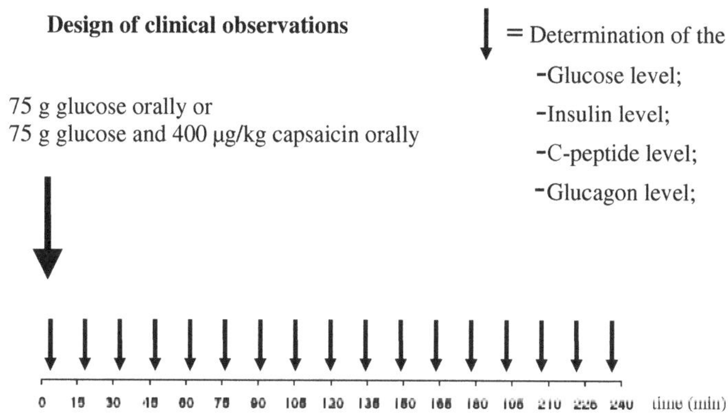

Fig. 9.7 Design of clinical observations with glucose observation and utilization in 14 healthy human subjects without and with (400 μg orally) capsaicin application. The measurement of glucose, insulin, C-peptide, glucagon was carried out from the plasma level in every 15 min period from the glucose application to 4 h. (After Dömötör et al. 2006a, b)

The absorption of glucose from the small intestine and glucagon release increased by capsaicin administration; however, no significant changes were obtained neither in insulin nor in C-peptide release under these observational circumstances (Fig. 9.7).

The plasma levels of glucose increased significantly 30–150 min and the plasma level of glucagon increased from 90 to 180 min after capsaicin administration in healthy human subjects given 75 g glucose orally. The plasma levels of insulin and C-peptide increased from 75 to 165 min after glucose administration; however, levels did not differ significantly.

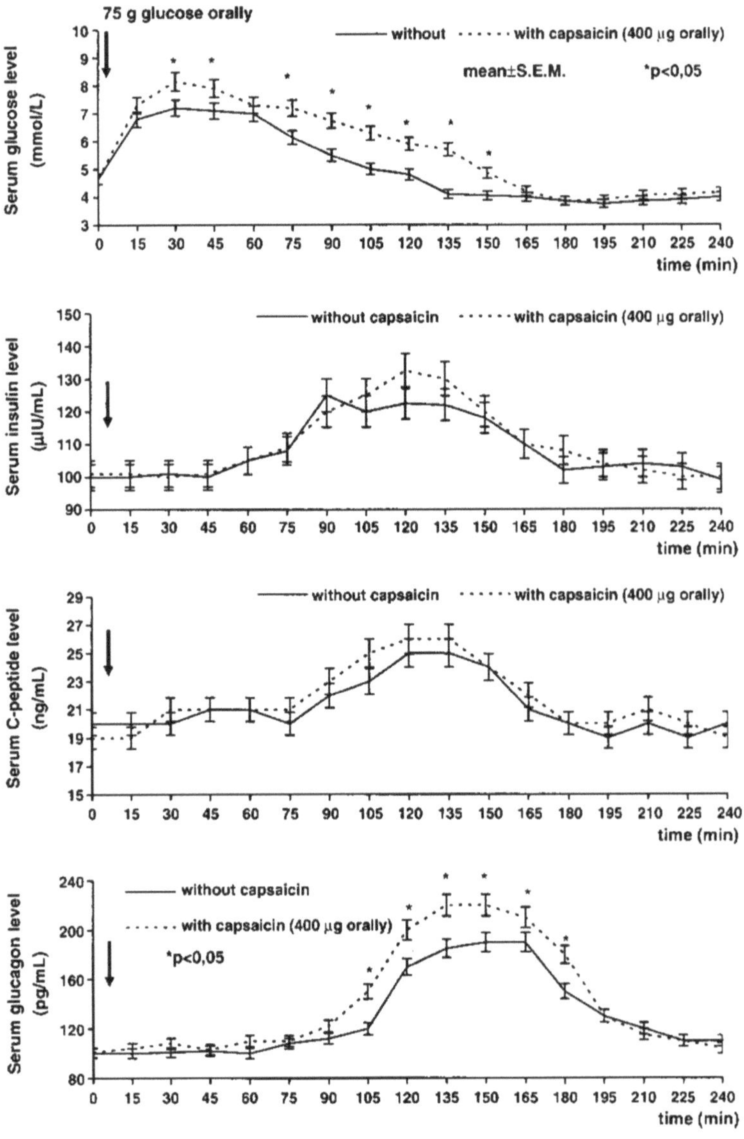

Fig. 9.8 Changes in plasma level of glucose, insulin, C-peptide, and glucagon after oral administration of glucose (75 g in 100 ml water) in 14 healthy human subjects. Capsaicin (400 μg) was orally given in gelatine capsule (Hungaropharma, Budapest, Hungary). The plasma levels of glucose, insulin, C-peptide, and glucagon were measured every 15 min for 4 h. The results are expressed as mean ± SEM. (After Dömötör et al. 2006a, b)

9.3.11 Results of the Immunohistochemical Examinations in the Human Gastric and Large Bowel Mucosa in Healthy Human Subjects and in Patients with Different Gastrointestinal Disorders

9.3.11.1 Demonstration of Capsaicin Receptors, CGRP, and SP in the Human Gastric and Large Bowel Mucosa in Healthy Human Subjects

The results of these observations were obtained in "healthy human subjects," who had different functional complaints and the endoscopic examinations were carried out to exclude the presence of any histologically proven disease (the clinical histological examinations were carried out by the independent pathologist) and the opinion of pathologist gave normal histology.

The immunohistochemical examination demonstrated the presence of capsaicin (TRVP1) receptors in the gastric and large bowel mucosa obtained from biopsy samples (Fig. 9.8). The location of capsaicin receptor could be demonstrated near the nerve endings, vascular vessel and in the epithelial layer (Fig. 9.9) (Dömötör et al. 2005).

The CGRP and SP could be observed in gastric mucosa and these parts of large bowel mucosa as well (Fig. 9.10) (Dömötör et al. 2005).

9.3.11.2 Demonstration of Capsaicin Receptor, CGRP, and SP in the Gastric and Large Bowel Mucosa in Patients with Different Disorders

The preliminary results of these observations were published by Dömötör et al. (2005).

These patients went over the clinical endoscopic and pathological examinations. The original pathological diagnosis was given by an independent pathologist.

The capsaicin receptor, and released neuropeptides (CGRP and SP) could be detected in all types of patients with different disorders (Table 9.3). The results of these preliminary clearly indicated the following: (1) capsaicin receptor could be demonstrated in patients with superficial gastritis, erosive gastritis, stomach polyps, stomach cancer, inflammation of large bowel disease, colon polyps with severe dysplasia, and colorectal cancers.

The CGRP could be demonstrated in most of the all of the above-mentioned diseases; meanwhile the SP could not be demonstrated in these diseases (Table 9.3).

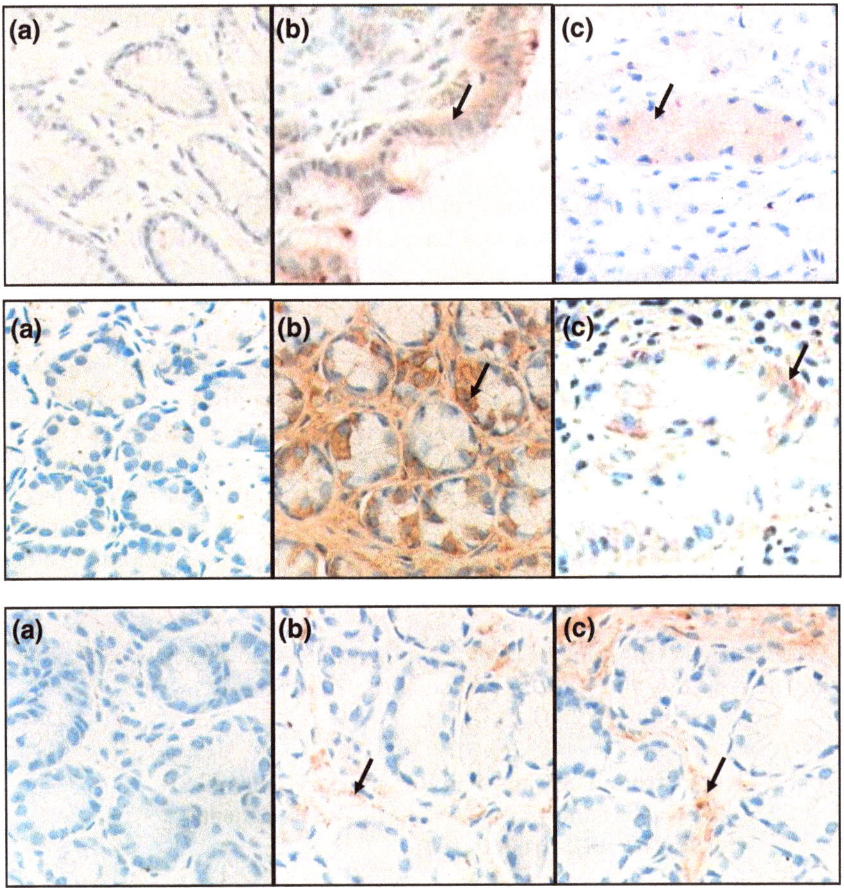

Fig. 9.9 The immune distribution of TRPV1 (*first row*), CGRP (*second row*), and of SP (*third row*) in the gastric mucosa of a healthy subject (**a**) and of patient with H. pylori negative (**b**) and H. pylori positive (**c**) chronic gastritis. *Arrows* show the immunosigns in the mucosa. (After Mózsik et al. 2007)

9.3.12 Capsaicin Receptor, CGRP, and SP in the Patients with Helicobacter Positive and Negative Chronic Gastritis

These observations were carried out in 57 patients with chronic gastritis (21 patients from them were Helicobacter positive and 30 patients were Helicobacter pylori negative).

The expression of capsaicin receptors and CGRP increased in the gastric mucosa with both bacteria positive and negative chronic gastritis, meanwhile SP increased with a limited extent determined by a semiquantitative scale (Fig. 9.9) (Dömötör et al. 2006a).

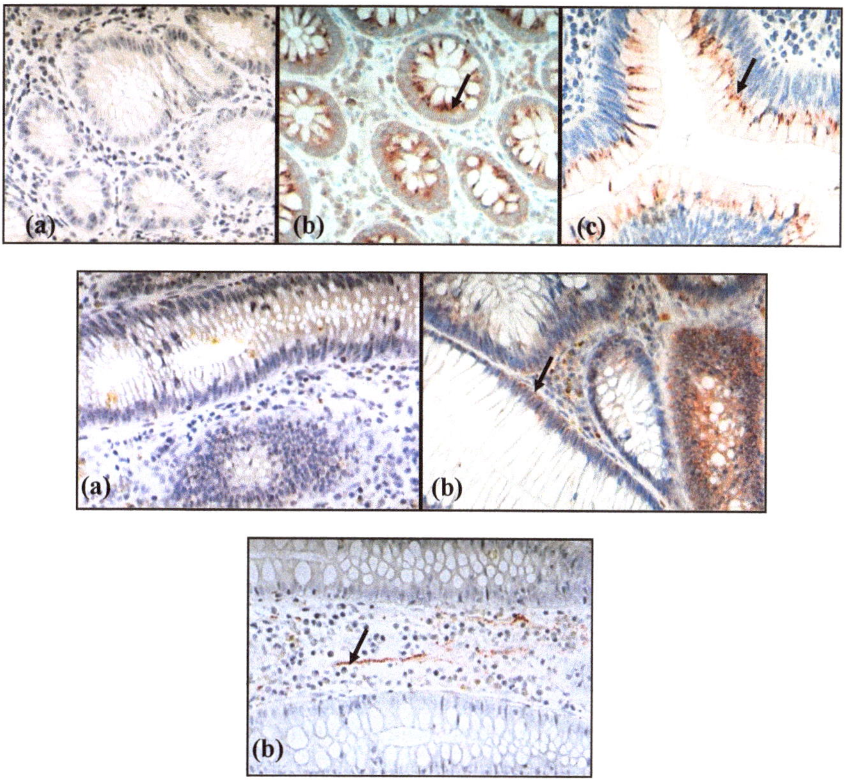

Fig. 9.10 The immundistribution of TRPV1 (*first line*), CGRP (*second line*), and of SP (*third line*) in the colon mucosa of control person (**a**) and of patient with inflammatory bowel disease (**b**) and with severe dysplastic polyp (**c**). *Arrows* show the immunsigns in the mucosa. (After Mózsik et al. 2007; with permission)

9.3.13 Measurements of the Gastric Microbleeding Before and After 2 Week Capsaicin Treatment: Testing of the Changes in Baseline, Indomethacin-Induced Acute Gastric Microbleeding and of Capsaicin-Stimulated Gastric Mucosal Protective Effect on the Indomethacin-Induced Acute Gastric Microbleeding in Healthy Human Subjects

9.3.13.1 Baseline Before and After 2 Weeks Indomethacin Treatment Without Application of any Drug and/or Compound

The baseline of gastric microbleeding was detected 2.1 ± 0.1 versus 2.0 ± 0.1 mL/day, before and after 2 weeks capsaicin treatment (without other drug/compound application).

Table 9.3 Immune distribution of capsaicin receptor (TRPV1), calcitonin gene-related peptide (CGRP), and substance P (SP) in the gastric and large bowel mucosa of patients with different GI disorders. (After Mózsik et al. 2007)*

	TRPV1	CGRP	SP
Stomach			
Superficial gastritis	+	+	–
Erosive gastritis	+	+	–
Gastric ulcer	±	±	±
Polyp	+	+	–
Carcinoma	+	+	–
Large bowel			
Inflammation	+	+	+
Polyp with moderate dysplasia	–	–	–
Poly with severe dysplasia	+Spot-like	–	–
Carcinoma	+Spot-like	+	–

*The signs of + or – indicate the trend of expression in the specific immunohistochemical examinations in the mucosa specimens (stomach and large bowel) in patients with different diseases

9.3.13.2 Measurement of Indomethacin-Induced Acute Gastric Mucosal Microbleeding: Before and After 2 weeks Capsaicin Treatment—in Healthy Human Subjects

The acute administration of indomethacin significantly increased the extent of gastric microbleeding versus baseline (without administration of indomethacin) ($P < 0.001$; $n = 14$) in healthy human subjects before (baseline vs. Ind., 2.1 ± 0.1 vs. 8.3 ± 0.2 mL/day) and after (baseline vs. Ind., 2.0 ± 0.1 vs. 7.8 ± 0.3 mL/day) 2 weeks capsaicin (3×400 μg orally given) treatment (Mózsik et al. 2005).

9.3.13.3 Measurement of Acutely Applied Capsaicin-Induced Gastric Mucosal Protective Effect on the Indomethacin-Induced Acute Gastric Microbleeding Before and After 2 Weeks Capsaicin Treatment in Healthy Human Subjects

The intragastrically applied capsaicin dose-dependently prevented the indomethacin-induced gastric mucosal damage (Mózsik et al. 2003, 2004a, 2005)—before ($Y = -0.0087X + 9.18$, $r = -0.99$: $P < 0.001$) and after ($Y = -0.0096X + 10.1$; $r = -0.99$; $P < 0.001$) 2 weeks capsaicin treatment—when capsaicin was acutely and intragastrically (in doses of 200 and 400 μg) given before the 1 day indomethacin treatment (see the description in the methods) (Mózsik et al. 2005) (Figs. 9.11 and 9.12).

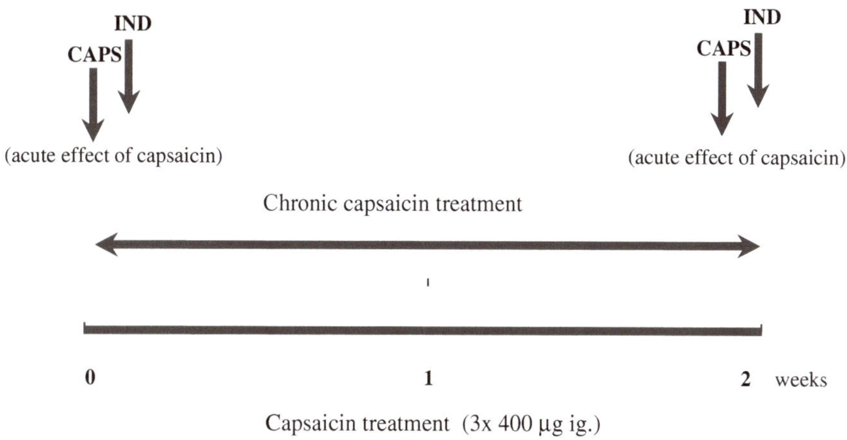

Fig. 9.11 Clinical study design of a chronic capsaicin treatment in healthy human subjects. Abbreviations: *CAPS* capsaicin, *IND* indomethacin

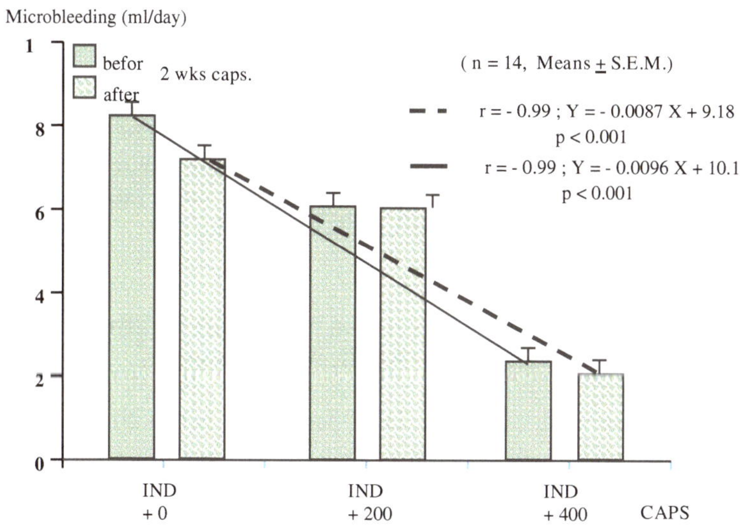

Fig. 9.12 Capsaicin (given 200 and 400 μg ig.)-induced gastric mucosal preventive effects on indomethacin (3 × 25 mg ig.)-produced gastric mucosal microbleeding before and after a chronic capsaicin (3 × 400 μg ig. for 2 weeks) in 14 healthy human subjects. The results were expressed as mean ± SEM)

9.3.14 Expression of Capsaicin Receptor, CGRP, and SP in Patients with Chronic Gastritis

9.3.14.1 Capsaicin-Sensitive Afferentation in H. pylori Positive and Negative Chronic Gastritis

The symptoms of patient's suffering from chronic gastritis with or without H. pylori infection (20 H. pylori positive and 30 H. pylori negative) were nonspecific including epigastric discomfort, nausea, loss of appetite, and vomiting. The patients underwent physical, laboratory, ultrasonographic, endoscopic, and histological (including special immunohistochemical) examinations. Twenty people with functional dyspepsia (all of them underwent the aforementioned medical, laboratory, iconographic, and histological examinations and all of these examinations indicated negative results) were taken as healthy controls. The age of patients was 39–68 years; there were 22 males and 29 females with chronic gastritis, and 10 males and 10 females in the functional dyspepsia group.

The H. pylori infection was detected by ^{14}C-urea breath test, rapid urease test, Warthinn-Starry silver staining, and specific histological examinations. The gastric tissue samples from the stomach and antrum were examined by an independent histologist and classified of chronic gastritis according to the Sydney System.

The immunohistochemical studies were carried out on formalin fixed, paraffin-embedded tissue samples of gastric mucosa using the peroxidase-labeled polymer method (Lab Vision Co., Fremont, USA). SP was detected by the NC1/34HL rat monoclonal antibody, the TRPV1 receptor, and CGRP were labeled using polyclonal rabbit antisera (all from Alcam Ltd., UK, Cambridge).

9.3.14.2 Capsaicin-Sensitive Afferentation in H. pylori Positive Chronic Gastritis Before and After Eradication Treatment

These observations were carried out in 38 persons, including 20 healthy subjects and 18 patients with H. pylori positive gastritis. The age of persons with histologically intact gastric mucosa (controls) were 41 to 67 years (mean = 52.2 years). The age of patients with chronic H. pylori positive gastritis (6 males, 12 females) was 39–68 years (mean = 56.4 years).

The time period between the first and control gastroscopy was 6 weeks after the starting of the examinations. The biopsies were taken from the corpus and antrum of patients with chronic gastritis, before and after eradication treatment and from healthy subjects.

The H. pylori positive patients underwent 7 days eradication treatment with a combination of double dose PPI (pantoprazole 2 × 40 mg/day), amoxicillin (1000 mg twice daily), and clarithromycin (500 mg twice daily) according to the European guidelines. After this 1 week combination treatment, the patients continued to take normal dose of PPI for another week.

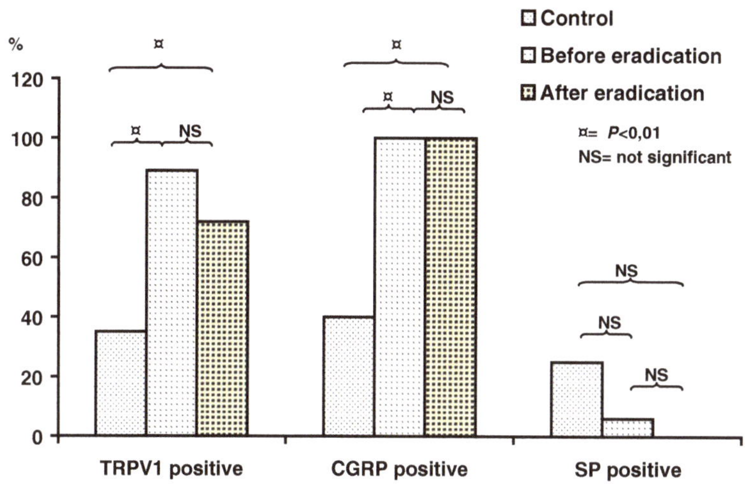

Fig. 9.13 Changes in the immunhistochemical distribution of capsaicin receptor (TRPV1), CGRP, and SP in patients with *H. pylori* positive chronic gastritis before and after eradication therapy (after Lakner et al. 2011)

The H. pylori infection was detected before and after treatment with ^{14}C-urea breath test, rapid urease test, gastroscopy, Warthinn-Starry silver staining, and specific histological and immunohistological examinations of gastric mucosa.

The results of eradication treatment was successful in 89 %, the gastric histology (by biopsy and by histology) indicated normal picture in 22 % of cases, and 78 % of patients showed moderate gastritis.

The expression of TRPV1 and CGRP increased significantly in the gastric mucosa of patients with chronic gastritis—independently on the presence of H. pylori positive or negative status and of successful eradication treatment in patients with H. pylori positive gastritis (Fig. 9.9), meanwhile on significant expressions obtained in SP of gastric mucosa in these groups) (Dömötör et al. 2005; Lakner et al. 2011; Mózsik et al. 2011, 2014; Czimmer et al. 2013; Vincze et al. 2004) (Figs. 9.9, 9.13, 9.14 and Table 9.4).

9.3.15 Clinical Pharmacological Challenges of the Natural Capsaicin for the Human Medical Treatments and Drug Processing

9.3.15.1 Chemistry of Natural Capsaicin with Respect to Spices of Capsaicin in Producing Plants in Over the World

The name of "capsaicin" is generally used in the medical physiological, pharmacological research; however, this material does not contain a clinical entity. The name of "capsaicin" covers 5 homologs (capsaicin, dihydrocapsaicin, nordihydrocapsaicin,

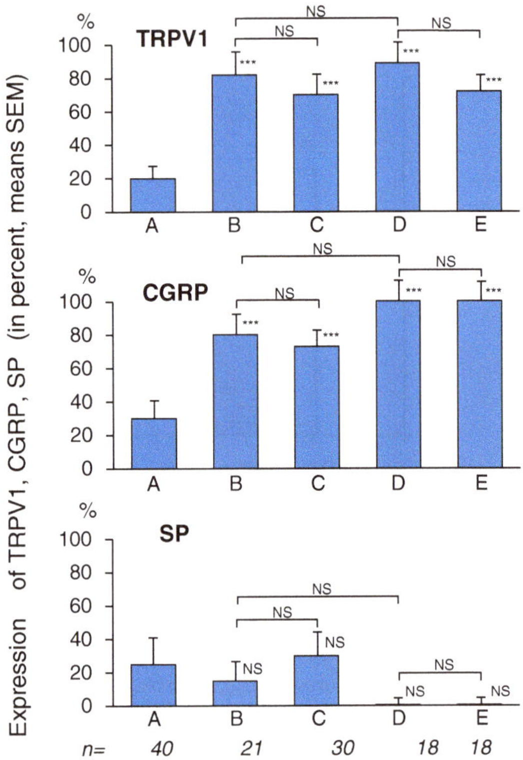

Fig. 9.14 Changes in the expression of capsaicin receptor (TRPV1), calcitonin gene-ralated peptide (CGRP), and substance P (SP) in the human gastric mucosa of healthy voluntaries (histologically intact) (**a**), *H. pylori* positive (**b**), *H. pylori* negative (**c**) and *H. pylori* positive before, (**d**) and after eradication (pantoprazole 40, amoxicillin 1000 and clarithromycin 500 mg, all two times per day, for 7 days) (n = number of patients). (After Mózsik et al. 2014)

homodihydrocapsaicin, homocapsaicin) and two analogs (nanonoid acid valilylamide and decanoid acid vanillylamide) (for further information, see Mózsik et al. 2009a, b).

The United States Pharmacopeia describes the list of capsaicins and their definitions, identifications, melting range, and also defines the content of capsaicin, dihydrocapsaicin, and other components as follows (USP 30-NP25, 2006, Edition pp. 1609): capsaicin contents not less than 90.0 % and not more 110.0 % of labeled percentage of total capsaicin. The content of capsaicin is not less than 55 %, and the sum of capsaicin and dihyrocapsaicin should not be less than 75.0 %. The content of other capsaicinoids cannot be more than 15 %, all these were calculated on the dried basis (see details in Ref. Mózsik et al. 2009a, b) These criteria were absolutely accepted by the Hungarian Authorities of Hungarian Institute of Pharmacy and, of course, by us during the our preclinical and clinical examinations.

9.3.15.2 International Requirements for Plant Origin Capsaicin for Orally Applicable Drug in Humans

Drug Master File (DMF)

To receive permission for human use of capsaicin preparation from the National and International Regulatory Authorities we have to show the following details: (1) Specification of capsicum species; (2) Climatic regulations of places of *Capsicum*

Table 9.4 The summary of the changes in the immunohistochemical distribution of capsaicin receptor, calcitonin gene-related peptide, and substance P in patient with chronic *H. pylori* positive gastritis before and after eradication therapy

	TRPV1		CGRP		Substance P	
	Positive	Negative	Positive	Negative	Positive	Negative
Before eradication ($n = 18$)	88.89 % (16)	11.11 % (2)	100 % (18)	0 % (0)	5.56 % (1)	94.44 % (17)
After eradication ($n = 18$)	72.22 % (13)	17.78 % (5)	100 % (18)	0 % (0)	0 % (0)	100 % (18)
Control group ($n = 20$)	35 % (7)	65 % (13)	40 % (8)	60 % (12)	75 % (15)	25 % (5)

cultivation; (3) Chemical treatments of *Capsicum* plants during their cultivation; (4) Details of treatment of *Capsicum* plants (their collections, drying, extractions, storages, etc.); (5) Analytical results supporting the chemical composition of the plant origin capsaicin extracts; (6) Chemical stability of natural capsaicin (capsainoids); (7) Analytical results showing the (possible) contamination of the natural capsaicin product with organic phosphates, pesticides, fusariums, aflatoxin; (8) International centification (including the Drug and Food Administration, FDA) on the capsaicin (capsaicinoids) content of the natural preparation.

Extremely important to mention that facts given by only internationally accredited laboratories.

The DMF of capsaicin originated from India is signed in the documentation of Food and Drug Administration (FDA) in the United States ("17856 A II 26.10.2004 Asian Herbex Ltd: Capsaicin USP as manufactured in Andhra Pradesh, India").

9.3.16 Human First Phase Examinations Based on the Permission of International and National Authorities

9.3.16.1 Necessary Permissions for Human Clinical First Phase Examinations from the Authorities in Healthy Human Subjects

We aimed to use capsaicin of natural origin (capsaicinoids) for the preparation of an orally applicable drug or for different drug combinations.

We compiled the documentations for the National Institute of Pharmacy (Budapest, Hungary) to ask permission for human clinical pharmacological studies with capsaicin: (1) Expert's opinion; (2) Results of toxicological studies (including those which were required by the National Institute of Pharmacy); (3) Chemical stability of the natural capsaicin preparation; (4) Results of pharmaceutical industrial formulation from the natural capsaicin; (5) Different permissions from the Medical Faculty of our University (Pécs, Hungary); (6) Documentation of health insurance of volunteers; (7) Preclinical dossiers; (8) Documented permission on the accreditation of Clinical Pharmacological Unit for human phase I and II (which accreditation was controlled by the National Institute of Pharmacy in Hungary; (9) Exact and accepted protocols by the National Institute of Pharmacy and National Clinical Pharmacological Ethical and Clinical Pharmacological Committee of Hungary; (10) Written information of volunteers on the planned examinations; (11) Request for authorization of a clinical trial on medical product for human use to competent authorities and for opinion of ethical committees in the community; (12) Data of investigators (CV, certificates) and participating institutes.

9.3.16.2 Three Protocols Authorized by the Hungarian Competent Authorities

(a) "Human phase I. Single-blind study comparing the pharmacokinetic properties of ASA after single oral dose administration alone and after co-administration of two different does of capsaicin (400 and 800 μg) and evaluating their safety in healthy male subjects" (protocol number: 1.4.1., EudraCT number: 2008-007048-32);
(b) "Human phase I. Single-blind study investigating the pharmacokinetic properties of diclofenac after single oral dose administration alone and after co-administration of two different doses of capsaicin (400 and 800 μg) and evaluating their safety and healthy male subjects" (protocol number: 1.4.2; EudraCT number: 2008-007050-36);
(c) "Human phase I. Single-blind study comparing the pharmacokinetic properties of naproxen after single oral dose administration and after co-administration of two different doses (400 and 800 μg) of capsaicin and evaluating their safety in healthy male subjects" (protocol number: 4.3; EudraCT number: 2008-007098-19).

The human phase I. exanimations of "a" and "b" were carried out in the 2012 at First Department of Medicine and Institute of Cardiology, Medical and Health Centre of Pécs University, Hungary.

Objectives of these studies were:

1. The primary objective of these trials was to investigate whether two different doses of capsaicin (400 and 800 μg) co-administered with ASA (or with diclofenac or naproxen) would influence the pharmacokinetic properties of ASA (diclofenac and naproxen) administered alone.
2. The secondary objective of these studies was to evaluate the safety and tolerability of both preparations administered alone and after co-administration.
3. Platelet aggregometry substudy: the aim was to confirm the presumption that giving capsaicin with ASA (diclofenac, naproxen) would not alter the inhibitory effect of ASA (diclofenac, naproxen) on platelet aggregation.

Study design: healthy male volunteers aged 18–55 years, body mass index between 18 and 29.2 kg/m^2, laboratory parameters were in normal range. All the inclusion criteria of the protocols were strictly kept by the healthy volunteers.

Fifteen healthy subjects participated in each of these randomized studies (according to random allocation of protocols). Monitoring of the vital signs (blood pressure, heart rate, temperature, ECG), physical examinations, routine laboratory tests, fecal occult blood test, continuous monitoring of adverse events were done. Pharmacokinetic measurements for ASA (acetylsalicylic acid, salicylic acid), diclofenac, naproxen, and capsaicinoids, as well as platelet aggregation were carried out.

The manufacturer of the study products was PannonPharma Ltd, Pécsvárad, Hungary.

The mathematical analysis of the study of ASA plus capsaicin were finished up to now.

The main results of ASA plus capsaicin examinations are to test that:

1. The product ASA plus 400 μg capsaicin, ASA plus 800 μg capsaicin and reference product ASA product are bioequivalent;
2. The combined ASA-therapies reach equivalent effectiveness on inhibiting platelet aggregation to that of ASA monotherapy;
3. Thus, 400 μg and 800 μg capsaicin did not influence the inhibitory effect of ASA on platelet aggregation;
4. Capsaicin (at doses of 400 and 800 μg) by itself did not have a significant effect on platelet aggregation;
5. Capsaicin (given in two different doses) did not significantly modify ASA absorption from the gastrointestinal tract, and did not change the pharmacokinetic characteristics of salicylic acid (transformed from ASA);
6. Neither capsaicin nor dihydrocapsaicin could be detected chemically in the sera of the volunteers (who participated in the classical clinical human phase I. examinations (employing orally applied doses of 400 μg or 800 μg capsaicin). *High pressure liquid chromatography (HPLC) has serum detection limit around 20 nanogram/mL and the value is 26 fentogram/mL serum by liquid chromatography–mass spectrometry (LC-MC).*

These results offered us to conclude the following:

1. The applications of capsaicin alone or in combination with ASA and diclofenac (up to now) are safety and well tolerable drug combinations in healthy subjects.
2. Since capsaicin (and dihydrocapsaicin) could not be detected in the healthy human subjects its actions appear to be dominantly on the GI mucosa.
3. Capsaicin alone is not able to modify the aggregation of platelets, however, it did not modify the ASA-induced inhibition of platelets.
4. The gastroprotective effect of capsaicin exists against the NSAIDs-induced GI mucosal damage in doses capable of stimulating capsaicin-sensitive afferentation; however, the platelet aggregation by NSAIDs remained unchanged.
5. These special human situations offered us to produce a new gastroprotective capsaicin containing drugs or drug combinations for the medical treatment in patients with gastrointestinal disorders and which would prevent the NSAID-induced side effects in patients who are needed to be treated with NSAIDs.

The number of patients with GI disorders and other medical conditions needed to be treated with NSAIDs is extremely big. We have no final conclusions on the possible role of capsaicin-sensitive afferentations in the treatment of H. pylori (or other factors)-caused gastritis (but this infection represents the biggest infection disease in over the World).

Our results encourage us to pursue further human observations for the successful actions of capsaicin described in this chapter will possibly stimulate the development of new candidate capsaicin containing drug combinations (like ASA plus capsaicin) to be used in the medical therapy (Clinical Study Reports to Protocol 1.4.1, Pécs and Pécsvárad, Hungary 2012). We are also aware that many other observations are needed in these fields.

9.4 Discussion

The vagal nerve plays a key role in the gastrointestinal physiology, pathology, and pharmacology. The nerve fibers of vagus can be divided into afferent (about 90 %) and efferent fibers (10 %) based on the results of animal observations. About 9–10 % of vagal afferent fibers are capsaicin-sensitive afferent fibers (Gabella and Pease 1973; Grijalva and Novin 1990).

Most observations on the gastrointestinal field were based on the modification of efferent fibers of vagal nerve, except the classical surgical vagotomy (both in the animal experiments and in the human therapy of peptic ulcer disease). This standpoint was emphasized in time period of application of different anticholinergic compounds acting at the level of muscarinic receptor.

Since histamine has an essential role in the gastric acid secretion and in many other immunological processes, various H_2 receptor antagonist compounds were developed like cimetidine, ranitidine, famotidine, and nizatidine.

After recognition of the H^+-K^+-ATPase as biochemical structure of gastric acid secretion, the so-called proton pump inhibitors (H^+-K^+-ATPase inhibitors) were developed and studied in clinical practice using great efforts (Mózsik 2006).

The principal problems for clinicians were that the research did not offer any possibilities for studying capsaicin-sensitive afferent fibers of the vagal nerve in the human physiology, pathology, pharmacology, and in human medical therapy.

The observations of Jancsó et al. (1967, 1968, 1970) opened a new gate for evaluation of the potential roles of capsaicin-sensitive afferent fibers independently from the other afferent nerves in various physiological, pharmacological, and pathological processes.

Szolcsányi and Barthó (1981) were the first authors, who clearly demonstrated the dual actions of capsaicin on the peptic ulcer in rat: capsaicin given in small doses prevented, meanwhile this compound given in higher doses aggravated the gastric ulcer in the rat. Later on, Holzer studied the details of capsaicin actions in the GI tract (see the reviews of Holzer 1998; 1999, 2013).

Our experimental studies with capsaicin have been carried out together with professor Szolcsányi (Department of Pharmacology and Pharmacotherapy, Medical and Health Centre, University of Pécs, Hungary) from 1980, understanding the actions of capsaicin in gastric mucosal damage and protection have been our main focus (Mózsik et al. 1997).

My work team started with the human clinical pharmacological studies from the years of 1960 in patients with peptic ulcer disease (Mózsik et al. 1965, 1967, 1969a, b). These studied tried to clear up the absorption, metabolism, and excretion of various anticholinergic agents in patients with peptic ulcer before the starting of chronic treatment, after the regular chronic treatment, and after cessation of these drugs. The application of anticholinergic agents to patients was used to approach the cholinergic-mediated processes both in the development and treatment of peptic ulcer diseases.

After the year 1970, the H_2 receptor blocking compounds were deeply studied in human GI physiology, pathology, and pharmacology. Many clinical pharmacological studies have been carried out in patients with peptic ulcer disease (Mózsik et al. 1994; Patty et al. 1984; Tárnok et al. 1979, 1983).

In the past two decades, the proton pump inhibitors were widely studied.

The problems, results, and difficulties of our clinical pharmacology practice put down the bases of a very clear research line for the observations with capsaicin. The results of different animal observations offered a new possibility for evaluation of capsaicin-sensitive afferent nerves (by the application of capsaicin) during physiological, pathological, pharmacological, and therapeutic events of the GI tract.

Results from animal experiments clearly indicated to us that the stimulatory doses of capsaicin on capsaicin-sensitive fibers produce gastric mucosal defensive actions and they are able to prevent the NSAID-induced gastric mucosal damage. These scientifically carried out studies with capsaicin in animals also offered a new tool to approach the capsaicin-sensitive afferent nerves in the healthy human beings, and in some patients with different GI disorders.

Our studies with capsaicin in healthy human subjects and in patients with different gastrointestinal disorders started from 1997. These studies were permitted by the Regional Ethical Committee of Pécs University, Hungary, and these observations were carried out according to GCP respecting the Helsinki Declaration.

The human observations were carried out according to the basic laws of human clinical pharmacology (inclusion and exclusion criteria, randomization, prospective studies, generally self-controlled group of healthy human subjects, etc.).

We had three aims in these studies with the capsaicin:

1. To understand the main mechanisms of capsaicin-sensitive afferent nerves on gastric functions.
2. To try to understand the potential role(s) of capsaicin-sensitive afferent nerves in the development of human physiological, pathological and pharmacological events.
3. To evaluate and even develop a new capsaicin containing drug or drug combinations to modify the capsaicin-sensitive afferentation in healthy human subjects and to treat patients with gastrointestinal mucosal damage against NSAIDs and Helicobacter pylori infection.

These aims led us to use a significant number of the methodologies applied in the human studies. However, we had to use classical molecular pharmacological methods to compare and to understand some details of capsaicin-induced changes in the human physiological, pathological parameters, and also for better understanding of the results of capsaicin observations.

The following main trends were applied in the capsaicin research:

1. To determine the dose-response curves for the various drugs and capsaicin.
2. To introduce the classical molecular pharmacological methods for understanding the capsaicin-induced action in comparison to others produced by anticholinergic drugs, H_2 receptor antagonists, or proton pump inhibitors.
3. The specific immunohistochemistry (for obtaining morphological evidence) was incorporated into the research.
4. Different parameters were simultaneously measured (e.g., plasma glucose, insulin, C-peptide, and glucagon were detected during the sugar loading test in the healthy human subjects).
5. Capsaicin studies were carried out not only following acute administration but also after a chronic capsaicin administration.
6. The immunohistochemical studies were carried out in the GI mucosa of patients with different GI disorders (acute gastric mucosal damage, chronic inflammation, precancerous state, and cancers in the stomach and in the large bowel);
7. The human pathological diagnosis was given by an independent pathologist.
8. The ED_{50} (necessary doses of drugs to produce 50 % inhibition) values were determined and expressed in (−) molar values (pD_2).
9. The possible role of capsaicin afferentation in the prevention or treatment of gastric mucosal damage produced by NSAIDs in healthy subjects and in patients who are treated with these drugs (as pain killers, platelet aggregation, anti-inflammatory compounds, etc.) was evaluated.
10. Protocols for human phase I. examinations with capsaicin alone and/or with combination of capsaicin plus NSAIDs to receive permission from national and international authorities were prepared.

9.4.1 Capsaicin-Sensitive Efferent Nerves Versus Gastric Secretion in Healthy Human Subjects

Capsaicin in a dose-dependent manner decreased the gastric basal secretion (basal acid output, BAO) (Mózsik et al. 1999, 2004a, 2005). Capsaicin was applied in very small doses (200–800 μg orally) which stimulate the capsaicin-sensitive afferent nerve.

When we applied the molecular pharmacological approach to the actions of capsaicin, anticholinergic agents, H_2R antagonists, or proton pump inhibitors, we were surprised that capsaicin was able to inhibit the gastric acid secretion at a smaller molar concentration than other clinically widely used drugs (Figs. 9.2 and 9.3). Analyzing the intrinsic activity of these drugs and capsaicin by the molecular pharmacological methods (intrinsic activity of atropine was taken to be 1.00), we found capsaicin's action to be lesser than atropine's (Fig. 9.3).

The affinity curves of different drugs and capsaicin were molecular pharmacologically determined and given as pD_2 (the necessary doses of drugs and capsaicin to produce 50 % inhibition of gastric acid secretion (basal acid output), which expressed in (−) molar value) and as intrinsic activity (pA_2) (the necessary doses of drugs and capsaicin to produce 50 % inhibition, also expressed in (−) molar) values (Table 9.1).

The results of these molecular pharmacological studies clearly indicated the sensitivity of the various regulatory targets of different drugs and capsaicin in comparison to possible physiological roles of the target organs and the drug actions influence their functional activities and states. There is no question that the stimulation of capsaicin-induced afferent-sensitive nerves plays a very significant effect in regulation of processes important for maintenance of gastric mucosal integrity in human beings (including in healthy subjects and patients with different GI disorders or treated with different drugs, especially with NSAIDs).

The decrease of gastric acid secretion was explained by the increased H^+ back diffusion after capsaicin application via the increased vasodilator processes induced by the release of the CGRP and SP in animal observations or by the increase of somatostatin secretion. The CGRP and SP together with capsaicin receptor (TRVP1) could be detected by inmunohistological methods in the gastric mucosa around the nerves, vascular spaces, parietal cells, and in epithelial layer.

The human observations with increased gastric secretory responses are present in all of increased gastric mucosal blood flow. On the other hand, the increased gastric acid (H^+) secretion is closely associated with the increase of K^+, Mg^{2+}, Ca^+, and albumin in gastric juice. However, the decrease of gastric acid secretion produced by antisecretory agents is associated with the decrease of H^+, K^+, Mg^{2+}, Ca^{2+}, and albumin (Myren 1968).

Human observations with capsaicin do not suggest presence of increased H^+ back diffusion during capsaicin action (except when capsaicin was given in high doses):

1. The increased H^+ back diffusion suggests the decreased level of albumin in the gastric juice. Our results cannot prove the existence of gastric H^+ back diffusion in healthy human subjects during the capsaicin action:
2. We calculated the "parietal" and "non-parietal "components of gastric juice after Hollander's original observation (Hollander 1934). Our results clearly indicate that the decrease of gastric H^+ concentration (and output) is closely associated with the increased extent of "non-parietal component" during the capsaicin action in the healthy human subjects. The "non-parietal component" of the gastric juice is a buffering part, which is not obtained in circumstance of passive metabolic processes. Earlier, the significant increase of buffering ("non-parietal component") secretion was obtained in 2–10 days after cessation of a prolonged atropine treatment in patients with peptic ulcer disease (Antal et al. 1965).
3. There are other arguments against the existence of the passive H^+ back diffusion in the stomach during capsaicin action in the healthy human subjects. When the capsaicin was directly given to gastric mucosa (using gastroscope) then the "gastric transmucosal potential difference" (GTPD) increased in a dose-dependent manner (Mózsik et al. 2005).

If ethanol was intragastrically given (using the biopsy channel), then this GTPD immediately decreased, which could be reversed by the topical application of capsaicin. This action of capsaicin is also dose-dependent after ethanol application in the healthy human subjects (Mózsik et al. 2005).

The capsaicin action on the gastric secretory responses can be explained by different ways:

1. Direct cellular action of capsaicin on the parietal cells;
2. Direct stimulatory action of capsaicin on the "non-parietal component" of gastric secretory responses;
3. Capsaicin (given in doses producing the stimulation of capsaicin-sensitive afferent nerves) results in direct neural (or hormonal) influences on the gastric mucosa;
4. Other yet not known mechanism(s) existing in the regulation of the human gastric secretion.

Capsaicin given in ED_{50} increased the gastric emptying (Debreceni et al. 1999; Mózsik et al. 2004a, b). This action of capsaicin on the gastric emptying can be explained at least by two pathways:

1. Decrease of gastric acid secretion;
2. Direct action on muscular function of the stomach (pylorus).

Up to now, the acute action of capsaicin was evaluated dominantly by measuring one or two parameters.

9.4.2 *Capsaicin Effect on Glucose Absorption from Small Intestine in Healthy Human Subjects and its Hormonal and Metabolic Backgrounds*

The sugar loading test was applied for measuring absolutely different physiological events, e.g., glucose absorption from the proximal part of the small intestine and consequently the produced hormonal regulations during the glucose loading test.

The response to glucose loading in healthy human subject can be divided into three different periods on the basis of physiological events after orally applied glucose in healthy human persons:

1. Absorption (first period, from 30 to 90 min);
2. Insulin (and other hormones) release (second period, from 60 to 150 min);
3. Glycogen mobilization by the liver (third period, from 150 to 180 min) under adrenergic neural influences.

The glucose can be absorbed from the proximal part of the small intestine by active transport mechanism (in presence of Mg^{2+}, mitochondrial ATP breakdown into ADP) (Dömötör et al. 2006b). The monitoring of the glucose level was used as biological marker for the equilibrium of the different physiological events.

In the first period, the plasma glucose level depends only on the glucose absorption; in the second period, the plasma level of glucose represents the equilibrium between the absorption and hormone release; and in the third, the glucose level represents the mobilization of glucose by the liver in healthy human subjects. It is also important that the insulin and glucagon act contra regulatory on glucose utilization in the serum.

By studying the time sequence of changes in plasma levels of glucose, insulin, C-peptide, and glucagon after glucose loading in healthy human subjects without and with capsaicin (400 μg orally), we found the followings:

1. The plasma level of glucose (from 30 to 150 min) and the glucagon (from 90 to 180 min) increased significantly after glucose plus capsaicin administration.
2. The plasma levels of insulin and C-peptide were increased from 90 to 165 min, however, no significant changes were observed between subjects without and with capsaicin.
3. No difference in timing of insulin and glucagon release was observed, which clearly excludes the existence of antagonism between insulin and glucagon release (short time).
4. The plasma level of glucagon was higher for longer than it was in case of insulin. It should be noted that capsaicin increased the glucagon level.

The results clearly indicate that capsaicin-sensitive afferent nerves have a key role in the regulation of glucose absorption from the small intestine (due to a local increase of blood flow), glucose utilization, and release of neuropeptide (presently the glucagon release). This human observation proved clear-cut active participation of capsaicin-sensitive afferent nerves in the carbohydrate metabolism (by the ways of modification of sugar absorption, hormone release). Till now, only the somatostatin release induced by capsaicin has been known (Szolcsányi 2004).

9.4.3 *Capsaicin (Given Orally in Small Doses of 200, 400, and 800 Mg) Prevents Indomethacin-Induced Gastric Microbleedings in Healthy Human Subjects*

Indomethacin (IND) was used in these studies, which is a nonselective COX inhibitor (the ratio of ED 50 of indomethacin on COX-1/COX-2 = 0.3 0) (Kawai et al. 1998) (Table 9.5). The extent of gastric microbleeding appears as a consequence of COX-1 and COX-2 inhibition.

The results of our observations (Sarlós et al. 2003; Mózsik et al. 2003, 2004a, 2005) were that capsaicin given intragastrically dose-dependently prevented the IND-induced gastric microbleeding (before and after 2 weeks of capsaicin treatment).

Under the results of Kawai et al. (1998), we calculated the extents of gastric microbleeding depending on COX-1 and COX-2 enzyme activity (Table 9.6). It was found that the capsaicin-induced gastric mucosal protection remained unchanged before and after the 2 weeks capsaicin treatment in both COX-1 and COX-2 enzyme parts of the COX system.

Table 9.5 Comparison of inhibitory effects (IC_{50}) by giving the COX-1 and of various NSAIDs using human platelet COX-1 and synovial cell COX-2 (After Kawai et al. 1998)*

NSAID	Ratio COX-1 : COX-2
Aspirin	0.12
Diclofenac	38.00
Etodolac	179.00
Ibuprofen	0.86
Indomethacin	*0.30*
Loxoprofen-SRS	3.20
NS-398	1263.00
Oxaprozin	0.061
Zaltoprofen	3.80

The orally given 200, 400, and 800 μg capsaicin dose-dependently reduced the indomethacin-induced gastric microbleeding. All the healthy persons included in this study received all the mentioned doses of capsaicin in random allocation.

9.4.4 Questions of Desensitization to Capsaicin Receptor to Capsaicin (in Doses Applied by us During the Studies)

9.4.4.1 Facts to Exclude the Presence of the Desensitization of Capsaicin Receptor to Applied Doses of Capsaicin in Acute Observation Circumstances

When we applied the capsaicin twice in doses of 800 μg ig. after 5 min interval (Fig. 9.5), then we received the same extents of increase in difference of GTPD, indicating a very active metabolic action under these observation circumstances.

The same extent of gastric mucosal protection was obtained in the IND-induced gastric mucosal damage in healthy human subjects. The actions of gastric mucosal prevention was dose-dependent on the indomethacin-induced gastric microbleedings (please note that these human observations were carried out in prospective, randomized and multiclinical studies) (Figs. 9.6 and 9.12).

The results of these mentioned observations clearly indicated that the doses of capsaicin in our studies could not produce desensitization of capsaicin receptors (these doses of capsaicin only were able to stimulate the capsaicin-sensitive afferent nerve).

9.4.4.2 Facts to Exclude the Presence of Desensitization to Capsaicin Receptor by Applied Doses of Capsaicin During 2 Weeks of Capsaicin Treatment

Capsaicin exerts gastro-protective effect on IND-induced gastric mucosal microbleeding that remained unchanged before and after 2 week capsaicin (3 × 400 μg orally given) treatment (Fig. 9.12).

Table 9.6 Correlation between the capsaicin actions, COX-1 and COX-2 systems and gastric microbleedings produced by indomethacin in healthy human subjects before and after the 2-week capsaicin (3 × 400 μg orally) treatment. (After Mózsik et al. 2007)*

• IC_{50} value of indomethacin to ratio of COX-1/COX-2 = 0.30 (1: 3.25)		
• Microbleeding in the stomach		
← 2 weeks capsaicin treatment →		
	Before	After
Baseline	2.1 ± 0.1 mL/day	2.0 ± 0.1 mL/day
After IND	8.25 ± 0.25 mL/day	7.8 ± 0.3 mL/day
Δ IND-induced	6.15 ± 0.2 mL/day	5.8 ± 0.3 mL/day
(=inhibition on COX-1 + COX-2) (=100 %)		
COX-1	1.447 ± 0.1 mL/day	1.364 ± 0.1 mL/day
COX-2	4.70 ± 0.2 mL/day	4.44 ± 0.2 mL/day
• 400 μg capsaicin (IG given) induced decrease of ind-gastric microbleeding		
	6 ± 0.2 mL/day	5.9 ± 0.2 mL/day

*mean ± SEM in 14 healthy human subjects

By other words, the gastric baseline microbleeding remained unchanged after the application of different doses of capsaicin (200, 400, and 800 μg orally) that induced gastric mucosal protection.

The registration of these facts (observations) are very important, since a very wide scale of capsaicin doses was applied in human observations, and of course they resulted very contradictory data (because capsaicin were applied in stimulatory doses to capsaicin-sensitive afferent nerve and much higher doses produce reversible and irreversible inhibitory actions in various animal experiments).

The capsaicin acts at the level of capsaicin receptor, which has been cloned (Caterina et al. 1997). It is true that the capsaicin action depends on its doses proved by animal experiments (Szolcsányi 1984; Mózsik et al. 2001). The small dose (400 μg = ED_{50}) was applied for two weeks (in dose of 400 μg × 3 orally) in healthy subjects. The gastric mucosal microbleeding was produced by orally given IND (Fig. 9.15).

The following results were obtained:

1. The extent of baseline gastric microbleeding before and after 2 weeks capsaicin (without application of any drug) remained unchanged.
2. The extent of acutely given indomethacin-induced gastric microbleeding was also unchanged.
3. The extent of capsaicin-induced gastric mucosal protection was also found to be the same (and dose-dependent) before and after the 2 weeks capsaicin treatment.

It has been concluded from these observations that the sensitivity of capsaicin receptor (TRVP1) was unchanged, and on the other hand, the orally applied capsaicin is capable to exert gastric mucosal protection against indomethacin.

Probably the applied small dose of capsaicin—used in our present studies—could not modify the TRVP1 receptor sensitivity. We have no knowledge in this field by using higher dose(s) of capsaicin in healthy human subjects.

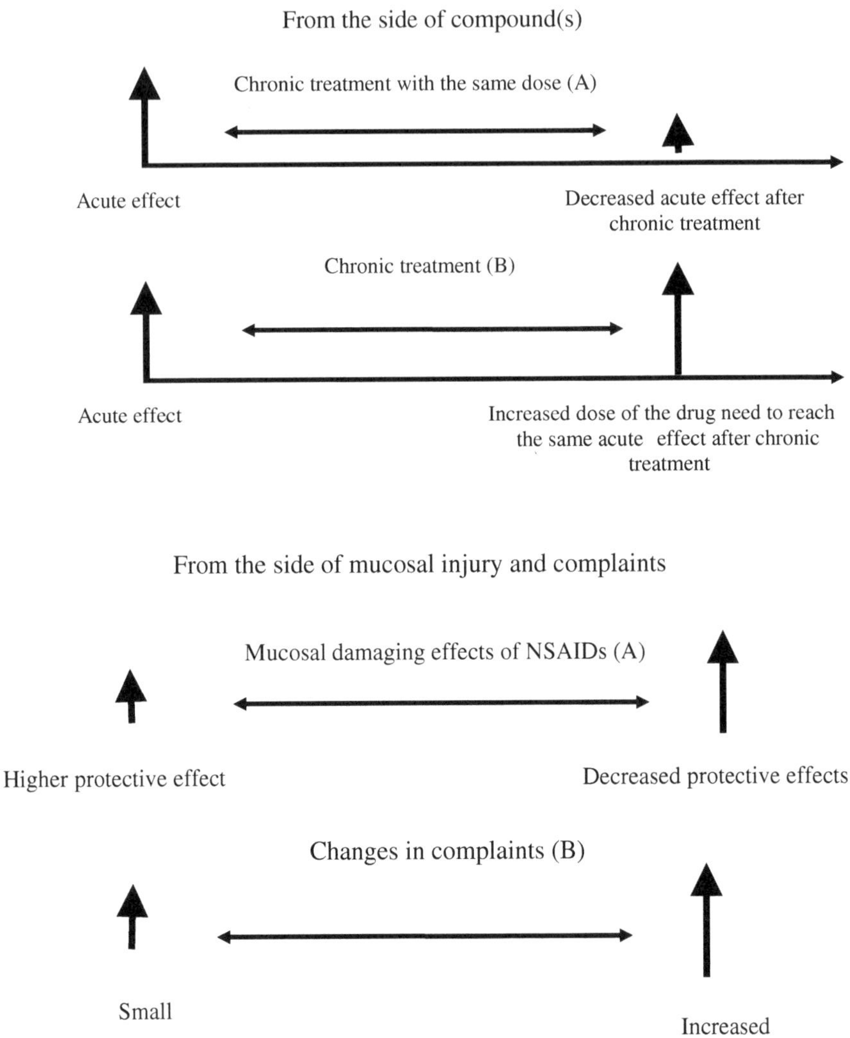

Fig. 9.15 Schematic demonstration the possible pathways in changes of chronic capsaicin treatment from the side of the compound (*upper part*) and from the side of mucosal injury and complaints (*lower part*) in healthy human subjects and in patients with different (including gastrointestinal) disorders

These facts are very important from the point of selection of capsaicin containing drug, because these dosages of capsaicin could exert beneficial effect (given orally in small doses), meanwhile the capsaicin in high doses can produce reversible or irreversible damage on the human gastric mucosa.

Earlier similar types of observations were carried out with atropine and other parasympatholytics (Mózsik et al. 1965, 1966, 1969a, b) and cimetidine (Wildersmith et al. 1990). Tolerance developed to the drugs applied chronically *in patients with peptic ulcer disease, and the "pharmacological denervation hypersensitivity*" occurred during clinically detectable tolerance (Mózsik et al. 1966, 1969a, b). These clinical pharmacological examinations modified the periodicity and dosage of applicable drugs (used in chronic treatment).

The careful analysis of the results with capsaicin actions, COX-1 and COX-2 systems and gastric microbleedings produced by IND in healthy human subjects before and after 2 weeks capsaicin (3×400 μg orally) treatment offered an excellent possibility to approach the capsaicin actions on the COX-1 and COX-2 enzyme system (Table 9.6).

9.4.5 Gastric (Gastrointestinal) Cytoprotection Versus Capsaicin Actions (Given in Stimulatory Doses of Capsaicin-Sensitive Afferent Nerves)

Observations with different chemical agents (drugs, mediators, and nutritive agents like retinoids, prostaglandins, and others) indicated a special gastric mucosal protection, which did not depend on the gastric acid inhibition (see the reviews Mózsik et al. 2010, 2011a, b). Later on many observations indicated that the so-called gastric cytoprotective agents are able to prevent the development of injuries of different organs (produced by different actions) and they can accelerate healing processes.

The existence of gastric cytoprotection was earlier proved in patients with peptic ulcer (Mózsik et al. 1965, 2010, 2011a, b) as it was nominated by André Robert (1979).

Only few points are interesting in our present position, namely: (1) The capsaicin-induced gastric mucosal protection in healthy human subjects is accompanied with the decrease of gastric acid secretion (that was one of the criteria differed from the of the existence of "classic" gastric cytoprotection); (2) both "classical cytopotective effects" *as well as capsaicin-produced gastric mucosal protection disappear after surgical vagotomy* (but not after chemical vagotomy); (3) gastric cytoprotective effects produced by different agents remained to be the same besides application of capsaicin (given in doses to produce stimulation of capsaicin-sensitive afferent nerves) (Mózsik et al. 1997). These results led us to suggest that: (1) some part a gastric mucosal (cyto) protection is very closely associated with the functional activity of capsaicin-sensitive afferent nerves; (2) increased extent of gastric mucosal damage might develop in consequence of surgical ablation of capsaicin-sensitive afferent nerves (Mózsik et al. 1982, 2011a, b).

These lines of capsaicin and cytoprotection protection in some sensses are similar but differ in others (Szabó et al. 2012; Mózsik et al. 2011a, b).

9.4.6 Immunohistochemical Distribution of Capsaicin Receptor (TRPV1), (CGRP), and Substance P (SP) in the Gastric and Large Bowel Mucosa of Patients with Different Gastrointestinal Disorders

The use of specific antisera against TRVP1 receptor, CGRP, and SP released by the stimulation of capsaicin-sensitive afferent nerve can immunohistochemically demonstrate their presence in the GI mucosa. Please note that mucosal biopsy cannot be performed in healthy human subjects due to ethical regulations. So "healthy subjects" are represented by human subjects with functional disorders having no endoscopic abnormalities and diagnosed by clinicians and independent pathologists. There is another problem, namely the regular biopsy can offer a small tissue sample for its regular pathological histological evaluation. Our specific immunohistochemical observations could be done only after successful routine histological examination.

We studied 178 patients with different gastrointestinal disorders (complaints), and the persons who had normal histology based on the opinion of independent pathologist were used as normal (healthy) human subjects (Dömötör et al. 2007; Mózsik et al. 2007).

The TRVP1 receptor, CGRP, and SP neuropeptides released by the stimulation of capsaicin receptor can be shown by immonohistochemistry both in the human gastric and colon mucosa. The TRVP1 receptors and neuropetides (CGRP and SP) could be demonstrated in the GI mucosa around the nerve endings, vascular vessels, parietal cells, however, in the epithelial layer also.

The capsaicin application and the immunohistochemical demonstration of TRVP1 receptor in the GI tract newly met in the healthy human subjects. We studied the immunohistochemical distribution of TRVP1, CGRP, and SP in the GI mucosa of patients with different disorders. The TRVP1 receptor, CGRP, and SP could be detected practically in all patients with different acute, chronic diseases (including benignant, precancerous, and cancerous diseases) (Dömötör et al. 2005). The results of these observations can be taken only as preliminary results. Their expression differed significantly in the GI mucosa of patients with acute and chronic disorders. Of course, the critical evaluation of these immunohistochemical observations is extremely hard, since we have only very limited information on the origin, stages, time periods of diseases, drug therapies, and suggested etiological backgrounds. The studies dealing with the changes of individual patients with chronic GI disorders—in this research respect—are in progress. We have to emphasize two different main points in these studies, namely (1) The changes of the expressions of TRVP1, CGRP, and SP are helpful from the point of development of GI mucosal injury and prevention, and (2) Probably the participations of TRVP1, CGRP, and SP differ in these GI pathological circumstances.

9.4.7 Immunohistochemical Examinations in Patients with Chronic H. pylori Positive and Negative Gastritis

In human observations, the possible participation of TRVP1, CGRP, and SP were studies in patients with chronic gastritis. The laboratory tests (quick urease test, urea breath test) and specific histological staining widely used in every day medical practice for demonstration of the presence of Helicobacter pylori infection were used, which suggested the presence of bacteria as the etiological for chronic gastritis.

Our studies were carried out in patients with H. pylori positive and negative chronic gastritis. The expression of TRVP1, CGRP, and SP increased significantly in the gastric mucosa with chronic gastritis; however, no difference was obtained on their expression in patients with H. pylori positive and negative chronic gastritis (Dömötör et al. 2006a).

The inflammation of the tissues does not represent a specific tissue reaction to provocation agents. This statement can be concluded from our results obtained in patients with H. positive and negative chronic gastritis due the potential role of capsaicin-sensitive afferent nerves. There is no question that the so-called "neurogenic inflammation" participated in the "general inflammatory processes" in patients with different gastrointestinal disorders.

9.4.8 Capsaicin-Sensitive Afferentation in Patients with Chronic H. pylori Positive Gastritis Before and After Eradication Treatment

The last step of our observations indicated that capsaicin-sensitive afferentation did not differ before and 6 weeks after successful eradication treatment in patients with chronic H. pylori positive gastritis (meanwhile the control biopsy was normal in 22–78 % indicated a moderate improvement of the histological picture of gastritis) (Lakner et al. 2011; Mózsik et al. 2011a, b, 2014; Czimmer et al. 2013).

After careful analysis of these results, it can be stated that the capsaicin-sensitive afferentation represents as an essential pathway in the healing of chronic gastritis (probably without and with Helicobacter pylori infection). These results suggest an independent mechanism in the healing of chronic gastritis which differs from the eradication treatment. By other words, besides the H. pylori infection other factors might exist. The H. pylori infection can be taken as one (but probably most important) exogenous factor, however, the capsaicin-sensitive afferent fibres of vagal nerve represents an endogenous factor in the injury and protection of gastric mucosa (Mózsik et al. 2014).

Our results with capsaicin (in healthy human subjects and in patients with different gastrointestinal disorders) are summarized in Fig. 9.9. The vagal nerve is able to modify the GI tract by regulatory steps at the central nervous system and at the level of target organ. The peripheral action of capsaicin is a dose-dependent action (Szolcsányi 1984; Mózsik et al. 2001) (Table 9.5). Capsaicin releases CGRP and SP (Inui et al. 1991; Dömötör et al. 2005), which modifies the vascular reactions in the gastrointestinal mucosa (Sipos et al. 2006) recently demonstrated that the existence of neuroimmune link between the CGRP, SP, and immune cells in the gastric mucosa of patients with chronic gastritis. Dömötör et al. (2006b) demonstrated the increased release of glucagon during a sugar loading test in healthy human subjects, indicated a new step of capsaicin-induced changes taking place between the capsaicin-sensitive afferent nerves and neurohormonal regulation. Dömötör et al. (2006b) gave a direct evidence for the role of capsaicin in the carbohydrates metabolism.

There were a few very surprising matters due to capsaicin from the point of human classical clinical pharmacology prior to our observations:

1. No permitted orally applicable capsaicin preparation available for humans;
2. No chronic toxicology to capsaicin in animal observations (two spices of animals—rodent and dog-treated with capsaicin for 6 months);
3. No direct clinical pharmacological study to germinative function;
4. Capsaicin (Sigma-Aldrich, USA) chemically is not uniform due to its content of dihydrocapsaicin, nordihydrocapsaicin, and some other capsaicinoids;
5. No classical human clinical pharmacological study (human phase I and phase II) was found in the literature;
6. No correct Drug Master File (DMF) for capsaicin preparations were developed for the commercially obtained capsaicin (except for a certain capsaicin preparation obtained from India and used by us);
7. No human pharmacokinetic observations were available for capsaicin (please remember that our capsaicin studies in healthy human subjects were started in 1997).

Bernard et al. (2008) were unable to create pharmacokinetic profile of capsaicinoids after administration of 15 and 30 mg of capsaicin/person; meanwhile, the detection limit was 10 ng/ml. Chaiyasit et al. (2009) applied orally 5 gram of C. frurenscens (equivalent to 26.6 mg pure capsaicin) indicated that the capsaicin could be detected in plasma after 10 min, and the peak concentration (C_{max}) was 2.47 ± 0.13 ng/mL, t max was 47.1 ± 2.0 min, and $t_{½}$ was 24.9 ± 5.0 min. After 90 min, capsaicin could not be detected in the plasma. Chaiyasit et al. (2009) explained the results of Bernard et al. (2008) by the time factor of pharmacokinetic behaviors of capsaicin in humans. The results of these observations were mentioned in the review paper by O'Neill et al. (2012).

We also received new information from the chronic toxicological studies in Beagle dogs (2008). These animals were treated with different doses (0.1, 0, 3, and 0.9 mg/kg body weight/day orally given) of capsaicin(noids) for 1 month. No toxic effects were observed in these dogs during the whole treatment periods. We noticed surprisingly that capsaicin and dihydocapsaicin could not be detected in the sera of Beagle dogs by either High Pressure Chromatography (HPLC) with the detection limit of 20 ng/mL serum or Liquid Chromatography—Mass Spectrometry (LC–MS) with the detection was 26 fg/mL in the serum at any time after the oral administration of capsaicin(oids) (Mózsik et al. 2008; Boros et al. 2008).

In our human phase I. examination (when we applied orally 400 or 800 μg capsaicinoid orally alone or in combination with aspirin or diclofenac) neither capsaicin nor dihydrocapsaicin could be detected in the sera of healthy volunteers of any time after the capsaicin(oids) application.

Our comments on the above-mentioned pharmacokinetic observations in healthy subjects are:

1. The applied dose of capsaicin was extremely high in human beings.
2. The exact chemical compositions of plant origin capsaicin preparations was not known.
3. Capsaicin concentration was measured in the sera of healthy subjects during these studies and no dihydrocapsaicin concentration mentioned.
4. There was no mentioning of the fact that capsaicin is transformed into dihydocapsaicin during metabolism.

In light of the results obtained in Beagle dogs and healthy human subjects, it is clear that capsaicin(oids) acts (act) primarily locally. This state was accepted in our human phase I. clinical pharmacological studies, when the capsaicin(oids) alone and in combination with aspirin, diclofenac, and naproxen were put in bioadhesive compounds during the industrial preparation, since we aimed at the enhance local actions of these drug candidate molecules in the stomach.

We never tested the actions of capsaicin(oids) in the gastrointestinal tract in any other application forms than oral.

9.4.9 Main Conclusion from Our Observations on Capsaicin Application in Healthy Human Subjects and in Patients with Different Disorders

1. Capsaicin (as a specific agent to stimulate the capsaicin-sensitive afferent nerves) plays a special role in the regulation the gastric functions (decrease of gastric acid secretion, increase of gastric emptying, increase in "buffering part" of the gastric secretion, increase of gastric transmucosal potential difference), absorption of glucose (and in its metabolism as well as in increase of glycagon release) in healthy human subjects, when it is applied in stimulatory doses.
2. Capsaicin (given orally in stimulatory doses) protects against the alcohol and NSAID-induced gastric mucosal damage in healthy human subjects.
3. Capsaicin given in stimulatory doses to capsaicin-sensitive afferent nerves did not produce desensitization of its receptor (neither in acute administrations nor in chronic administrations) in healthy human subjects.
4. The presence of capsaicin receptor (also CGRP and SP, which are very close in physiological relation) can be shown by specific immunohistochemical methods in various gastrointestinal disorders.

5. Capsaicin-induced gastroprotection differs from the eradication treatment in patients with chronic H. pylori positive gastritis (and probably the roles of capsaicin receptor and CGRP differ from the SP).
6. It is very important to note that these gastroprotective actions can be obtained only by administration of capsaicin in stimulatory doses to its sensitive afferent nerves.
7. The human phase I. examinations clearly indicated that the capsaicin and dihydrocapsaicin cannot be detected in the serum of volunteers; and the examined person tolerated well the orally given capsaicin in doses of 400 and 800 μg or in co-administration with ASA and diclofenac. Furthermore, it is also important, that the administration of capsaicin (in different doses) will not modify the absorption and metabolism of ASA and diclofenac; meanwhile, the inhibition of platelet aggregation remained the same.

After looking at this conclusion list, there are clear evidences that the capsaicin is an orally applicable drug either alone or in combinations with different NSAIDs to healthy human subjects and to patients. Its indications are wide from the prevention of drug-induced gastric mucosal damage in from patients under long-term aspirin treatment (due to cardiovascular disease, thrombophilia, and rheumatoid arthritis), in pain killer treatment, and pin patients having chronic H. pylori positive gastritis and in patient with different carbohydrate disorders.

We are of the opinion that we can scientifically put down the clinical pharmacological bases of the oral capsaicin or drug combination use. Of course, we are aware that many other observations are needed to be carried out in accordance to the regulations of international drug development, production, and marketing for a capsaicin containing drug for the everyday medical treatment.

Acknowledgments This study was supported by the National Office for Research and Technology, "Pázmány Péter" Programme, RET-II 08/2005 (2005–2008), and by Baross Grant Programme (REG-DG-09-2-2009-0087,CAPSATAB) (2011–2012).

References

Abdel- Salam OME, Debreceni A, Mózsik Gy (1999) Capsaicin-sensitive afferent sensory nerves in modulating gastric mucosal defense against noxious agents. J Physiol Paris 93:443–454

Abdel- Salam OME, Czimmer J, Debreceni A, Mózsik Gy (2001) Gastric mucosal integrity: Gastric mucosal blood flow and microcirculation. An overview. J Physiol Paris 95:105–127

Aijoka H, Miyake H, Matsuura N (2000) Effect of FRG-8813, a new-type histamine H_2-receptor antagomist, on the recurrence of gastric ulcer healing by drug treatment. Pharmacology 61:83–90

Aijoka H, Matsuura N, Miyake H (2002) High quality of ulcer healing in rats by lafutidine and new-type histamine H_2-receptor antagonist: involvement of capsaicin of sensitive sensory neurons. Inflammopharmacology 10:483–493

Antal L, Mózsik Gy, Jávor T, Krausz M (1965) The electrolyte content of gastric juice after prolonged atropine treatment. In: Magyar I (ed) Acta tertii conventus medicinae internae hungarici. Gastroenterologia. Akadémiai Kiadó, Budapest, pp 167–169

Bernard BK,Tsubuku S, Kayhara T, Maeda K, Hanada M, Nakamura T, Shirai Y, Nakayaha A, Ueno S, Mihara H (2008) Studies of the toxicological potential of capsaicinoids.X. Safety assessment and pharmacokinetics of capsaicinoids in healthy male vlonteers after single oral ingestion of CH-19 sweet extract. Int J Toxicol 27(Suppl 3):137–147

Boros B, Dornyei Á, Felinger A (2008) Determination of capsaicin and dihydrocapsaicin in dog plasma by liquid chromatography- Mass Spectography (analytical method report). PTE TTK Analitikai Kémiai Tanszék, Pécs

Buck SH, Burks TF (1986) The neuropharmacology of capsaicin: a review of some recent observation. Pharmacol Rev 38:179–226

Caterina MJ, Schumacher MA, Tominaga H, Rosen TA, Levine JD, Julius D (1997) The capsaicin receptor: a heat-activated ion channel in the pain pathway. Nature 389:816–824

Chaiyasit E, Khovidhunkit W, Wittayertpanya S (2009) Pharmacokinetic and the effect of capsaicin in Capsicum flourescens on decreasing plasma glucose level. J Med Assoc Thai 92:108–113

Csáky TZ (1969) Introduction to general pharmacology. Appleton–century-craft educational division. Meredith Corporation, New York, pp 17–34

Czimmer J, Szabó IL, Szolcsányi J, Mózsik Gy (2013) Capsaicin-sensitive afferentation represents a new mucosal defensive neural pathway system in the gastric mucosa in patients with chronic gastritis. In: Mozsik Gy (ed) Current topics in gastritis–2012. INTECH Publishers, Rijeka, pp 61–75

Debreceni A, Abdel-Salam OME, Figler M, Juricskay I, Szolcsányi J, Mózsik Gy (1999) Capsaicin increases gastric emptying rate in healthy human subjects measured by ^{13}C-labeled octanoid acid breath test. J Physiol Paris 93:455–460

Dömötör A, Zs Peidl, Vincze Á, Hunyady B, Szolcsányi J, Gy Szekeres, Mózsik Gy (2005) Immunohistochemical distribution of vanilloid receptor, calcitonin- gene related peptide and substance P in gastrointestinal mucosa of patients with different gastrointestinal disorders. Inflammopharmacology 13:161–177

Dömötör A, Kereskay L, Gy Szekeres, Hunyady B, Szolcsányi J, Mózsik Gy (2006a) Participation of capsaicin sensitive afferent nerves in the gastric mucosa of patients with helicobacter pylori-positive or –negative chronic gastritis. Dig Dis Sci 52:411–417

Dömötör A, Szolcsányi J, Mózsik Gy (2006b) Capsaicin and glucose absorption and utilization in healthy human subjects. Eur J Pharmacol 534:280–283

Fisher MA, Hunt JN (1976) A sensitive method for measuring haemoglobin in the gastric juice. Digestion 14:409–414

Gabella G, Pease H (1973) Number of axons in the abdominal vagus of the rat. Brain Res 58:465–469

Grijalva CV, Novin D (1990) The role of hypothalamus and dorsal vagal complex in gastrointestinal function an pathophysiology. Ann N Y Acad Sci 597:207–221

Hollander F (1934) The component of gastric secretion. Am J Dig Dis Sci 1:319–329

Holzer P (1998) Neural emergency system in the stomachs. Gastroenterology 114:823–839

Holzer P (1999) Capsaicin cellular targets. Mechanisms of action, as selectivity for thin sensory neurons. Phamacol Rev 43:143–201

Holzer P (2013) Transient receptor potential (TRP) channels as drug targets for disesases of the gastrointestional system. Pharmacol Ther 131: 142–170

Holzer P, Lippe IL (1988) Stimulation of afferent nerve endings by intragastric capsaicin against ethanol-induced damage of gastric mucosa. Neuroscinece 27:981–987

Holzer P, Sametz W (1986) Gastric mucosal protection against ulcerogenic factors in the rat mediated by capsaicin-sensitive afferent neurones. Gastroenterology 91:975–981

Hossenbocus A, Fitzpatrick P, Colin-Jones DG (1975) Measurement of gastric potential difference at endoscopy. Gut 14:410–415

Inui T, Kinoshita J, Yamahuchi A, Yamatani T, Chiba T (1991) Linkage between capsaicin-stimulated calcitonin gene-related peptide and somatostatin release in the rat stomach. Am J Physiol 261:G770–G774

Jancsó N, Jancsó- Gábor A, Szolcsányi J (1967) Direct evidence for neurogenic inflammation and its prevention by denervation and by pretreatment with capsaicin. Brit J Pharmacol 31:138–151

Jancsó N, Jancsó- Gábor A, Szolcsányi J (1968) The role of sensory nerves endings in the neurogen inflammation induced in human skin and in the eye and paw of the rat. Brit J Pharmacol 33:32–41

Jancsó-Gábor A, Szolcsányi J, Jancsó N (1970) Irreversible impairment of the irregulation induced by capsaicin and similar pungent substances in rat and guinea-pigs. J Physiol London 206:495–507

Karádi O, Mózsik Gy (2000) Surgical and Chemical Vagotomy on the Gastrointestinal Mucosal Defense. Akadémiai Kiadó, Budapest

Kawai S, Nishida S, Kato M, Furumaya Y, Okamoto R, Koshino T, Mizushima Y (1998) Comparison of cyclooxygenase-1 and -2 inhibitory activities of various nonsteroidal anti-inflammatory drugs using human platelets and synovial cells. Eur J Pharmacol 347:87–94

Lakner L, Dömötör A, Cs Tóth, Szabo IL, Mecker Á, Hajós R, Kereskay L, Gy Szekeres, Döbrönte Z, Mózsik Gy (2011) Capsaicin-sensitive afferentation represents an indifferent defensive pathway from eradication in patients with helicobacter pylori positive gastritis. World J Gastrointest Pharmacol Ther 2:36–41

Marfertheimer P, Megraud F, 0'Morain C, Bazzoli F, El-Omar E, Graham D, Hunt R, Rokkas T, Vakil N, Kuipers EJ (2007) Current concept in the management of Helicobacter pylori infection: the Maastricht III consensus report. Gut 56: 772–781

Mózsik Gy (2006) Molecular pharmacology and biochemistry of gastroduodenal mucosal damage and protection. In: Mózsik Gy (ed) Discoveries in gastroenterology: from basic research to clinical perspectives (1960–2005). Akadémiai Kiadó, Budapest, pp 139–224

Mózsik Gy (2010) Gastric cytoprotection 30 years after its discovery by André Robert: a personal perspective. Inflammopharmacology 18:209–221

Mózsik Gy, Jávor T, Dobi S (1965) Clinical-pharmaological analysis of long term parasympatholytic treatment. In: Magyar I (ed) Acta tertii conventus medicinae internae Hungarici. Gastroenterologia. Akadémiai Kiadó, Budapest, pp 709–715

Mózsik Gy, Abdel-Salam OME, Szolcsányi J (1997) Capsaicin-sensitive afferent nerves in gastric mucosal damage and protection. Akadémiai Kiadó, Budapest

Mózsik Gy, Sarlos P, Racz I, Szolcsányi J (2003) Evidence for the direct protective effect of capsaicin in human healthy subjects. Gastroenterology 124(Suppl 1):A-454

Mózsik Gy, Belágyi J, Szolcsányi J, Pár G, Pár A, Rumi Gy, Rácz I (2004a) Capsaicin-sensitive afferent nerves and gastric mucosal protection on human healthy subjects. A critical overview. In: Takeuchi K, Mozsik Gy (eds) Mediators in gastrointestinal protection and repair. Research Signpost, Kerala, pp 43–62

Mózsik Gy, Pár A, Pár G, Juricskay I, Figler M, Szolcsányi J (2004a) Insight into the molecular pharmacology to drugs acting on the afferent and efferent fibres of vagal nerve in the gastric mucosal protection. In: Sikirič P, Seiwerth P, Mózsik Gy, Arakawa T, Takeuchi K (eds) Proceedings of the 11th international conference on ulcer research. Monduzzi, Bologna, pp 163–168

Mózsik Gy, Past T, Perjési P, Szolcsányi J (2008) Determination of capsaicin and dihydrocapsaicin content of dog's plasma by HPLC-FLD method. In: Mózsik Gy, Past T, Pejési P, Szolcsány J (eds) Original reports on toxicology of capsaicin.VII. 8 day oral tocicity study of test item capsaicin natural USP 37 in beagle dogs (final report). LAB International research Centre Hungary Ltd. Veszprém, Hungary by the date of final repot 13 June 2008. Study Code: 07/496–100 K, pp 1–35 text and 190 pages in Appendices (Appendix 2.11) pp 1–37

Mózsik Gy, Szabó IL,Dömötör A (2011b) Approach to role of capsaicin-sensitive afferent nerves in the development and healing in patients with chronic gastritis. In: Tonito P (ed) Gastritis and gastric cancer. New Insights in gastroprotection, diagnosis and treatments. INTECH Publishers, Rijeka, pp 25–46

Mózsik Gy, Szabó IL, Czimmer J (2014) Vulnerable points of the Helicobacter pylori story—based on animal and human observations (19752012). In: Buzas Gy (ed) Helicobacter pylori—a Worldwide Perspective 2013. Bentham Science Publishers, Oak Park (in press)

Mózsik Gy, Jávor T (1969b) Development of drug cross-tolerance in patients treated chronically with atropine. Eur J Pharmacol 6:169–174

Mózsik Gy, Jávor T, Dobi S, Petrássy K, Szabó A (1966) Development of "pharmacological denervation phenomenon" in patients treated with atropine. Eur J Pharmacol 1:391–395

Mózsik Gy, Berstad A, Myren J, Setekleiv J (1969a) Absorption and urinary excretion oxyphencyclamin HCI in patients before and after a prolonged oxyphencyclimide treatment. Med Exp 19:10–16

Mózsik Gy, Moron F, Jávor T (1982) Cellular mechanisms of the development of gastric mucosal damage and of gastro protection induced by prostacyclin in rats. A pharmacological study. Prostagland Leukot Med 9:71–84

Mózsik Gy, Hunyady B, Garamszegi M, Németh A, Pakodi F, Vincze A (1994) Dynamism of cytoprotective and antisecretory drugs in patients with unhealed gastric and duodenal ulcers. J Gastroenterol Hepatol 9:S88–S92

Mózsik Gy, Debreceni A, Abdel-Salam OME, Szabó I, Figler M, Ludány A, Juricskay I, Szolcsányi J (1999) Small doses capsaicin given intragastrically inhibit gastric basal gastric secretion in healthy human subjects. J Physiol Paris 93:433–436

Mózsik Gy, Vincze Á, Szolcsányi J (2001) Four responses of capsaicin sensitive primary afferent neurons to capsaicin and its analog. Gastric acid secretion, gastric mucosal damage and protection. J Gastroenterol Hepatol 16:193–197

Mózsik Gy, Rácz I, Szolcsányi J (2005) Gastroprotection induced by capsaicin in human healthy subjects. World J Gastroenterol 11:5180–5184

Mózsik Gy, Szolcsányi J, Dömötör A (2007) Capsaicin research as a new tool to approach of the human gastrointestinal physiology, pathology and pharmacology. Inflammopharmacology 15:232–245

Mózsik Gy, Dömötör A, Past T, Vas V, Perjési P, Kuzma M, Gy Blazics, Szolcsányi J (2009a) Capsaicinoids: from the plant cultivation to the production of the human medical therapy. Akadémiai Kiadó, Budapest

Mózsik Gy, Past T, Abdel-Salam OME, Kuzma M, Perjési P (2009b) Interdisciplinary review for correlation between the plant origin capsaicinoids, nonsteroidal antiinflammatory drugs, gastrointestinal mucosal damage and prevention in animals and human beings. Inflammopharmacology 17:113–150

Mózsik Gy, Past T, Dömötör A, Kuzma M, Perjési P (2010) Production of orally applicable new drug or drug combinations from natural origin capsaicinoids for human medical therapy. Curr Pharm Des 16:1197–1208

Mózsik Gy, Szabo IL, Czimmer J (2011a) Approaches to gastrointestinal cytoprotection: from isolated cell, via animal experiments to healthy human subjects and patients with different gastrointestinal disorders. Curr Pharm Des 17:1556–1572

Myren J (1968) Gastric secretion following stimulation with histamine, histology and gastrin in man. In: Semb L, Myren J (eds) The physiology of gastric secretion. Universitetforlaget, Oslo, pp 413–428

Nagy L, Mózsik Gy, Feledi É, Cs Ruzsa, Zs Vezekényi, Jávor T (1984) Gastric microbleeding measurements during 1 day treatment with indomethacin and indomethacin plus sodium salicylate (1:10) in patients. Acta Physiol Hung 64:373–377

O'Neill J, Brock C, Olesen E, Andersen T, Nilsson M, Dickenson AH (2012) Unravelling the mystery of capsaicin: a tool to understand and treat pain. Pharmacol Rev 64:939–997

Onodera S, Shibata M, Tanaka M (1999) Gastroprotective mechanisms of lafutidine, a novel anti-ulcer drug with histamine H_2-receptor antagonist activity, Artneim. Forsch. Drug Res 49:519–526

Patty I, Tárnok F, Simon L, Jávor T, Deák G, Sz Benedek, Kenéz P, Nagy L, Mózsik Gy (1984) A comparative dynamic study of the effectiveness of gastric cytoprotection by the vitamin A, De-Nol, sucralfate and ulcer healing by pirenzepine in patients with chronic gastric ulcer (A multiclinical and randomized study). Acta Physiol Hung 64:379–384

Robert A, Nemazis JE, Lancastter C, Hanchar A (1979) Cytoprotection by prostaglandins in rats. Prevention of gastric necrosis by alcohol, HCl, NaOH, hypertonic NaCl and thermal injury. Gastroenterology 77:4433–4443

Sarlós P, Rumi Gy, Szolcsányi J, Mózsik Gy, Vincze Á (2003) Capsaicin prevents the indomethacin-induced gastric mucosal damage in human healthy subject. Gastroenterology 124(Suppl 1):A-511

Sipos G, Altdorfer K, Pongor É, Chen LP, Fehér E (2006) Neuroimmune link in the mucosa of chronic gastritis with Helicobacter pylori infection. Dig Dis Sci 51:1810–1817

Szabo S, Taché Y, Tarnawski A (2012) The "Gastric Cytoprotection" concept of André Robert and the origins of a new series of international symposia. In: Filaretova LP, Takeuchi K (eds) Cell/Tissue injury and cytoprotection/organoprotection in the gastrointestinal tract. Front gastrointest res, vol 30. Karger, Basel, pp 1–23

Szabo IL, Czimmer J, Szolcsányi J, Mózsik Gy (2013) Molecular pharmacological approaches to effects of capsaicinoids and of classical antisecretory drugs on gastric basal acid secretion and on indomethacin-induced hastric mucosal damage in human healthy subjects (mini review). Curr Pharm Des 19:84–89

Szállasi A, Blumberg M (1999) Vanilloid (capsaicin) receptors and mechanisms. Pharmacol Rev 51:159–211

Szolcsányi J (1984) Capsaicin sensitive chemoprotective neural system with dual sensory-afferent function. In: Chalh LA, Szolcsányi J, Lembeck F (eds) Antidromic vasodilatation and neurogenic inflammation. Budapest, Akadémiai Kiadó, pp 27–56

Szolcsányi J (1997) A pharmacological approach to elucidation of the role of different nerve fibres and receptor endings in mediation of pain. J Physiol Paris 73:251–259

Szolcsányi J (2004) Forty years in capsaicin research for sensory pharmacology and physiology. Neuropeptide 38:377–384

Szolcsányi J, Barthó L (1981) Impaired defense mechanisms to peptic ulcer in the capsaicin-desensitized rat. In: Mózsik Gy, Hänninen O, Jávor T (eds) Advances in physiological sciences, gastrointestinal defense mechanisms, vol 29. Pergamon Press, Oxford-Akadémiai Kiadó, Budapest, pp 39–51

Takeuchi K (2006) Unique profile of Lafutidine: a novel histamine H_2-receptor antagonist: mucosal protection throughout GI mucosal mediated by capsaicin-sensitive afferent nerves. Acta Pharmacol. (Sinica Suppl):27–35

Tárnok F, Jávor T, Mózsik Gy, Nagy L, Patty I, Gy Rumi, Solt I (1979) A prospective multiclinical study comparing the effects of placebo, carbenoxolone, atropine cimetidine in patients with duodenal ulcer. Drugs Exp Clin Res 5:157–166

Tárnok F, Deák G, Jávor T, Mózsik Gy, Nagy L, Patty I (1983) Effect of combination atropine and cyproheptadine and atropine + carbenoxolone in duodenal ulcer therapy. Int J Tiss React 5:315–321

Vincze A, Szekeres Gy, Király Á, Bódis B, Mózsik Gy (2004) The immunohistochemical distribution of capsaicin receptor, CGRP and SP in the human gastric mucosa in patients with different gastric disorders. In: Sikirič, Seiwert S, Mózsik Gy, Arakawa T, Takeuchi K (eds) Proceedings of 11th international congress of ulcer resarch. Monduzzi, Bologna, pp 149–153

Wildersmith CH, Ernst T, Gennoni M, Zeyen B, Halter F, Merki HS (1990) Tolerance to H_2-receptor antagonist. Dig Dis Sci 35:976–983

Chapter 10
Capsaicin Receptor as Target of Calcitonin Gene-Related Peptide in the Gut

Stefano Evangelista

Abstract Calcitonin gene-related peptide (CGRP), a 37 aminoacid-residue peptide, is a marker of afferent fibers in the upper gastrointestinal tract, being almost completely depleted following treatment with the selective neurotoxin capsaicin that targets these fibers via transient receptor potential vanilloid type-1 (TRPV-1). It is widely distributed in the peripheral nervous system of mammals where it is present as α isoform, while intrinsic neurons of the enteric nervous systems express predominantly CGRP-β. Many gastrointestinal functions involve CGRP-containing afferent fibers of the enteric nervous system such as defense against irritants, intestinal nociception, modulation of gastrointestinal motility and secretion, and healing of gastric ulcers. The main effects on stomach homeostasis rely on local vasodilator actions during increased acid-back diffusion. In humans, release of CGRP through the activation of TRPV-1 has been shown to protect from gastric damage induced by several stimuli and to be involved in gastritis. In both dyspepsia and irritable bowel syndrome the repeated stimulation of TRPV-1 induced an improvement in epigastric pain of these patients. The TRPV-1/CGRP pathway might be a novel target for therapeutics in gastric mucosal injury and visceral sensitivity.

10.1 Molecular Biology

In the central and peripheral nervous systems, the RNA transcript from the calcitonin gene yields an mRNA, which encodes the 37 aminoacid-residue peptide calcitonin gene-related peptide (CGRP), proved to be an important physiologic mediator (Wimalawansa 1996; van Rossum et al. 1997). CGRP is the first

S. Evangelista (✉)
Department of Preclinical Development, Menarini Ricerche SpA,
Via Sette Santi 1, 50131 Florence, Italy
e-mail: sevangelista@menarini-ricerche.it

O. M. E. Abdel-Salam (ed.), *Capsaicin as a Therapeutic Molecule*, Progress in Drug Research 68, DOI: 10.1007/978-3-0348-0828-6_10, © Springer Basel 2014

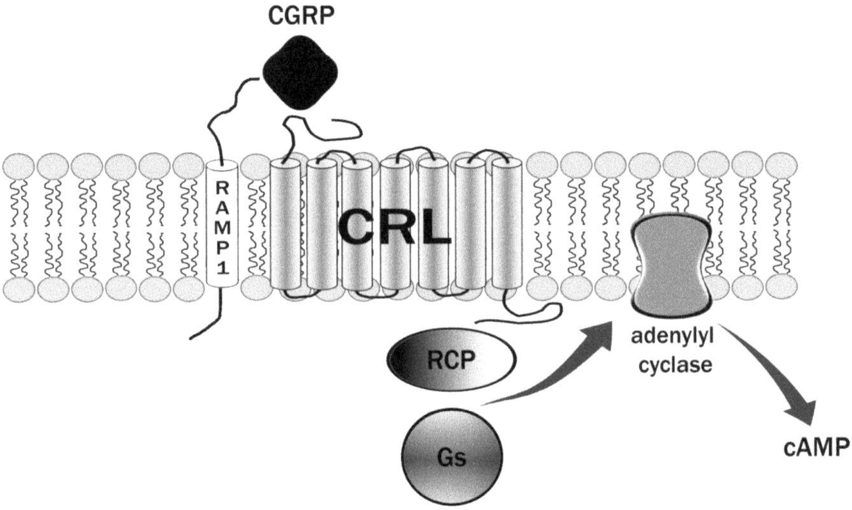

Fig. 10.1 Schematic view of the CGRP receptor that consists of calcitonin receptor-like peptide (CLR), receptor activity modifying protein 1 (RAMP1), and receptor component protein (RCP)

biologically active neuropeptide identified through the molecular biology approach (Rosenfeld et al. 1983) and can be found in two forms as CGRP-α, which is generated by transcription and alternative splicing of the calcitonin (CT)/CGRP-α gene, and as CGRP-β, which is encoded by the CGRP-β gene. The two forms differ by one and three amino acids in rats and humans respectively. CGRP-β has been shown to have a pattern of expression that overlaps, but is nonidentical to that of CGRP-α, with CGRP-α having a higher level of expression in most neurons of the central and peripheral nervous system (Mulderry et al. 1988). One exception is the intrinsic neurons of the enteric nervous systems, which express predominantly CGRP-β mRNA.

CGRP is a member of a family of peptides that share sequence homology and have some overlapping biological activities. The members of the family include amylin, adrenomedullin, and CGRP (Barwell et al. 2012).

Receptors to this peptide have been divided into two classes in the past, CGRP1 and CGRP2, on the basis of functional tests. After the cloning of calcitonin receptor-like receptor (CLR) and receptor activity-modifying proteins (RAMPs), it became clear that the CGRP1 receptor was a complex between CLR and RAMP1 (Fig. 10.1). It is now apparent that the CGRP2 receptor phenotype is the result of CGRP acting at receptors for amylin and adrenomedullin and therefore, the term "CGRP2" receptor should no longer be used, and the "CGRP1" receptor should be known as the "CGRP" receptor. The CGRP receptor consists of a seven-transmembrane-spanning protein designated RAMP1 and an intracellular component protein (RCP) (Fig. 10.1). RAMP1 is involved in receptor trafficking and is required for CGRP binding to CLR, whereas the interaction of CLR with other RAMP proteins forms adrenomedullin receptors (Evans et al. 2000).

The human C-terminal fragment of the peptide, $hCGRP_{8-37}$, was the first and widely used tool for determining whether the action of CGRP as well as that of CT is mediated via specific CGRP receptors or CT receptors. It selectively antagonizes CGRP activity, being also an agonist for CT receptor (van Rossum et al. 1997). So far some CGRP antagonists are in development as a potential treatment for acute migraine attacks (Negro et al. 2012). This new class of drugs is designed to block and/or reverse CGRP-mediated dilation of intracranial vessels induced by activation of the main sensory nerves in the brain. CGRP is also thought to play a role in cardiovascular homeostasis and nociception (Wimalawansa 1996; van Rossum et al. 1997).

10.2 Distribution

CGRP is widely distributed in both peripheral and central neurons. The function and expression of CGRP may differ depending on the location of synthesis in the spinal cord. CGRP is derived mainly from the cell bodies of motor neurons when synthesized in the anterior horn of the spinal cord and may contribute to the regeneration of nervous tissue after injury. When synthesized in the posterior horn of the spinal cord, CGRP came from posterior root ganglion and may be linked to the transmission of pain. In the trigeminal vascular system, the cell bodies on the ganglion are the main source of CGRP. High levels of CGRP-like immunoreactivity (LI) have been found in the rat (Sternini et al. 1987) and human (Tani et al. 1999) stomach and the absence of CGRP-LI in endocrine cells suggests that it is more important as a neurotransmitter than as a circulating hormone. Further to dorsal root ganglia, gastric muscle, and mucosa are innervated by vagal afferent from nodose ganglia, another source of CGRP playing important functional role of the stomach (Young et al. 2008) (Fig. 10.2). Since no positive CGRP cells are found in the stomach, most gastric CGRP is of extrinsic origin and is contained and released from peripheral endings of capsaicin-sensitive afferents (Holzer 2007).

In the enteric nervous system CGRP-β is expressed in a subset of Dogiel type II, intrinsic primary afferent neurons that are not sensitive to capsaicin, while CGRP-α is the primary isoform expressed in the sensory afferent neurons of the extrinsic nervous system originating from the dorsal root and vagal ganglia (Fig. 10.2).

10.3 Target of TRPV-1 Agonists and Antagonists

Capsaicin is the main capsaicinoid in chili peppers, followed by dihydrocapsaicin. These two compounds are also about twice as potent to the taste and nerves as compared to the minor capsaicinoids such as nordihydrocapsaicin, homodihydrocapsaicin, and homocapsaicin (Table 10.1). Capsaicin is believed to be synthesized in the interlocular septum of chili peppers by addition of a branched-chain

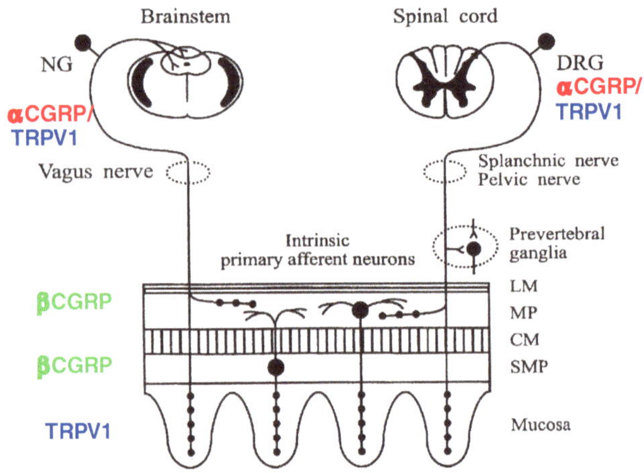

Fig. 10.2 Schematic representation of the extrinsic and intrinsic CGRP-containing neurons and TRPV-1 distribution in the gastrointestinal tract. Extrinsic spinal afferents have their cell bodies in the dorsal root ganglia and contain only α-CGRP. CGRP-containing extrinsic nerve terminals innervate the circular and longitudinal smooth muscle layers, the myenteric plexus and the submucosal plexus, where they densely innervate vascular structures and the mucosa. CGRP-containing intrinsic enteric neurons express only β-CGRP that are localized in the submucosal and myenteric plexuses. Submucosal neurons innervate the mucosa, whereas myenteric neurons project orally and aborally, both within the myenteric plexus and to the circular muscle layer. TRPV-1 was found in both DGR and NG and in the latter coexpressed with CGRP only in 10 % of the neurons. TRPV-1 is present also in the parietal cells of the mucosa. *CM* circular smooth muscle; *DRG* dorsal root ganglion; *LM* longitudinal smooth muscle; *MP* myenteric plexus; *NG* nodose ganglia; *SMP* submucosal plexus

fatty acid to vanillylamine; specifically, capsaicin is made from vanillylamine and 8-methyl-6-nonenoyl CoA. Biosynthesis depends on the gene *AT3*, which resides at the *pun1* locus, and which encodes a putative acyltransferase. Besides the six natural capsaicinoids, the synthetic capsaicinoid vanillylamide of n-nonanoic acid (VNA, also PAVA) is used as a reference substance for determining the relative pungency of capsaicinoids (Table 10.1).

From the pioneering work of Jancsò (1960) it has been shown that capsaicin is a selective neurotoxin for sensory nerves, and this has led the exploration of the functional role of these neurons, e.g., at the gastrointestinal level and to the hypothesis of dual "sensory-efferent" functions mediated by capsaicin-sensitive neurons (Holzer 1991, 2007). Capsaicin affects the afferent neurons by two distinct phases: an initial excitation followed by a long-lasting refractory state during which the neurons are not responsive to the neurotoxin and other stimuli. The refractory state (also called desensitization) is usually reversible in terms of weeks, but the systemic administration of high doses of the neurotoxin causes permanent neurotoxicity (Holzer 1991). These neurons are important to transmit sensory information toward the central nervous system but also to release their neurotransmitters toward the periphery, playing a local effector role in several regulatory processes. CGRP is considered the likely mediator of sensory neurons in the stomach and their marker in the upper gastrointestinal tract. Recent studies have shown that capsaicin specifically targets these afferent nerves via

Table 10.1 Names and characteristics of the natural capsacinoids and the synthetic one (PAVA) used as reference for pungency

Capsaicinoid name	Abbreviations	Typical relative amount (%)	Chemical structure
Capsaicin	C	69	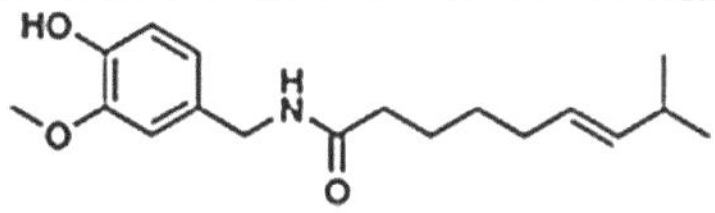
Dihydrocapsaicin	DHC	22	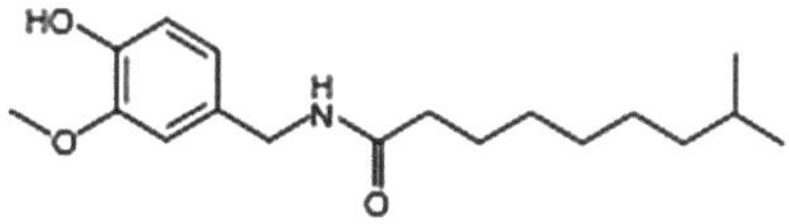
Nordihydrocapsaicin	NDHC	7	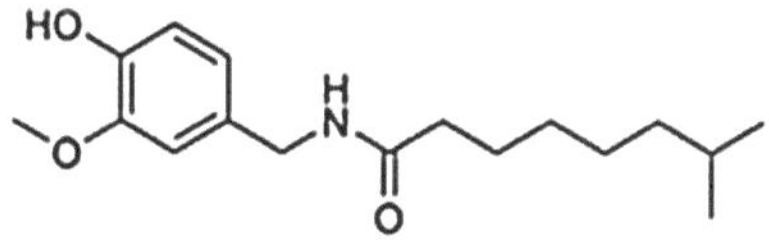
Homodihydrocapsaicin	HDHC	1	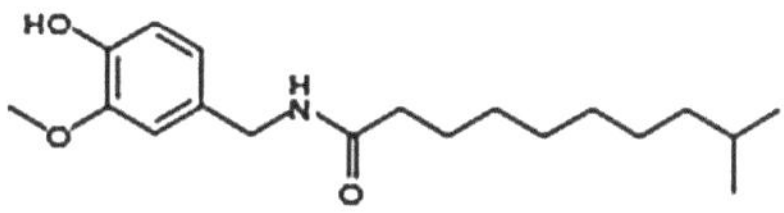
Homocapsaicin	HC	1	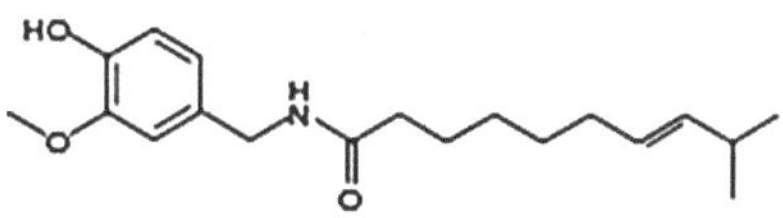
Nonivamide	PAVA		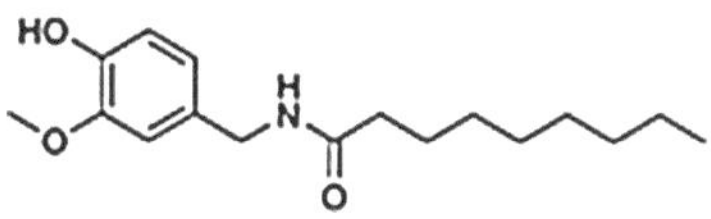

transient receptor potential vanilloid of type-1 (TRPV-1), a non selective cation channel with high permeability for Ca^{++} (Holzer 2007). TRPV-1 belongs to a family of store operated Ca^{++} channels and acts as a polymodal detector of potentially harmful stimuli including capsaicin, resiniferatoxin, noxious heat, H^{+} ions, anandamide, and several lipoxygenase products (Holzer 2007). Gingerol, piperine, and zingerone are other spices that might act as TRPV-1 agonists. TRPV-1 and CGRP coimmunoreactivity was found in almost all the dorsal root ganglia and in 10 % of the nodose ganglia (Zhong et al. 2008; Fig. 10.2).

The dual "sensory-efferent" functions can be envisaged with gastric ulcers: animals pretreated with high doses of capsaicin show an aggravation of experimentally induced ulceration because of depletion of protective neurotransmitters. On the other hand, local application of low doses of capsaicin affords gastric protection through the release of neuropeptides (among them: substance P and CGRP) in the periphery (Holzer 1991, 1998; Abdel-Salam et al. 1999; Szolcsànyi and Bartho 2001; Evangelista 2009). This was confirmed by the use of agonists and antagonists of the TRPV-1 (Peng and Li 2010). Functional TRPV-1 antagonists such as ruthenium red and capsazepine produced aggravation of gastric antral ulcers and inhibited the gastroprotective effects of low doses of capsaicin (Yamamoto et al. 2001). Resiniferatoxin is a naturally occurring, ultrapotent capsaicin analog that activates the vanilloid receptor in a subpopulation of primary afferent sensory neurons involved in nociception. Resiniferatoxin causes an ion channel in the plasma membrane of sensory neurons to become permeable to cations, most particularly the calcium cation; this evokes a powerful irritant effect followed by desensitization and analgesia. Neurochemical and functional studies were carried out to investigate and to compare the effects of resiniferatoxin and capsaicin in the rat stomach (Tramontana et al. 1994). Neonatal administration of resiniferatoxin (0.6–1.6 μmol/kg s.c.) produced a marked decrease in gastric CGRP-LI in both secretory and nonsecretory region of the stomach. Almost complete depletion of the peptide was determined by neonatal administration of capsaicin (164 μmol/kg s.c.). Vasoactive intestinal polypeptide-LI was concomitantly unaffected by resiniferatoxin or capsaicin, thus showing the selectivity of action of the neurotoxins on gastric afferent fibers. Oral administration of an equimolar dose (0.3 nmol/kg) of resiniferatoxin or capsaicin together with 50 % ethanol reduced at similar extent gastric haemorrhagic lesions produced by the mucosal barrier-breaker agent. These findings provide evidence that resiniferatoxin and capsaicin may act on a common neuronal target in the rat stomach and that the acute exciting (protective) effect is of the same magnitude (Mòzsik et al. 2006). In order to study compounds less pungent than capsaicin, a group of analogs named capsinoids (the natural capsiate, dihydrocapsiate, dihydrocapsiate, and the synthetic capsiate analog vanillyl nonanoate) with similar chemical structure of lead compound and TRPV-1 agonistic properties were developed (Luo et al. 2011). Both capsiate and its analog vanillyl nonanoate protected rat gastric mucosa from ethanol-induced injury by the release of CGRP and this effect was reverted by prior administration of the TRPV-1 antagonist capsazepine (Luo et al. 2011; Li et al. 2012). The gastroprotection of capsinoids was parallel to a decrease in cellular apoptosis and caspase-3 activity and to an increase of antioxidant activity seen as superoxide dismutase and malondialdehyde activity. Rutaecarpine, an alkaloid found in certain herbs including *Evodia rutaecarpa*, protects the gastric mucosa against injury induced by ASA and stress, and its gastroprotective effect is related to a stimulation of endogenous CGRP release via activation of the vanilloid receptor being reverted by pretreatment with capsaicin or capsazepine (Wang et al. 2005). Another TRPV-1 agonist such as anandamide was found able to protect gastric mucosa from injury induced by restrain stress in rats, and this effect was partially mediated by sensory nerves (Warzecha et al. 2011).

10.4 Biological Actions

CGRP, being a very potent vasodilator, is able to produce positive inotropic activity and vasorelaxation. Due to its wide distribution in the gastrointestinal tract CGRP has been the target of many studies summarized in some reviews

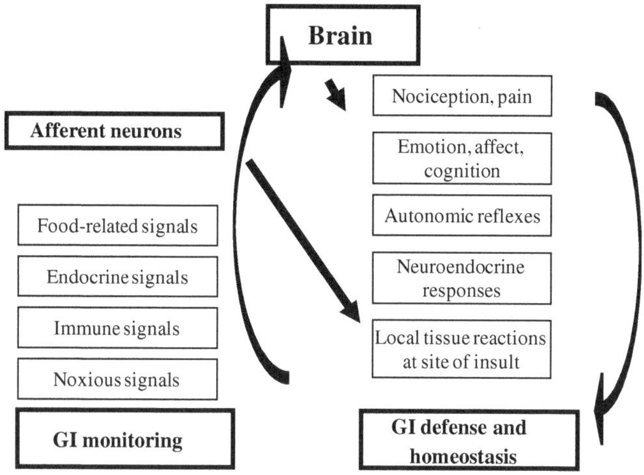

Fig. 10.3 Role of afferent neurons in gastrointestinal (GI) defense. The figure shows how primary afferent neurons monitor the chemical and physical environment within the GI tract and the various modalities of the response in order to maintain homeostasis: via brain-mediated reactions and reflexes and through local neuropeptides release at the site of the insult

(Holzer 1992, 2007; Bartho et al. 2008; Evangelista 2009). CGRP-containing pathways of the enteric nervous system have been shown to be involved in intestinal nociception, modulation of gastrointestinal motility and secretion (Fig. 10.3).

As regards the motility, two distinct effects appear important for CGRP action on intestinal smooth muscle: a direct relaxant effect, observed in the longitudinal and circular muscles of intestinal segments from various species and an indirect effect, produced via stimulation of neuronal receptors leading to the release of other transmitters which, in turn, affect intestinal motility (Bartho et al. 2008). The human gut (especially the circular musculature) is relaxed by capsaicin, but this effect seems to be under the control of different neurotransmitter agents, nitric oxide (NO), and VIP, neither of them of intrinsic neuronal origin. The "local efferent" effect of extrinsic afferent neurons can also be demonstrated in vivo, both in animals and man. Yet, nearly normal motility of the small and large intestines is maintained in animals with functionally inhibited capsaicin-sensitive nerves. CGRP is involved also in the peristaltic reflex elicited by muscle stretch and mucosal stimulation (Grider 1994). Peristaltic reflex are subjected to the activity of several neurotransmitters: both the 5-HT4 receptor antagonists and the CGRP antagonist $hCGRP_{8-37}$ inhibit ascending contraction and descending relaxation. Thus, the reflex in mouse, like that in rat and human intestine, is initiated by mucosal release of 5-HT and activation of 5-HT4 receptors on CGRP sensory neurons and is relayed via somatostatin and opioid interneurons to VIP/nitric-oxide synthase inhibitory motor neurons and via cholinergic interneurons to acetylcholine/tachykinin excitatory motor neurons. The importance of this system in regulating GI movements may be exaggerated under pathophysiological conditions, first of all inflammation. The afferent function of capsaicin-sensitive nerves plays a role in sympathetic reflexes, such as the inhibition of GI motility after laparotomy or by peritoneal irritation and diabetic gastroparesis (Bartho et al. 2008).

CGRP is a potent suppressor of basal and secretagogues-stimulated gastric acid and pepsin secretion in humans, dogs, rabbits, and rats (Ren et al. 1998; Evangelista 2009). Multiple mechanisms seem to be involved in the CGRP antisecretory activity such as the release of somatostatin from D cells (Ren et al. 1998), where CL and RAMP1 mRNAs has been found, the direct inhibition of gastrin- and cholinergic-dependent stimulatory effects and the stimulation of mucus and bicarbonate from gastroduodenal mucosa (Evangelista 2009).

Concerning the ion and fluid intestinal transport, CGRP exhibited concentration-dependent dual actions upon rat colonic epithelia acting directly on colonic enterocytes. At low concentrations (i.e., 0.03–10 nM) CGRP produces antisecretory effects that are abolished by pretreating tissues with tetrodotoxin (TTX). At higher concentrations (30–200 nM) secretory responses predominate, and these effects were not abolished by TTX (Cox et al. 1989). In guinea-pig colon, CGRP depolarizes myenteric neurons that are synaptically coupled to submucosal neurons. Cholinergic neurons using nicotinic and muscarinic synapses for transmission of information to the epithelium are involved in inducing chloride secretion. CGRP is also present in human epithelia but it is not known whether the described secretory effects are of physiological relevance. It should be observed that in human volunteers the intraluminal capsaicin application did not affect electrolyte absorption and fluid secretion (Hammer et al. 1998). During inflammation the activation of CGRP receptors may result in effects on tight junction permeability not observed in normal tissue (Holzer 2007).

It is known that the vascular system of the gastrointestinal tract is innervated by both sympathetic vasoconstrictor and parasympathetic vasodilator neurons but splanchnic blood vessels receive also a dense supply of fibers containing CGRP (Sternini et al. 1987; Green and Dockray 1988). These fibers innervate blood vessels of the entire body and their density is greater around arteries than veins. In the gastrointestinal tract, CGRP-containing nerve fibers are surrounding the mucosa and submucosa blood vessels and species differences are known concerning their presence, being scarce in human and porcine stomach (Green and Dockray 1988). CGRP exerts also a potent vasodilator and past studies have shown it as a non-cholinergic and nonadrenergic transmitter able to dilate mesenteric artery after periarterial stimulation (Holzer 1992). When released from extrinsic afferent nerve fibers in acid-threatened stomach, CGRP causes a NO-dependent vasodilation that has been shown to be a defensive signal in the face of pending acid injury in the gastric mucosa (Holzer 1998) (Fig. 10.3). The vasodilator effect of CGRP has been widely studied in the upper gastrointestinal tract (see below) and is working under pathological conditions.

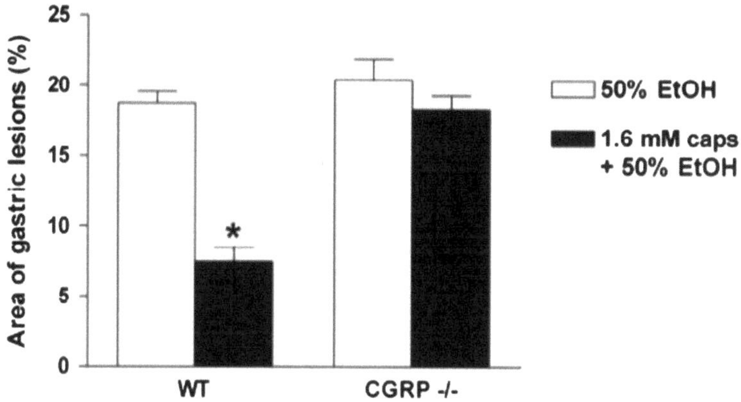

Fig. 10.4 Lack of capsaicin (caps)-induced gastric mucosal protection against 50 % ethanol-induced lesions in mice knockout to CGRP (CGRP−/−). Means ±S.E values of 5–6 mice for group. * = $P < 0.01$ between wild type (WT) groups. Modified from (Ohno et al. 2008)

10.5 Pathophysiology

10.5.1 CGRP in Gastrointestinal Defence

10.5.1.1 Experimental Evidences

Both indomethacin- or ethanol-induced mucosal lesions were enhanced by systemic administration of $hCGRP_{8-37}$ while low dose of capsaicin and/or TRPV-1 agonists have clearly shown to exert gastroprotection via the stimulation of sensory nerves and the local release of CGRP (Holzer 2007) indicating that endogenous CGRP plays a trophic role on mucosal defense of the stomach. Further, gastroprotection by capsaicin was dose-dependently antagonized by the CGRP antagonist, $hCGRP_{8-37}$, and by a monoclonal antibody to CGRP (Evangelista 2009). Recent studies using CGRP-knockout mice (Ohno et al. 2008) have strongly confirmed these findings: the protective action of capsaicin against ethanol-induced lesions was completely abolished in CGRP−/− mice (Fig. 10.4). The authors also showed that the adaptive gastroprotection induced by previous exposure of the stomach to mild irritants was mediated by CGRP being completely absent in CGRP knockout mice (Ohno et al. 2008).

Furthermore, several studies have reported a depletion of tissue CGRP-LI during the formation of several gastric ulcers (Evangelista 2009). Decreased levels of gastric CGRP-LI were observed after acetic acid-, cysteamine-, concentrated ethanol- or water-immersion stress-ulcers, and the ulcerogens did not affect the tissue content of other peptides (Evangelista 2009) suggesting that reduction in gastric CGRP-LI cannot be attributed only to damage of the tissue.

On the other hand, restoration of CGRP-LI was observed in animals bearing ulcers during healing (Evangelista 2009), and intense CGRP immunostaining was observed in the ulcer margin of patients with gastric ulcers (Tani et al. 1999). Healing of ulcer elicited by acetic acid in CGRP knockout mice was markedly delayed as compared with wild type mice as well as the granulation tissue, and neovascularization at the base of these ulcers was poor in CGRP−/− animals (Ohno et al. 2008). Furthermore, in isolated rat stomachs exposed to hyperosmolar concentrations of sodium chloride, the addition of CGRP enhanced the recovery of mucosal integrity after mild but not severe damage produced by the lesioning agent (Miller et al. 1995). These findings and the observation that there is a tonic flow of CGRP toward the peripheral endings of sensory fibers suggest that the peptide is restored in connection with the healing of ulcers after its release produced by the ulcerogen.

As regards the known CGRP antisecretory effect (Evangelista 2009) along with somatostatin releasing activity from gastric D cells (Ren et al. 1998), other mechanisms have been explored to explain the CGRP protective role in the stomach. It is known that hyperemia induced by an injury is a physiological response to tissue damage and limits the extent of injury in the stomach (Holzer 1992, 1998). Modulation of this response is an important defense mechanism and it has been reported that CGRP released by capsaicin-sensitive fibers is involved in gastric hyperemic protective effects (Holzer 1998).

Local application of low doses of capsaicin or TRPV-1 agonists able to stimulate gastric nerve endings (Szolcsànyi and Bartho 2001; Holzer 2007) enhance gastric blood flow through the mucosa, dilate submucosal arterioles, and reduce concomitantly gross mucosal lesions produced by ethanol (Holzer 1998; Szolcsànyi and Bartho 2001; Mòzsik et al. 2006). Afferent nerve endings originating from dorsal root ganglia and passing through the celiac/superior mesenteric ganglion complex have been reported to modulate these effects, which are abolished by chemical ablation induced by the pretreatment with high doses of capsaicin (Holzer 1998; Szolcsànyi and Bartho 2001).

It is noteworthy that the gastric hyperemic responses to acid back diffusion (Holzer 1998) or hypertonic solution (Matsumoto et al. 1991) depend on sensory innervation of the tissue. On the other hand, it has been shown that exposure of isolated tissues of the rat stomach to low pH solution produces a selective release of CGRP (Geppetti et al. 1991). Hydrogen ions diffusing into the gastric wall of disrupted mucosal barrier may promote protective vasodilation by activating the "efferent" function of capsaicin-sensitive afferent nerves and activating TRPV-1 that are sensible to acidosis of the tissue (Holzer 2011).

A mediator role of CGRP in this protective hyperemia induced by afferent fibers is largely proved. In fact, capsaicin released CGRP from isolated tissues of the rat stomach (Holzer 1998; Evangelista 2009), an effect that was abolished after disruption of capsaicin-sensitive neurons (Holzer 1998) or in CGRP−/− animals (Ohno et al. 2008); intravascular application of capsaicin induced a release of CGRP into the vascular bed of the rat stomach followed by a marked vasodilator effect (Holzer 1998; Szolcsànyi and Bartho 2001) and gastric vasodilating response to topical application of capsaicin was blocked, at least in part, by the antagonist $hCGRP_{8-37}$ (Li et al. 1991). Further, low doses of locally applied CGRP dilated submucosal arterioles and enhanced gastric blood flow (Holzer 1998, 2007) and CGRP-induced vasodilation is in keeping with the distribution of this peptide around blood vessels in the stomach (Sternini et al. 1987) and the high number of vascular CGRP receptors in this region (Gates et al. 1989).

Taken together, these observations strongly suggest that CGRP is the likely mediator of the protective function of sensory nerves in the stomach.

Similarly other gastrointestinal disorders involving inflammation, infection, or ulceration were reported to be correlated to change in CGRP innervation (Holzer 2007). Experimental colitis induced by trinitrobenzensulfonic acid (TNB) as well inflammatory bowel diseases were associated with tissue CGRP decrease (Reinshagen et al. 1998) and upregulation of TRPV-1 in nerve fiber of the colon (Yiangou et al. 2001). Silencing of CLR or the use of the CGRP antagonist increased the severity of the TNB lesions (Reinshaghen et al. 1998; Clifton et al. 2007). This is only an example of how CGRP innervation can be used as a surveillance system that along other ones (immune, endocrine, etc.) can coordinate the defense of all gastrointestinal tracts from injury (Fig. 10.3).

10.5.1.2 Clinical Findings

In humans, TRPV-1 labeling was localized in parietal cells of stomach from surgical specimens as assessed by immunohistochemistry, in situ hybridization, and Western blot analysis (Faussone-Pellegrini et al. 2005). These authors found TRPV-1 labelling in the parietal cells and in neurons and nerve fibers in the mucosa and submucosa (Fig. 10.5) confirming its potential capability to influence gastric secretion and protection. Intragastric application of small doses of capsaicin (1–8 μg/ml corresponding to 3–26 μM) in healthy humans decreased in a dose-dependent manner basal gastric acid secretion (Mòzsik et al. 2005; Szabó et al. 2013). In the same study, it was shown that low concentrations of capsaicin protect against gastric injuries induced by ethanol or indomethacin as evaluated by micro-bleeding and transmucosal potential difference (Mòzsik et al. 2005), and a suspension of 20 g chili was able to protect the human gastroduodenal mucosa from the damage induced by a high dose of acetylsalicylic acid (Yeak et al. 1995). Gastric microbleeding induced by indomethacin was not affected by repeated daily doses (3 × 400 μg i.g.) of capsaicin given for 2 weeks (Mòzsik et al. 2005). In humans the TRPV-1 receptor and CGRP were detected in patients with different gastric diseases (Tani et al. 1999; Dömötör et al. 2005; Mózsik et al. 2007). In gastritis patients, CGRP and TRPV-1 were enhanced as compared to controls but both are not dependent on the presence of *H. pylori* (Dömötör et al. 2007).

Taken together, these findings indicate that stimulation of TRPV-1 with low doses of capsaicin is protective for human stomach in terms of decreased acid secretion and reduction of injury induced by irritants and might be a potential tool to develop gastroprotective drugs.

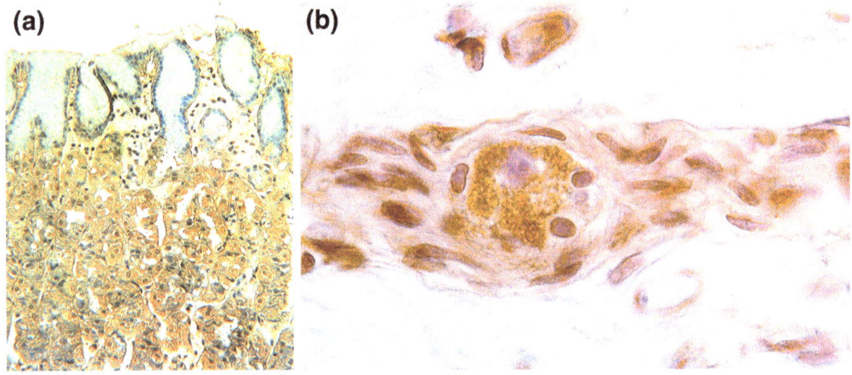

Fig. 10.5 TRPV-1 distribution in gastric human samples. DAB reactions; counterstaining with haematoxylin, bright field microscopy. For methodology see Faussone-Pellegrini et al. (2005). **a** Gastric mucosa: the parietal cells are labelled by anti-capsaicin receptor antibody and no other epithelial cell types are positive. Calibration bar = 100 μm. **b** Gastric submucosa: anti-capsaicin receptor-positive neurons and nerve fibres in a submucous ganglion. Calibration bar = 15 μm. From Faussone-Pellegrini and Vannucchi, University of Florence, Italy

10.5.2 CGRP in Gastrointestinal Motility Disorders and Visceral Sensitivity

10.5.2.1 Experimental Evidences

Infection, inflammation, intestinal anaphylaxis, trauma, and stress are known to induce change in motility and all have been reported to be associated to the activity and release of tachykinins and CGRP from extrinsic afferents. Peptides are released from central endings of afferent neurons in the spinal cord and brainstem and mediate transmission to the efferent reflex arc. Likewise, CGRP released within the gut in response to an irritant may facilitate the excitation of afferents and participate to transmission of nociceptive traffic between afferent neurons and second-order neurons in the spinal cord and brainstem (Bueno et al. 1997). As an example the induction of colonic inflammation by acetic acid instillation facilitates the pain reaction to rectal distension, changing the pain threshold, and this hypersensitivity can be blocked by a CGRP antagonist (Bueno et al. 1997; Plourde et al. 1997). The precise site at which CGRP and also tachykinin receptors mediate colonic hyperalgesia seems to be the spinal cord since CGRP was found enhanced there after colonic irritation and its antagonist is more effective if given by intrathecal than intravenous route (Bueno et al. 1997; Plourde et al. 1997). Since irritation, immune challenge, and inflammation release tachykinin and CGRP from extrinsic afferents and from intrinsic neurons inside the gut, these peptides may either increase the peripheral sensory gain of extrinsic afferents or contribute to the afferent transmission of algesic signal within the central nervous system. As extrinsic afferents of the gut do not possess receptors for CGRP, it is probable that peptide-induced sensitization or excitation of sensory neurons is an indirect consequence of peptide action on gastrointestinal effectors (Holzer 2007). In this context, TRPV-1 has been shown to play a role in gastroesophageal (Bielefeldt and Davis 2008), small intestinal (Rong et al. 2004) and colonic (Jones et al. 2005, 2007) visceral mechanosensitivity or neonatal irritation of the colon (Winston et al. 2007). TRPV-1 was shown to be upregulated in nociceptive visceral afferents of rodents with TNB-induced colitis (Miranda et al. 2007; De Schepper et al. 2008a). De Schepper et al. (2008a) showed that acute TNB-induced colitis increased the response to colorectal distention in rat pelvic afferent C fibres but not in Aδ fibres. This inflammation-induced increase in mechanosensitivity was reduced by the TRPV-1 antagonist BCTC (*N*-(4-*tert*-butylphenyl)-4-(3-chloropyridin-2-yl)tetrahydropyrazine-1(2*H*)-carboxamide monohydrochloride; De Schepper et al. 2008b). Due to different experimental conditions and irritant used, Phillis et al. (2009) showed that mechanosensitivity of nociceptive serosal and mesenteric colonic splanchnic afferents to graded stimuli was unaffected during dextran sulfate sodium colitis in rats (Phillis et al. 2009). However, TRPV-1 seems to be an important amplifier of noxious stimuli as the antagonist SB-750364 inhibited mechanosensitivity and spontaneous neuronal discharge only during inflammation but not in healthy conditions (Phillis et al. 2009). Taken together, it could well be that the effect of TRPV-1 antagonists may only become significant after TRPV-1 upregulation, which is not necessarily associated with obvious inflammation. In rats, stress-induced visceral hypersensitivity that is dependent on mast cell degranulation and subsequent TRPV-1 activation also occurs in the absence of overt inflammation (van den Wijngaard et al. 2009), but preceding inflammation is a trigger to enhance expression and function of TRPV-1, a change that persists once inflammation disappears. In fact, persistent hyperalgesia is observed after resolution of dextran sulfate (Ejkelkamp et al. 2007) and zymosan (Jones et al. 2005) colitis or in adults rats exposed when neonated to chemical irritation of the colon with acetic acid (Winston et al. 2007).

10.5.2.2 Clinical Findings

Application of capsaicin to the human jejunum induced abdominal pain similar to that induced by distension (Schmidt et al. 2004). Capsaicin did not stimulate jejunal motility neither did it affect mechanosensitivity, therefore the altered pain sensitivity is due to stimulation of chemoreceptors probably by the TRPV-1 activation. On the other hand, capsaicin load can be considered as a valuable test to investigate hypersensitivity (van Wanrooii et al. 2014). In trial involving 116 outpatients suffering from dyspepsia, the median perception score after ingestion of capsule containing 0.75 mg of capsaicin was significantly higher than placebo (Fuhrer et al. 2011). In heartburn patients, 5 mg of capsaicin mixed to the meal significantly decreased the peak to the heartburn. When refluxed, capsaicin probably sensitized the oesophagus and primed it to noxious stimuli such as

Table 10.2 Percentage of area of immunoreactivity of vanilloid receptor 1 (TRPV-1), substance P, and CGRP in rectal samples from patients characterized by rectal hypersensitivity and controls

	Rectal hypersensitivity	Control	p
Mucosa			
TRPV-1	0.44 (0.30–0.59)	0.11 (0.00–0.21)	0.0005
Substance P	0.45 (0.29–0.85)	0.39 (0.29–0.61)	0.43
Submucosa			
TRPV-1	3.50 (2.20–3.90)	0.80 (0.62–1.30)	0.002
CGRP	24.3 (14.2–42.8)	4.30 (0.10-10.0)	0.0009
Circular muscle			
TRPV-1	2.30 (1.20–3.00)	0.78 (0.19–1.62)	0.002
Longitudinal muscle			
TRPV-1	1.13 (0.70–2.20)	0.32 (0.14–0.80)	0.01

Values are median with a 95 % range. Modified from (Chan et al. 2003)

acid (Rodriguez-Stanley et al. 2000). Intraesophageal capsaicin infusion has been found to lower sensory and pain thresholds to oesophageal balloon distension, again presumably through direct activation of TRPV-1 and release of neurotransmitters (Gonzalez et al. 1998).

Another study has analyzed the impact of acute ingestion of red chili powder (capsaicin equivalent of 14 mg) on men diagnosed with irritable bowel syndrome (IBS) and volunteers. Chili did not alter small bowel and colonic transit in both groups but increased the rectal threshold for pain in healthy volunteers (Agarwal et al. 2002). Similarly in IBS and healthy men the repeated ingestion of 5 g chili daily did not affect rectosigmoid motility (Shah et al. 2000).

It is noteworthy that rectal biopsy samples taken from patients with well-characterized rectal hypersensitivity showed a marked increase in TRPV-1 in muscle, submucosal, and mucosal layers as compared with controls (Chan et al. 2003) (Table 10.2). Submucosal immunoreactive CGRP expressed in ganglion cells but not SP was increased as well (Table 10.2). The increase in TRPV-1 significantly correlated with the decrease in heat and distension sensory thresholds confirming that both afferent and intrinsic fibers take part in the change in signaling pathways of visceral hypersensitivity. Likewise, Akbar et al. (2008, 2010) and Keszthelyi et al. (2013) showed that increased TRPV-1 transcription and nerve fibers were present in quiescent inflammatory bowel disease patients with IBS-like symptoms with a correlation to pain severity. These authors observed that also substance P immunoreactivity, CD3 lymphocytes, and mast cells staining for c-kit were more prevalent in IBS patients (Akbar et al. 2008). As shown in Fig. 10.3, mediators released by endocrine and immune cells can sensitize afferent nerve endings and activate TRPV-1 since this activation is attenuated in TRPV-1 knockout mice (Jones et al. 2007).

In a recent placebo controlled study performed in 50 IBS patients diagnosed according to Rome II criteria, the repeated administration of 600 mg/daily by enteric coated capsules of red pepper for 6 weeks significantly decreased the intensity of abdominal pain and bloating, improving visceral sensitivity (Bortolotti and Porta 2011). On the other hand, a study performed in healthy volunteers with the repeated ingestion of capsaicin (0.25 mg tid for 4 weeks) desensitized both chemonociceptive and mechanonoceciptive pathways (Fuhrer and Hammer 2009). In a double-blind, placebo-controlled study, 30 individuals with dyspepsia were given either 2.5 g daily of red pepper powder (divided up and taken prior to meals) or placebo for 5 weeks (Bortolotti et al. 2002). By the third week of treatment, individuals taking red pepper were experiencing significant improvements in pain, bloating, and nausea as compared to placebo, and these relative improvements lasted through the end of the study.

These positive results were attributed to the desensitizing effect of repeated administration of capsaicin. It produced a long-lasting refractory state during which the neurons affected are not responsive. Therefore the repeated stimulation of TRPV-1 induced an excess of the influx of Ca^{++} and other cations, sensory neurons are thus defunctionalized and depleted of their transmitter for a period of time which is the base of improvement of epigastric pain recorded. The potential clinical application of TRPV-1 agonists have to be confirmed by large clinical trials but the mechanism of action described seems to be interesting for developing drugs in functional gastrointestinal diseases. Agents that are able to block TRPV-1-bearing nociceptors, without an initial excitatory effect, might add to the actual limited pharmacological armamentarium for functional gastrointestinal disorders and might affect both chemoreceptors and mechanoreceptors in the gut by desensitizing these two perception pathways.

Acknowledgments We would like to thank Dr. Stefania Meini for drawing of the figures.

References

Abdel-Salam OM, Debreceni A, Mòzsik G, Szolcsànyi J (1999) Capsaicin-sensitive afferent sensory nerves in modulating gastric mucosal defence against noxious agents. J Physiol Paris 93:443–454

Agarwal MK, Bhatia SJ, Desai SA, Bhure U, Melgiri S (2002) Effect of red chillies on small bowel and colonic transit and rectal sensitivity in men with irritable bowel syndrome. Ind J Gastroenterol 21:179–182

Akbar A, Yiangou Y, Facer P, Walters JRF, Anand P, Gosh S (2008) Increased capsaicin receptor TRPV-1 expressing sensory fibres in irritable bowel syndrome and their correlation with abdominal pain. Gut 57:923–929

Akbar A, Yiangou Y, Facer P et al (2010) Expression of the TRPV-1 receptor differs in quiescent inflammatory bowel disease with or without abdominal pain. Gut 59:767–774

Bartho L, Benko R, Holzer-Petsche U, Holzer P, Undi S, Wolf M (2008) Role of extrinsic afferent neurons in gastrointestinal motility. Eur Rev Med Pharmacol Sci 12(Suppl 1):21–31

Barwell J, Wootten D, Simms J, Hay DL, Poyner DR (2012) RAMPs and CGRP receptors. Adv Exp Med Biol 744:13–24

Bielefeldt K, Davis BM (2008) Differential effects of ASIC3 and TRPV-1 deletion on gastroesophageal sensation in mice. Am J Physiol Gastrointest Liver Physiol 294:G130–G138

Bortolotti M, Coccia G, Grossi G, Miglioli M (2002) The treatment of functional dyspepsia with red pepper. Aliment Pharmacol Ther 16:1075–1082

Bortolotti M, Porta S (2011) Effect of red pepper on symptoms of irritable bowel syndrome: preliminary study. Dig Dis Sci 56:3288–3295

Bueno L, Fioramonti J, Delvaux M, Frexinos J (1997) Mediators and pharmacology of visceral sensitivity: from basic to clinical investigations. Gastroenterology 112:1714–1743
Chan CLH, Facer P, Davis JB et al (2003) Sensory fibres expressing capsaicin receptor TRPV-1 in patients with rectal hypersensitivity and faecal urgency. Lancet 361:385–391
Clifton MS, Hoy JJ, Chang J et al (2007) Role of calcitonin receptor-like receptor in colonic motility and inflammation. Am J Physiol Gastrointest Liver Physiol 293:G36–G44
Cox HM, Ferrar JA, Cuthbert AW (1989) Effects of alpha- and beta-calcitonin gene-related peptides upon ion transport in rat descending colon. Br J Pharmacol 97:996–998
De Schepper HU, De Man JG, Ruyssers NE et al (2008a) TRPV-1 receptor signaling mediates afferent nerve sensitization during colitis-induced motility disorders in rats. Am J Physiol Gastrointest Liver Physiol 294:G245–G253
De Schepper HU, De Winter BY, Van Nassauw L et al (2008b) TRPV-1 receptors on unmyelinated C-fibres mediate colitis-induced sensitization of pelvic afferent nerve fibres in rats. J Physiol 586:5247–5258
Dömötör A, Kereskay L, Szekeres G, Hunyady B, Szolcsányi J, Mózsik G (2007) Participation of capsaicin-sensitive afferent nerves in the gastric mucosa of patients with *Helicobacter pylori*-positive or-negative chronic gastritis. Dig Dis Sci 52:411–417
Dömötör A, Peidl Z, Vincze A et al (2005) Immunohistochemical distribution of vanilloid receptor, calcitonin-gene related peptide and substance P in gastrointestinal mucosa of patients with different gastrointestinal disorders. Inflammopharmacology 13:161–177
Ejkelkamp N, Kavelaars A, Elsenbruch S et al (2007) Increased visceral sensitivity to capsaicin after DSS-induced colitis in mice: spinal cord c-Fos expression and behaviour. Am J Physiol 293:1075–1082.k
Evans BN, Rosenblatt MI, Mnayer LO, Oliver KR, Dickerson IM (2000) CGRP-RCP, a novel protein required for signal transduction at calcitonin gene-related peptide and adrenomedullin receptors. J Biol Chem 275:31438–31443
Evangelista S (2009) Role of calcitonin-gene related peptide in gastric mucosal defence and healing. Curr Pharm Des 15:3571–3576
Faussone-Pellegrini MS, Taddei A, Bizzoco E, Lazzeri M, Vannucchi MG, Bechi P (2005) Distribution of the vanilloid (capsaicin) receptor type 1 in the human stomach. Histochem Cell Biol 124:61–68
Fuhrer M, Hammer J (2009) Effect of repeated, long term capsaicin ingestion on intestinal chemo- and mechanosensation in healthy volunteers. Neurogastroenterol Motil 21:521–527
Fuhrer M, Vogelsang H, Hammer J (2011) A placebo-controoled trial of an oral capsaicin load in patients with functional dyspepsaia. Neurogastroenterol Motil 23:918–e397
Gates T, Zimmermann RP, Mantyh CR, Vigna SR, Mantyh PW (1989) Calcitonin gene-related peptide-α receptor binding sites in the gastrointestinal tract. Neuroscience 31:757–770
Geppetti P, Tramontana M, Evangelista S et al (1991) Differential effect of neuropeptide release of different concentrations of hydrogen ions on afferent and intrinsic neurons of the rat stomach. Gastroenterology 101:1505–1511
Gonzalez R, Dunkel R, Koletzko B, Shusdziarra V, Allescher HD (1998) Effect of capsaicin-containing red pepper sauce suspension on upper gastrointestinal motility in healthy volunteers. Dig Dis Sci 43:1165–1171
Green T, Dockray GJ (1988) Characterization of the peptidergic afferent innervation of the stomach in the rat, mouse and guinea-pig. Neuroscience 25:181–193
Grider JR (1994) CGRP as a transmitter in the sensory pathway mediating peristaltic reflex. Am J Physiol 266:G1139–G1145
Hammer J, Hammer HF, Eherer AJ, Petritsch W, Holzer P, Kreis GJ (1998) Intraluminal capsaicin does not affect fluid and electrolyte absorption in the human jejunum but does cause pain. Gut 43:252–255
Holzer P (1991) Capsaicin: cellular targets, mechanisms of action, and selectivity for thin sensory neurons. Pharmacol Rev 43:143–201
Holzer P (1992) Peptidergic sensory neurons in the control of vascular functions: mechanisms and significance in the cutaneous and splanchnic vascular beds. Rev Physiol Biochem Pharmacol 121:49–146

Holzer P (1998) Neural emergency system in the stomach. Gastroenterology 114:823–829

Holzer P (2007) Role of visceral afferent neurons in mucosal inflammation and defense. Curr Opin Pharmacol 7:563–569

Holzer P (2011) Acid sensing by visceral afferent neurons. Acta Physiol (Oxf) 201:63–75

Jancsò N (1960) Role of nerve terminals in the mechanism of inflammatory reactions. Bull Millard Fillmore Hosp 7:53–77

Keszthelyi D, Troost FJ, Jonkers DM et al (2013) Alterations in mucosal neuropeptides in patients with irritable bowel syndrome and ulcerative colitis in remission: a role in pain syntom generation? Eur J Pain 17:1299–1306

Jones RC 3rd, Xu L, Gebhart GF (2005) The mechanosensitivity of mouse colon afferent fibers and their sensitization by inflammatory mediators require transient receptor potential vanilloid 1 and acid-sensing ion channel 3. J Neurosci 25:10981–10989

Jones RC 3rd, Otsuka E, Wagstrom E, Jensen CS, Price MP, Gebhart GF (2007) Short-term sensitization of colon mechanoreceptors is associated with long-term hypersensitivity to colon distention in the mouse. Gastroenterology 133:184–194

Li D-S, Raybould HE, Quintero E, Guth PH (1991) Role of calcitonin gene-related peptide in gastric hyperemic response to intragastric capsaicin. Am J Physiol 261:G657–G661

Li N-S, Luo X-J, Dai Z et al (2012) Beneficial effects of capsiate on ethanol-induced mucosal injury in rats are related to stimulation of calcitonin gene-related peptide release. Planta Med 78:24–30

Luo X-J, Li N-S, Zhang Y-S et al (2011) Vanillyil nonanoate protects rat gastric mucosa from ethanol-induced injury through a mechanism involving calcitonin gene-related peptide. Eur J Pharmacol 666:211–217

Matsumoto J, Ueshima K, Takeuchi K, Okabe S (1991) Capsaicin-sensitive afferent neurons in adaptive responses of the rat stomach induced by a mild irritant. Jpn J Pharmacol 55:181–185

Miller CA, Nakashima M, Gittes G, Debas HT (1995) Calcitonin gene-related peptide (CGRP) upregulates the restitution of rat gastric mucosa in vitro. J Surg Res 58:421–424

Miranda A, Nordstrom E, Mannem A, Smith C, Banerjee B, Sengupta JN (2007) The role of transient receptor potential vanilloid 1 in mechanical and chemical visceral hyperalgesia following experimental colitis. Neuroscience 148:1021–1032

Mòzsik G, Domotor A, Abdel-Salam OM (2006) Molecular pharmacological approach to drug actions on the afferent and efferent fibres of the vagal nerve involved in gastric mucosal protection in rats. Inflammopharmacology 14:243–249

Mózsik G, Szolcsányi J, Dömötör A (2007) Capsaicin research as a new tool to approach of the human gastrointestinal physiology, pathology and pharmacology. Inflammopharmacology 15:232–245

Mòzsik G, Szolcsànyi J, Racz I (2005) Gastroprotection induced by capsaicin in healthy human subjects. World J Gastroenterol 11:5180–5184

Mulderry PK, Ghatei MA, Spokes RA et al (1988) Differential expression of alpha-CGRP and beta-CGRP by primary sensory neurons and enteric autonomic neurons of the rat. Neuroscience 25:195–205

Negro A, Lionetto L, Simmaco M, Martelletti P (2012) CGRP receptor antagonists: an expanding drug class for acute migraine? Expert Opin Investig Drugs 21:807–818

Ohno T, Hattori Y, Komine R et al (2008) Roles of calcitonin gene-related peptide in maintenance of gastric mucosal integrity and in enhancement of ulcer healing and angiogenesis. Gastroenterology 134:215–225

Peng J, Li Y-J (2010) The vanilloid receptor TRPV1: role in cardiovascular and gastrointestinal protection. Eur J Pharmacol 627:1–7

Phillis BD, Martin CM, Kang D et al (2009) Role of TRPV-1 in high-threshold rat colonic splanchnic afferents is revealed by inflammation. Neurosci Lett 459:57–61

Plourde V, St-Pierre S, Quirion R (1997) Calcitonin gene-related peptide in viscerosensitive response to colorectal distension in rats. Am J Physiol 273:G191–G196

Reinshagen M, Flämig G, Ernst S et al (1998) Calcitonin gene-related peptide mediates the protective effect of sensory nerves in a model of colonic injury. J Pharmacol Exp Ther 286:657–661

Ren J, Dunn ST, Tang Y et al (1998) Effects of calcitonin gene-related peptide on somatostatin and gastrin gene expression in rat antrum. Regul Pept 73:75–82
Rodriguez-Stanley S, Collings KL, Robinson M, Owen W, Miner PB Jr (2000) The effects of capsaicin on reflux, gastric emptying and dyspepsia. Aliment Pharmacol Ther 14:129–134
Rong W, Hillsley K, Davis JB, Hicks G, Winchester WJ, Grundy D (2004) Jejunal afferent nerve sensitivity in wild-type and TRPV-1 knockout mice. J Physiol 560:867–881
Rosenfeld MG, Mermod J, Amara SG et al (1983) Production of a novel neuropeptide encoded by the calcitonin gene via tissue-specific RNA processing. Nature 304:129–135
Schmidt B, Hammer J, Holzer P, Hammer HF (2004) Chemical nociceptionin the jejunum induced by capsaicin. Gut 53:1109–1116
Shah SK, Abraham P, Mistry FP (2000) Effect of cold pressor test and a high-chilli diet on rectosigmoid motility in irritable bowel syndrome. Ind J Gastroenterol 19:161–164
Sternini C, Reeve JR, Brecha N (1987) Distribution and characterization of calcitonin gene-related peptide immunoreactivity in the digestive system of normal and capsaicin-treated rats. Gastroenterology 93:852–862
Szabó IL, Czimmer J, Szolcsányi J, Mózsik G (2013) Molecular pharmacological approaches to effects of capsaicinoids and of classical antisecretory drugs on gastric basal acid secretion and on indomethacin-induced gastric mucosal damage in human healthy subjects (mini review). Curr Pharm Des 19:84–89
Szolcsànyi J, Bartho L (2001) Capsaicin-sensitive afferents and their role in gastroprotection: an update. J Physiol (Paris) 95:181–188
Tani N, Miyazawa M, Miwa T, Shibata M, Yamaura T (1999) Immunohistochemical localization of calcitonin gene-related peptide in the human gastric mucosa. Digestion 60:338–343
Tramontana M, Renzi D, Panerai C, Surrenti C, Nappi F, Abelli L, Evangelista S (1994) Capsaicin-like effect of resiniferatoxin in the rat stomach. Neuropeptides 26:29–32
van den Wijngaard RM, Klooker TK, Welting O et al (2009) Essential role for TRPV-1 in stress-induced (mast cell-dependent) colonic hypersensitivity in maternally separated rats. Neurogastroenterol Motil 21:1107–e94
van Rossum D, Hanisch UK, Quirion R (1997) Neuroanatomical localization, pharmacological characterization and functions of CGRP, related peptides and their receptors. Neurosci Biobehav Rev 21:649–678
van Wanrooii SJ, Wouters MM, Van Oudenhove L et al (2014) Sensitivity testing in irritable bowel syndrome with rectal capsaicin stimulations: role of TRPV-1 upregulation and sensitization in visceral hypersensitivity? Am J Gastroenterol 109:99–109
Wang Y, Hu CP, Deng PY et al (2005) The protective effects of rutaecarpine on gastric mucosa injury in rats. Planta Med 71:416–419
Warzecha Z, Dembinski A, Ceranowicz P (2011) Role of sensory nerves in gastroprotection effect of anandamide in rats. J Physiol Pharmacol 62:207–217
Wimalawansa SJ (1996) Calcitonin gene-related peptide and its receptors: molecular genetics, physiology, pathophysiology and therapeutic potential. Endocr Rev 17:533–535
Winston J, Shenoy M, Medley D, Naniwadekar A, Pasricha PJ (2007) The vanilloid receptor initiates and maintains colonic hypersensitivity induced by neonatal colon irritation in rats. Gastroenterology 132:615–627
Yamamoto H, Horie S, Uchida M et al (2001) Effects of vanilloid receptor agonists and antagonists on gastric antral ulcers in rats. Eur J Pharmacol 432:203–210
Yeak KG, Kang JY, Yap I et al (1995) Chili protects against aspirin-induced gastroduodenal mucosal injury in humans. Dig Dis Sci 40:580–583
Yiangou Y, Facer P, Dyer NH et al (2001) Vanilloid receptor 1 immunoreactivity in inflamed human bowel. Lancet 357:1338–1339
Young RL, Cooper NJ, Blackshaw LA (2008) Chemical coding and central projections of gastric vagal afferent neurons. Neurogastroenterol Motil 20:708–718
Zhong F, Christianson JA, Davis BM, Bielefeldt K (2008) Dichotomizing axons in spinal and vagal afferents of the mouse stomach. Dig Dis Sci 53:194–203

Chapter 11
Capsaicin for Osteoarthritis Pain

Laura L. Laslett and Graeme Jones

Abstract Capsaicin appears to be effective for osteoarthritis pain but it is uncertain whether the effect has a dose response, is consistent across joints, or changes over time. Methods: Randomized controlled trials of topical capsaicin use in OA were identified from PubMed, EMBASE, and ISI Web of Knowledge. Effect on pain scores, patient global evaluation of treatment effectiveness and application site burning were assessed by standardised mean differences (SMD), using RevMan. Results: Five double–blind randomized controlled trials and one case–crossover trial of topical capsaicin use were identified. Formulations ranged from 0.025 to 0.075 %, and trial durations from 4 to 12 weeks. Trials assessed OA of the knee ($n = 3$), hand ($n = 1$), and a mix of joints ($n = 2$). Capsaicin treatment efficacy (vs. placebo) for change in VAS pain score was moderate, at 0.44 (95 % CI 0.25–0.62) over 4 weeks of treatment. There was no heterogeneity between studies, indicating no between-study differences, including effect of OA site or treatment concentration. Two studies reported treatment beyond 4 weeks, with divergent results. One study reported an effect size of −9 mm after 12 weeks, and maximal between-group differences at 4 weeks. A second study reported that between-group differences increased over time, up to 20 weeks. Capsaicin was reported as being safe and well–tolerated, with no systemic toxicity. Mild application site burning affected 35 100 % of capsaicin treated patients with a risk ratio of 4.22 (95 % CI 3.25–5.48, $n = 5$ trials); incidence peaked in week 1, with incidence rates declining over time. Conclusions: Topical capsaicin treatment four times daily is moderately effective in reducing pain intensity up to 20 weeks regardless of site of application and dose in patients with at least moderate pain and clinical or radiologically defined OA, and is well tolerated.

L. L. Laslett · G. Jones (✉)
Musculoskeletal Unit, Menzies Research Institute Private bag 23,
Hobart, TAS 7000, Australia
e-mail: g.jones@utas.edu.au

O. M. E. Abdel-Salam (ed.), *Capsaicin as a Therapeutic Molecule*, Progress in Drug Research 68, DOI: 10.1007/978-3-0348-0828-6_11, © Springer Basel 2014

11.1 What is Osteoarthritis?

Osteoarthritis (OA) is the most common joint disorder. Research suggests OA is a complex collection of heterogeneous pathologies which result in a common outcome (Dieppe and Lohmander 2005), rather than a single disease entity. The lack of a common causal pathway has hampered development of effective treatments for modifying the natural history of the disease. Most existing treatments focus on relieving pain and improving function, and there are few examples of therapies which modify disease. The pathogenesis of pain in OA is complex and multifactorial, involving local nociception, inflammatory mediators, and central sensitization (Dieppe and Lohmander 2005; Kidd et al. 1996; Schaible and Grubb 1993).

11.2 Existing Treatments for Osteoarthritic Pain

Treatment of osteoarthritic pain includes a wide range of therapies, from non-pharmacological treatments (e.g. education, weight reduction, physiotherapy), pain medications (e.g. paracetamol, NSAIDs (non-steroidal anti-inflammatory drugs), opioids), nutraceuticals (e.g. glucosamine, chondroitin sulphate), and surgical therapies (e.g. joint replacement). The effect sizes of these treatments vary, but are typically small (Zhang et al. 2010) and fall far short of the levels of pain relief desired by patients. Most pharmacological therapies for osteoarthritis are taken orally e.g. paracetamol, but topical preparations of various medications have been used, including NSAIDS, comfrey, and capsaicin. When capsaicin is used for arthritic pain it is typically used topically, in concentrations of 0.025 or 0.075 %, and sold under trade names including Zostrix and Capzasin-P.

11.3 Capsaicin, and Putative Mechanisms in Osteoarthritic Pain

Capsaicin is the active ingredient in hot chilli peppers. It is a excitatory neurotoxin that selectively destroys primary afferent nociceptors in vivo and in vitro (Jancso et al. 1977; Wood et al. 1988). Capsaicin and related vanilloid compounds produce burning pain by activating the transient receptor potential vanilloid receptor 1 (TRPV1) (Caterina et al. 1997) (formerly known as VR1), which is a member of the transient release potential (TRP) channel superfamily (Szallasi and Blumberg 2007). Capsaicin–sensitive fibres are polymodal nociceptors which respond to capsaicin with discharge and subsequent desensitization to chemical, mechanical and thermal stimuli (Kenins 1982), including exposure to capsaicin itself (Baron 2000; Fusco and Giacovazzo 1997). Neural messages in capsaicin–sensitive fibres are thought to be transmitted transynaptically by the neurotransmitter substance P (Theriault et al.

1979), an 11 amino acid peptide belonging to the tachykinin family (Pernow 1983). This effect is reversible with treatment cessation (Nolano et al. 1999). This is particularly relevant to osteoarthritis as nociceptive fibres have been found in cartilage (Fortier and Nixon 1997; Wojtys et al. 1990) as well as the subchondral bone (Wojtys et al. 1990) in patients with osteoarthritis, but they are absent in the cartilage and bone of persons without osteoarthritis (Wojtys et al. 1990), suggesting that these fibres are involved in the signaling and maintenance of pain associated with OA. There has also been additional evidence from genetic studies supporting the association between pain sensitivity and OA. The Ile585Val variant of TRPV1 gene (thought to be involved in lower peripheral pain sensitivity) has been associated with reduced risk of painful knee OA, compared to non-painful knee OA or controls (Valdes et al. 2011).

This chapter will discuss the use of topical capsaicin in the therapy of painful osteoarthritis in adults.

11.4 Search Strategy

Literature databases (PubMed, EMBASE, ISI Web of Knowledge) were searched for randomized controlled trials of capsaicin use in OA, using the following keywords: "capsaicin", "osteoarthritis" "double-blind method", "randomized controlled trial (publication type)" or "controlled clinical trial (publication type)" up to 2012. This was supplemented by manually searching the bibliographies of relevant published reviews and papers. We required studies to include at least a subpopulation of adult patients with osteoarthritis. Any participants with other conditions (e.g. rheumatoid arthritis) have been omitted from this review. Studies not in English were excluded.

11.5 Identified Capsaicin Trials

We identified five double–blind randomized controlled trials (Deal et al. 1991; McCarthy and McCarty 1992; Altman et al. 1994; Deal 1994; McCleane 2000; Schnitzer et al. 2012) and one case–crossover trial (Kosuwon et al. 2010) (Table 11.1) in which capsaicin or capsaicin–like therapies were used in formulations ranging from 0.025 to 0.075 % as a topical therapy for painful osteoarthritis. Capsaicin was applied topically to the affected area(s) four times daily.

Studies included in Table 11.1 assess the effect of treatment with capsaicin (or capsaicin–like compounds) for 4–12 weeks in older adults with OA of the knee (Deal et al. 1991; Schnitzer et al. 2012; Kosuwon et al. 2010), hand (McCarthy and McCarty 1992), and a mixture of joints (Altman et al. 1994; McCleane 2000). Inclusion and exclusion criteria varied between trials but patients were typically required to have at least moderate pain and either radiological evidence of OA or be clinically diagnosable as having OA, or both.

Table 11.1 Double blind randomized controlled trials of capsaicin

Study, duration	*n*	Age (years)	Sex (M:F)	OA site	Formulation	Outcomes	Rate of application site burning
Deal 1991 (Deal et al. 1991) 4 weeks	70	61	25M:45F	Knee	0.025 % capsaicin	*VAS pain* −13.9 %, $p = 0.061$ *Pain (categories)* −0.35, $p = 0.053$ *Global evaluation* −0.39, $p = 0.051$	23/52 (44 %) capsaicin; 1/49 (0.02 %) placebo patient$^{\Omega}$
McCarthy 1992 (McCarthy and McCarty 1992) 4 weeks	14	65 ± 2	5M:9F	Hand	0.075 % capsaicin	*Pain VAS* ~−40 % ($p < 0.02$) *Tenderness scores* ~ −30 % $p < 0.02$. No effect on grip strength, joint swelling, duration of morning stiffness or function	7/7 capsaicin; 0/7 placebo

(continued)

Table 11.1 (continued)

Study, duration	*n*	Age (years)	Sex (M:F)	OA site	Formulation	Outcomes	Rate of application site burning
Altman 1994 (Altman et al. 1994) 12 weeks	113	62 ± 12[¥]		Knee	0.025 % capsaicin	*Pain VAS* Significant differences by week 4, effect size −9 mm at week 12 *Tenderness* Less tenderness in capsaicin group by week 8 ($p = 0.03$) *Global assessment* (physician) significant improvement by week 4 ($p = 0.042$). Patient assessment by week 4 ($p = 0.023$) *Pain severity (categorical)* and HAQ: no differences	26/36 (46 %) of capsaicin users

(continued)

Table 11.1 (continued)

Study, duration	*n*	Age (years)	Sex (M:F)	OA site	Formulation	Outcomes	Rate of application site burning
McCleane 2000 (McCleane 2000) 5 weeks	200	~49 ± 14	78M:89F	Hip, knee, shoulder, hand	0.025 % capsaicin ± 1.33 % GTN	*VAS pain scores* Difference between GTN + capsaicin and GTN or capsaicin alone $p < 0.05$ *Analgesic use* Difference between any actives and placebo $p < 0.05$, Adding GTN to capsaicin has additive effect. GTN application reduced burning sensation when combined with capsaicin	Not reported

(continued)

Table 11.1 (continued)

Study, duration	*n*	Age (years) Sex (M:F)	OA site	Formulation	Outcomes	Rate of application site burning
Schnitzer 2012 (Schnitzer et al. 2012) 12 weeks + extension	695	61 33 %:67 %	Knee	0.075 % civamide Placebo 0.01 % civamide	*Primary outcomes (12 weeks) using TWA WOMAC pain* $p = 0.009$. WOMAC physical function: $p \leq 0.001$ *Subject global evaluation* $p = 0.008$. Pain and physical function effect sizes greater in patients with higher pain scores	35 % in capsaicin group, 11 % in placebo $p \leq 0.001$
Kosuwon 2010 (Deal et al. 1991) 4 weeks treatment	70	61 (44–82) years 0M:61F	Knee	0.025 % capsaicin	*VAS pain*−0.72, $p \leq 0.05$ *WOMAC pain* −3.42, $p \leq 0.05$ *WOMAC function* −8.97, $p \leq 0.05$	66.6 % of patients during the capsaicin phase versus 16.6 % patients during placebo phase; $p \leq 0.05$

¥No data on sex ratios in Altman 1994 (3)

ΩData given only for whole cohort (rheumatoid arthritis and osteoarthritis)

VAS visual analog scale; *GTN* glycerol trinitrate; *IA* intra–articular; *OA* osteoarthritis; *NSAIDs* non–steroidal anti–inflammatory drugs; *ACR* American College of Rheumatology criteria; *KL* Kellgren and Lawrence classification; *WOMAC* Western Ontario and McMaster University Osteoarthritis Index; *HAQ* Health Assessment Questionnaire; *BMI* body mass index; *TWA* mean time weighted average (area under the curve/days of observation)

KL Kellgren and Lawrence classification

JSW Joint space width

11.6 Treatment Efficacy Within Placebo–Controlled Trials

Studies described in Table 11.1 show the efficacy of capsaicin (vs. placebo) on a range of outcomes, including pain using a visual analog scale (VAS), either a 0–100 scale or a 0–10 scale, as well as other outcomes including Western Ontario and McMaster Universities Index (WOMAC) pain, function and stiffness scales, patient and physician global evaluation, tenderness, grip strength, joint swelling, duration of morning stiffness, analgesic use, and adverse events.

VAS pain is the most commonly assessed outcome, and therefore we have further summarized the effect of capsaicin on pain intensity as assessed by visual analog scores (VAS) in Table 11.2. VAS scores have been compared using standardized mean differences in studies with available data (Deal et al. 1991; McCarthy and McCarty 1992; Altman et al. 1994; McCleane 2000; Kosuwon et al. 2010), using Review Manager (Revman) version 5.2 (The Cochrane Collaboration, Copenhagen). By convention (Cohen 1988), the standardized mean difference values of 0.2, 0.5, and 0.8 are considered small, medium, and large. Table 11.2 shows that capsaicin has a medium sized effect (SMD = 0.44) on pain intensity in patients with painful OA over 4 weeks of treatment. Results were remarkably consistent across trials with no heterogeneity, suggesting no dose response from different doses of capsaicin, and no difference in the effect of capsaicin on OA of different sites (e.g. hand vs. knee).

Most studies report capsaicin use over 4 weeks, with only, two studies continued treatment beyond 4 weeks (Altman et al. 1994; Schnitzer et al. 2012), both of which reported that continuing use was associated with beneficial effects. The study reported by Altman et al. (1994) demonstrated that the maximum difference between groups occurred at 4 weeks, and differences between groups remained similar between weeks 4 and 12. Schnitzer et al. (2012) report that differences in groups increase over time, even up to 20 weeks. These studies demonstrate that treatment with capsaicin is associated with benefits for treatment periods exceeding 4 weeks but that 4 weeks is probably sufficient for a therapeutic trial.

Two studies reported assessments of how patients reported the overall impression of treatment effectiveness (symptoms better, much better or completely gone) after 4 weeks. Capsaicin treated patients had a 40 % increased likelihood of reporting that their symptoms were at better after 4 weeks of treatment (Table 11.3). Schnitzer's study reported that after 12 weeks, the Osteoarthritis Research Society International (OARSI) simplified response was 10 % greater in civamide-treated patients (Schnitzer et al. 2012), suggesting that response to treatment continues up until at least 12 weeks.

Schnitzer et al. (2012) also identified interactions between baseline WOMAC pain and function scores and treatment effect, in that civamide treatment had greater efficacy in patients with more severe pain intensity and worse physical function at baseline. This suggests that capsaicin treatments may be more effective in patients with more painful OA.

In summary, the available evidence shows that treatment with capsaicin is effective in reducing pain intensity in older adults with painful osteoarthritis, conferring a medium sized effect.

Table 11.2 Forest plot comparing changes in VAS pain score over 4 weeks of treatment with capsaicin in patients with painful osteoarthritis

Study or subgroup	Capsaicin			Placebo			Weight (%)	Std. mean difference	Year	Std. mean difference
	Mean	SD	Total	Mean	SD	Total		IV random, 95 % CI		IV random, 95 % CI
Deal 1991	33.4	18	36	19.5	23	34	14.3	0.67 [0.19, 1.15]	1991	
Mc Carthy 1992	55	31.7	7	19	29.1	7	2.5	1.11 [−0.05, 2.26]	1992	
Altman 1994	29	15.1	57	20	18.7	56	23.7	0.53 [0.15, 0.90]	1994	
McCleane 2000	0.49	2.37	40	0.08	2.05	40	17.3	0.18 [−0.26, 0.62]	2000	
Kosuwon 2010	2.04	1.93	99	1.3[illegible]	1.97	99	42.2	0.37 [0.09, 0.65]	2010	
Total (95 % CI)			239			236	100.0	0.44 [0.25, 0.62]		

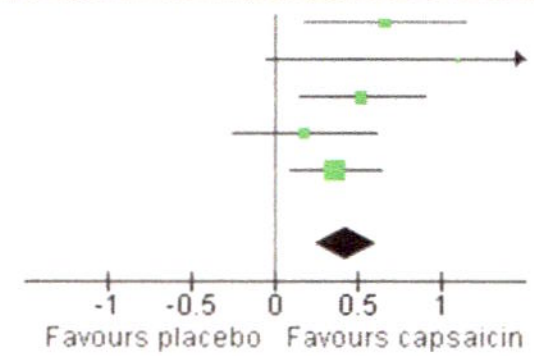

Heterogeneity $Tau^2 = 0.00$; $Chi^2 = 3.88$, df $= 4 (P = 0.42)$; $I^2 = 0$ %
Test for overall effect $Z = 4.69$ ($P < 0.00001$)

Table 11.3 Forest plot of patient global evaluation of treatment effectiveness after 4 weeks of treatment

Study or subgroup	Capsaicin		Placebo		Weight (%)	Risk ratio	Year	Risk ratio
	Events	Total	Events	Total		M-H, Fixed, 95 % CI		M-H, Fixed, 95 % CI
Deal 1991	26	36	17	34	33.1	1.44 [0.98, 2.14]	1991	
Altman 1994	49	57	35	56	66.9	1.38 [1.09, 1.73]	1994	
Total (95 % CI)		93		90	100.0	1.40 [1.14, 1.71]		
Total events	75		52					
Heterogeneity $Chi^2 = 0.05$, df = 1 ($P = 0.83$); $I^2 = 0$ %								
Test for overall effect $Z = 3.27$ ($P = 0.001$)								

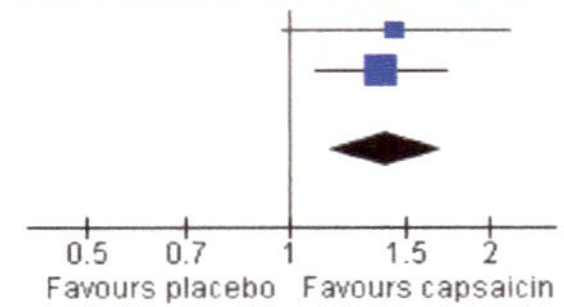

A treatment was considered "effective" if patients reported feeling "better" "much better" or their symptoms had "completely gone"

11.7 Safety of Capsaicin in Placebo–Controlled Trials

In concordance with studies investigating the use of capsaicin in other painful conditions, these studies reported that capsaicin was safe and well–tolerated. There have been no reports of systemic toxicity with the use of topical capsaicin in osteoarthritis.

Mild application site burning was the most comment adverse event associated with topical use of capsaicin, being more common in patients using capsaicin (35–100 %), and causally associated with capsaicin use, but rapidly ameliorates with continuing use. Proportion of participants reporting application site burning are shown in Tables 11.1 and 11.4. The risk ratio for application site burning is 4.22 (Table 11.4).

Most studies reported rates of burning over the entire study duration. However, two studies reported temporal trends in reports of incident application site burning over 12 weeks (Altman et al. 1994; Schnitzer et al. 2012). Both studies reported peak incidence in week 1, with incidence declining over time, and this had not plateaued by 12 weeks of treatment. Altman's study showed that incidence had diminished and almost plateaued by 12 weeks, but Schnitzer's data showed that incidence plateaued earlier, after 2 weeks. Regardless of the time at which reports of incident burning slow, this data suggests that overall, burning diminishes with continued use.

While most studies described the intensity of the burning sensation qualitatively, one study (McCleane 2000) specifically asked patients (at baseline only) to rate the discomfort scores on a 0–10 VAS. Predictably, the capsaicin treated patients reported a greater mean application discomfort score (2.41; 95 % CI 1.52–3.30) compared to placebo (0.90; 95 % CI 0.21–1.59), the difference being statistically significant ($p < 0.001$).

This localized application site burning provides challenges for treatment blinding, as it has the potential to unblind study participants. One study attempted to reduce this potential source of confounding by including a very low dose of capsaicin-like treatment into the placebo in order to mimic the burning effect (Schnitzer et al. 2012). If the burning sensation was associated with clinical response, this may have further implications for blinding, as well as predicting which patients might benefit from capsaicin use. However, Altman et al. (1994) found no significant difference in pain reduction amongst capsaicin treated patients who reported burning or stinging at the application site at week 12 compared to capsaicin patients not reporting burning (45 % reduction, $n = 16$ vs. 57 % reduction, $n = 27$; $p = 0.39$).

In summary, transient application site burning is more common in patients randomized to receive topical capsaicin compared to placebo. This is reported to be mostly mild in intensity, and there have been no reports of systemic toxicity with the use of topical capsaicin in osteoarthritis.

Cotherapy may influence toxicity. McCleane (2000) added a glycerol trinitrate (GTN) arm and GTN plus capsaicin arms to capsaicin alone and placebo. They found that the addition of GTN to capsaicin reduced the discomfort of the burning sensation associated with capsaicin use compared to capsaicin alone, and this combination provided an additive effect on pain outcomes, with human receiving capsaicin and GTN having greater reduction in pain intensity than either capsaicin or GTN alone.

Table 11.4 Forest plot of reports of application site burning

Study or subgroup	Capsaicin		Placebo		Weight (%)	Risk ratio	Year	Risk ratio
	Events	Total	Events	Total		M-H, Fixed, 95 % CI		M-H, Fixed, 95 % CI
Deal 1991	23	36	0	34	0.9	44.46 [2.81, 704, 39]	1991	
Mc Carthy 1992	7	7	0	7	0.9	15.00 [1.02, 220.92]	1992	
Altman 1994	26	57	2	56	3.5	12.77 [3.18, 51.28]	1994	
Kosuwon 2010	66	99	16	99	27.8	4.13 [2.58, 6.60]	2010	
Schnitzer 2012	120	344	39	351	67.0	3.14 [2.26, 4.36]	2012	
Total (95 % CI)		543		547	100.0	4.22 [3.25, 5.48]		
Total events	542		57					

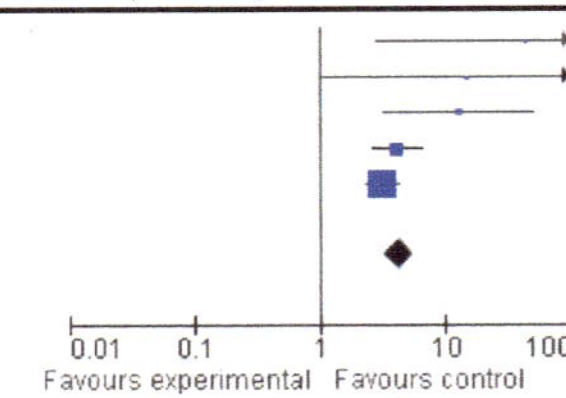

Heterogeneity Chi^2 = 9.20; df = 4 (P = 0.06); I^2 = 57 %
Test for overall effect Z = 10.80 (P < 0.00001)

Note Duration of capsaicin use ranges from 4 to 12 weeks

Capsaicin can be hazardous when applied to mucous membranes, (for example, its' use in pepper spray by law enforcement), and therefore capsaicin should not be ingested, inhaled, or applied to the eyes. Therefore, caution should be advised when applying capsaicin preparations topically, that patients take care to avoid touching eyes, mouth, nose, abraded skin or genitals. As capsaicin is a neurotoxin, neurotoxicity is theoretically possible, either via specific (via TRPV1) or nonspecific mechanism (Szallasi and Blumberg 1999).

Overall, the safety profile of topically applied capsaicin is good.

11.8 Patient Preference

Topical therapies enable the active ingredient to be absorbed through the skin to a localized area, thereby conferring benefit to that specific area and reducing the amount of medication that is systemically absorbed. This reduces the potential for drug interactions or drug-related systemic adverse events. This may be more suited for patients with small numbers of affected joints rather than generalized osteoarthritis. Also, capsaicin may be more effective in patients with neuropathic components to their arthritis.

In a study asking older patients with knee OA to weight their treatment preferences based on effectiveness, risk of side-effects and other factors (including cost), capsaicin was the preferred treatment from a range of other oral medications (non–selective NSAIDs, COX-2 (cyclooxygenase–2) inhibitors, opioids, glucosamine and chondroitin sulphate) (Fraenkel et al. 2004). This suggests that patients might be willing to accept less effective treatments in exchange for a lower risk of adverse effects. The controversy surrounding the use of the COX–2 inhibitor class of NSAIDs and heightened cardiovascular risk (Bombardier et al. 2000; Bresalier et al. 2005; Caughey et al. 2011; Solomon et al. 2005), highlights the importance of safe treatment options to minimize adverse side effects.

11.9 Areas of Uncertainty

The longest clinical trial of capsaicin for osteoarthritis pain is 12 weeks, with a long–term open label extension. However, osteoarthritis symptoms often fluctuate so it is uncertain how efficacy and toxicity would be affected by intermittent use or by continuous use for longer than 12 weeks. There is the possibility of tachyphylaxis with the latter; although the trial of Schnitzer et al. (2012) does not support this, demonstrating increasing efficacy over time. The effect sizes seem consistent for the hand and knee but there is very limited data at other sites and it seems less likely that it will be effective for non–superficial joints such as the hip.

Different trials used different formulations of capsaicin ranging from 0.025 to 0.075 %. It is possible that both efficacy and side effects may vary by strength of formulation, yet no studies have compared different formulations to determine the optimal combination of efficacy and side effects and the magnitude of benefit seemed similar across trials. Clinicians would typically start with the lower concentration and titrate upwards depending on response.

Further elucidation of which patients may benefit most from capsaicin therapy is required, such as early versus late OA, localized versus generalized OA, and those with and without neuropathic pain.

11.10 Summary

In conclusion, data from placebo-controlled trials show that topical capsaicin treatment four times daily is moderately effective in reducing pain intensity over 12 weeks and possibly longer. The most common adverse effect is localized burning sensations of mild to moderate intensity, which is causally associated with capsaicin use, but diminishes with continuing use. Overall, this suggests that capsaicin should be used early in the OA treatment algorithm especially for superficial joints like the hand and knee.

References

Altman RD, Aven A, Holmburg CE, Pfeifer LM, Sack M, Young GT (1994) Capsaicin cream 0.025% as monotherapy for osteoarthritis: a double-blind study. Semin Arthritis Rheum 23(6 (Suppl 3)):S25–33

Bombardier C, Laine L, Reicin A, Shapiro D, Burgos-Vargas R, Davis B, Day R, Ferraz MB, Hawkey CJ, Hochberg MC, Kvien TK, Schnitzer TJ (2000) Comparison of upper gastrointestinal toxicity of rofecoxib and naproxen in patients with rheumatoid arthritis. VIGOR study group. N Engl J Med 343(21):1520–1528. doi:10.1056/nejm200011233432103

Baron R (2000) Capsaicin and nociception: from basic mechanisms to novel drugs. Lancet 356(9232):785–787. doi:10.1016/s0140-6736(00)02649-0

Bresalier RS, Sandler RS, Quan H, Bolognese JA, Oxenius B, Horgan K, Lines C, Riddell R, Morton D, Lanas A, Konstam MA, Baron JA (2005) Cardiovascular events associated with rofecoxib in a colorectal adenoma chemoprevention trial. N Engl J Med 352(11):1092–1102. doi:10.1056/NEJMoa050493

Caughey GE, Roughead EE, Pratt N, Killer G, Gilbert AL (2011) Stroke risk and NSAIDs: an Australian population-based study. Med J Aust 195(9):525–529

Cohen J (1988) Statistical power analysis for behavioral sciences, 2nd edn. Lawrence Erlbaum Associates Incorporated, New Jersey

Caterina MJ, Schumacher MA, Tominaga M, Rosen TA, Levine JD, Julius D (1997) The capsaicin receptor: a heat-activated ion channel in the pain pathway. Nature 389(6653):816–824. doi:10.1038/39807

Dieppe PA, Lohmander LS (2005) Pathogenesis and management of pain in osteoarthritis. Lancet 365(9463):965–973. doi:10.1016/s0140-6736(05)71086-2

Deal CL (1994) The use of topical capsaicin in managing arthritis pain: a clinician's perspective. Semin Arthritis Rheum 23(6 Suppl 3):48–52

Deal CL, Schnitzer TJ, Lipstein E, Seibold JR, Stevens RM, Levy MD, Albert D, Renold F (1991) Treatment of arthritis with topical capsaicin: a double-blind trial. Clin Ther 13(3):383–395

Fraenkel L, Bogardus ST Jr, Concato J, Wittink DR (2004) Treatment options in knee osteoarthritis: the patient's perspective. Arch Intern Med 164(12):1299–1304. doi:10.1001/archinte.164.12.1299
Fusco BM, Giacovazzo M (1997) Peppers and pain. The promise of capsaicin. Drugs 53(6):909–914
Fortier LA, Nixon AJ (1997) Distributional changes in substance P nociceptive fiber patterns in naturally osteoarthritic articulations. J Rheumatol 24(3):524–530
Jancso G, Kiraly E, Jancso-Gabor A (1977) Pharmacologically induced selective degeneration of chemosensitive primary sensory neurones. Nature 270(5639):741–743
Kidd BL, Morris VH, Urban L (1996) Pathophysiology of joint pain. Ann Rheum Dis 55(5):276–283
Kenins P (1982) Responses of single nerve fibres to capsaicin applied to the skin. Neurosci Lett 29(1):83–88
Kosuwon W, Sirichatiwapee W, Wisanuyotin T, Jeeravipoolvarn P, Laupattarakasem W (2010) Efficacy of symptomatic control of knee osteoarthritis with 0.0125% of capsaicin versus placebo. J Med Assoc Thai 93(10):1188–1195
McCleane G (2000) The analgesic efficacy of topical capsaicin is enhanced by glyceryl trinitrate in painful osteoarthritis: a randomized, double blind, placebo controlled study. Eur J Pain 4(4):355–360. doi:10.1053/eujp.2000.0200
McCarthy GM, McCarty DJ (1992) Effect of topical capsaicin in the therapy of painful osteoarthritis of the hands. J Rheumatol 19(4):604–607
Nolano M, Simone DA, Wendelschafer-Crabb G, Johnson T, Hazen E, Kennedy WR (1999) Topical capsaicin in humans: parallel loss of epidermal nerve fibers and pain sensation. Pain 81(1–2):135–145
Pernow B (1983) Substance P. Pharmacol Rev 35(2):85–141
Schaible HG, Grubb BD (1993) Afferent and spinal mechanisms of joint pain. Pain 55(1):5–54
Schnitzer TJ, Pelletier JP, Haselwood DM, Ellison WT, Ervin JE, Gordon RD, Lisse JR, Archambault WT, Sampson AR, Fezatte HB, Phillips SB, Bernstein JE (2012) Civamide cream 0.075% in patients with osteoarthritis of the knee: a 12-week randomized controlled clinical trial with a longterm extension. J Rheumatol 39(3):610–620. doi:10.3899/jrheum.110192
Szallasi A, Blumberg PM (1999) Vanilloid (Capsaicin) receptors and mechanisms. Pharmacol Rev 51(2):159–212
Szallasi A, Blumberg PM (2007) Complex regulation of TRPV1 by vanilloids. TRP ion channel function in sensory transduction and cellular signaling cascades. CRC Press, Boca Raton
Solomon SD, McMurray JJ, Pfeffer MA, Wittes J, Fowler R, Finn P, Anderson WF, Zauber A, Hawk E, Bertagnolli M (2005) Cardiovascular risk associated with celecoxib in a clinical trial for colorectal adenoma prevention. N Engl J Med 352(11):1071–1080. doi:10.1056/NEJMoa050405
Theriault E, Otsuka M, Jessell T (1979) Capsaicin-evoked release of substance P from primary sensory neurons. Brain Res 170(1):209–213
Valdes AM, De Wilde G, Doherty SA, Lories RJ, Vaughn FL, Laslett LL, Maciewicz RA, Soni A, Hart DJ, Zhang W, Muir KR, Dennison EM, Wheeler M, Leaverton P, Cooper C, Spector TD, Cicuttini FM, Chapman V, Jones G, Arden NK, Doherty M (2011) The Ile585Val TRPV1 variant is involved in risk of painful knee osteoarthritis. Ann Rheum Dis 70(9):1556–1561. doi:10.1136/ard.2010.148122
Wood JN, Winter J, James IF, Rang HP, Yeats J, Bevan S (1988) Capsaicin-induced ion fluxes in dorsal root ganglion cells in culture. J Neurosci 8(9):3208–3220
Wojtys EM, Beaman DN, Glover RA, Janda D (1990) Innervation of the human knee joint by substance-P fibers. Arthroscopy 6(4):254–263
Zhang W, Nuki G, Moskowitz RW, Abramson S, Altman RD, Arden NK, Bierma-Zeinstra S, Brandt KD, Croft P, Doherty M, Dougados M, Hochberg M, Hunter DJ, Kwoh K, Lohmander LS, Tugwell P (2010) OARSI recommendations for the management of hip and knee osteoarthritis: part III: changes in evidence following systematic cumulative update of research published through January 2009. Osteoarthr Cartil 18(4):476–499. doi:10.1016/j.joca.2010.01.013

Chapter 12
The Role of Capsaicin in Dermatology

Katherine Boyd, Sofia M. Shea and James W. Patterson

Abstract Neurogenic pain and pruritus are the common chief complaints at dermatology office visits. Unfortunately, they are also notoriously difficult conditions to treat. Topical capsaicin used as a single therapy or as an adjuvant offers a low-risk option for patients who do not achieve control on other therapies. This chapter presents the evidence behind topical capsaicin use in dermatologic conditions characterized by neurogenic pain or pruritus, including postherpetic neuralgia, notalgia paresthetica, brachioradial pruritus, lichen simplex chronicus, prurigo nodularis, pruritus ani, pruritus of hemodialysis, aquagenic pruritus, apocrine chromhidrosis, lipodermatosclerosis, alopecia areata, and psoriasis. It presents the most common capsaicin formulations, dosages, and durations of treatment for each condition. Additionally, the chapter addresses various adverse effects and limitations in the use of topical capsaicin in dermatology.

12.1 Introduction

In a 2006 study by McDermott et al., patients who experienced neuropathic pain had greater unemployment status, reported missing from work more than 5 days per month, and had decreased daily functioning as a result of their pain (McDermott et al. 2006; Tolle et al. 2006). This occurred despite more frequent visits to their physician and management with a variety of prescription medications (McDermott et al. 2006; Tolle et al. 2006). A more recent study from Europe demonstrated that neuropathic pain is associated with increased rates of insomnia, anxiety, and depression (Langley et al. 2013). Neuropathic pain and itch are common reasons for dermatology office visits, and the burden that results from these

K. Boyd · S. M. Shea · J. W. Patterson (✉)
Department of Pathology, University of Virginia Health System,
Charlottesville, VA 22908-0214, USA
e-mail: JWP9E@hscmail.mcc.virginia.edu

O. M. E. Abdel-Salam (ed.), *Capsaicin as a Therapeutic Molecule*, Progress in Drug Research 68, DOI: 10.1007/978-3-0348-0828-6_12, © Springer Basel 2014

conditions may be due in part to suboptimal treatment. Capsaicin represents a viable topical treatment option for patients experiencing neuropathic pain and itch who may fail to achieve relief from more commonly prescribed analgesics, antidepressants, antiepileptics, and other sedatives (Tolle et al. 2006).

While capsaicin has been used for medicinal purposes for centuries, its early documented use as a topical analgesic for treatment of neuropathic pain or itch is sparse. Native Americans used pepper pods as topical relief on their gums for toothaches, in addition to topical use as an aphrodisiac (Szallasi and Blumberg 1999). The analgesic effect of capsaicin was recognized in literature as early as 1850, when it was documented in the Dublin Free Press for relief of sore teeth (Szallasi and Blumberg 1999).

Since that time, topical use of capsaicin in the field of dermatology has expanded to include many conditions with a component of pain or itch. In this chapter, we will discuss the use of capsaicin in each of the following dermatologic conditions (Table 12.1):

- Postherpetic neuralgia
- notalgia paresthetica
- Brachioradial pruritus
- Lichen simplex chronicus and prurigo nodularis
- Pruritus ani, vulvae, and scroti
- Pruritus of hemodialysis
- Aquagenic pruritus
- Apocrine chromhydrosis
- Lipdermatosclerosis
- Alopecia areata
- Psoriasis

12.2 Dermatologic Conditions Responsive to Capsaicin Therapy

12.2.1 Post-Herpetic Neuralgia

Postherpetic neuralgia is defined as pain persisting more than 90 days following the occurrence of herpes zoster infection. It is the most common complication of HZV infection and occurs in 10–30 % of cases. The incidence and severity of herpes zoster infection increases with age, as does the likelihood of postherpetic neuralgia. Trigeminal neuralgia refers to postherpetic neuralgia occurring in the distribution of one of the branches of the trigeminal nerve (Pellissier et al. 2007).

Post-herpetic neuralgia and trigeminal neuralgia are conditions characterized by both neuropathic pain and neuropathic pruritus. As such, these conditions are particularly challenging to treat. Traditional treatment regimens include early high dose antiviral medications, oral analgesics such as nonsteroidal anti-inflammatory

Table 12.1 Dermatologic conditions responsive to capsaicin therapy

Dermatologic condition	Clinical manifestations
Post-herpetic neuralgia	Pain persisting more than 90 days following the occurrence of herpes zoster infection
Notalgia paresthetica	Focal pruritus typically located unilaterally on the mid- or upper back
	No primary lesion can be identified
	Often there is evidence of chronic rubbing or scratching seen as hyperpigmentation or mild lichenification in the area where the patient experiences the itch
Brachioradial pruritus	Unilateral or bilateral pruritus of the distal, and less commonly, proximal arms
	No primary lesion can be identified
	Often there is evidence of chronic rubbing or scratching seen as hyperpigmentation or mild lichenification in the area where the patient experiences the itch
Lichen simplex chronicus and prurigo nodularis	Thickened, erythematous or hyperpigmented scaly plaques that may also show evidence of excoriation
	Distribution is variable, and depends on the underlying source of pruritus. Lesions are in areas that the patient can reach
Pruritus ani, vulvae, and scroti	Intractable itching in the perianal or genital area, often with secondary lichenification
Pruritus of hemodialysis	Systemic pruritus
	May be associated with underlying neuropathy
Aquagenic pruritus	Rare condition characterized by itching sensation of the skin following exposure to water of any temperature or salinity
Apocrine chromhidrosis	Apocrine sweat is pigmented, usually yellow, green, or black
Lipodermatosclerosis	A manifestation of chronic venous insufficiency
	Painful panniculitis that typically presents on the medial lower legs in women over 40 years of age, as a result of chronic venous insufficiency
	Erythema progressing to hyperpigmentation, warmth, and induration
Alopecia areata	Most commonly, discrete round to oval areas of non-scarring hair loss
	Other, more rare forms include loss all scalp hair (alopecia totalis) or all of body hair (alopecia universalis)
Psoriasis	Classic form: variably sized erythematous and scaly plaques distributed on the extensor extremities, buttocks, and scalp
	Other forms:
	• Gutatte: eruptive, small plaques
	• Erythrodermic: total body erythema
	• Pustular: eruptive form, often in patients with unstable chronic psoriasis, may be associated with systemic symptoms

drugs, and high dose anti-epileptics, particularly gabapentin. Additionally, oral corticosteroids are often given to decrease inflammation-related pain. Topical analgesics, specifically lidocaine and capsaicin have also shown efficacy in pain and itch amelioration (Watson et al. 1993).

A 6-week randomized, double-blinded, vehicle-controlled study with 2-year open label follow-up demonstrated some amount of pain relief in 64 % of patients with postherpetic neuralgia treated with 0.075 % capsaicin cream compared to only 25 % of patients on placebo. A more recent Phase III trial of topical synthetic capsaicin (8 % transcapsaicin patch) documented a 30 % decrease in pain scores after 2–12 weeks when compared with placebo after 1 h exposure (Backonja et al. 2008). Although effect on pruritus was not mentioned, it may be speculated that itch was relieved to a similar extent.

The 8 % transdermal patch formulation is relatively new with limited data; however, this higher concentration preparation shows promise as a useful adjuvant therapy for the persistent pain of postherpetic neuralgia, particularly with repeat applications over the course of 2 years (Backonja et al. 2008).

12.2.2 Notalgia Paresthetica

Notalgia paresthetica is a common condition, presenting most frequently in middle-aged or older adults as focal pruritus typically located unilaterally on the mid or upper back. Usually, no primary lesion can be identified on examination, but often there is evidence of chronic rubbing or scratching seen as hyperpigmentation or mild lichenification in the area where the patient experiences the itch. Rare cases may have a bilateral and symmetric presentation. More extensive secondary changes may result from chronic scratching.

The pathogenesis of notalgia paresthetica is related to entrapment of the posterior rami of spinal nerves originating at T2–T6. Patients may have a history of back injury or complain of back and/or neck pain. Additionally, there is often evidence of spinal column degeneration or other vertebral pathology on imaging. Although pruritus may improve in many of these patients with surgical correction of their vertebral disease, a less invasive method for treating itch is preferred for patients who do not otherwise require surgery. Systemic therapy with gabapentin has shown some benefit, but topical therapy may be satisfactory in some cases without the side effects associated with gabapentin. Topical therapies include local anesthetics, corticosteroids, and capsaicin.

Both topical capsaicin cream (0.025 %) and the 8 % capsaicin patch have been shown to be efficacious in this condition. In a double-blind, vehicle-controlled crossover study with topical capsaicin, 20 patients with notalgia paresthetica were randomized to capsaicin 0.025 % cream or vehicle control group with crossover after 4 weeks of treatment and a 2 week washout period. Overall, 70 % of patients experienced improvement in their symptoms with capsaicin therapy while 30 % of patients had improvement with vehicle. While most patients experienced some relapse after 1 month of no treatment, repeat use of topical capsaicin cream 0.025 % again resulted in remission of their pruritus (Wallengren and Klinker 1995).

Additionally, a report of two cases of notalgia paresthetica treated with a 8 % capsaicin patch resulted in complete remission of itch in both patients immediately following removal of the patch. The patient who was able to tolerate the complete goal duration of therapy (60 min) remained symptom-free at 12 weeks. The other patient was able to tolerate the patch for only 20 min and experienced recurrence of pruritus after few days. While the authors admit that data for use of the capsaicin patch for neuropathic itch is currently limited, their experience does show efficacy of this formulation in the treatment of notalgia paresthetica with ease and convenience of application as a benefit over the cream (Metz et al. 2011).

12.2.3 Brachioradial Pruritus

Patients with brachioradial pruritus present with unilateral or bilateral pruritus of the distal, and less commonly, proximal arms. The pruritus is often felt to be worse during the summer months or after prolonged sun exposure and is most common in middle-aged or older patients with fair skin. As with notalgia paresthetica, there is no identifiable primary lesion, though secondary changes associated with chronic scratching and rubbing may be present.

The etiology of brachioradial pruritus is not completely understood. Because it apparently worsens with sun exposure in many patients, one theory suggests that brachioradial pruritus is a result of sun damage to peripheral nerve fibers in the sun-exposed skin of the arm. One study demonstrated a decrease of sensory nerve fibers in the distal arms of patients with brachioradial pruritus at the end of the summer season compared to number of nerve fibers during a symptom-free period (Wallengren and Sundler 2005). A second theory proposes that cervical spine disease causing entrapment of cervical nerve rami results in neuropathic itch in the distal arm distribution, analogous to the theoretical cause of notalgia paresthetica. Indeed, many patients complain of neck pain and have evidence of spinal column disease in the C5–C6 distribution on imaging. Current thinking is that cervical vertebral disease may predispose patients to brachioradial pruritus while ultraviolet light is an eliciting factor (Wallengren and Sundler 2005).

As with notalgia paresthetica, surgical treatment of cervical vertebral disease may result in amelioration of pruritus in some patients with brachioradial pruritus. Gabapentin has also been used with some success in treatment of this condition. Unfortunately, brachioradial pruritus is often resistant to topical or oral corticosteroids and antihistamines.

Topical capsaicin has been used successfully in some cases. Two studies done in tropical latitudes demonstrated 12 of 15 (80 %) patients experienced improvement of symptoms when treated with topical capsaicin (Knight and Hayashi 1994; Goodless and Eaglstein 1993). In another study carried out in a temperate climate, all patients experienced relief of itch during the treatment period but found that capsaicin 0.025 % cream was no better than vehicle. The authors postulate that one reason for this outcome is the difficulty in distinguishing laterality in pruritus. They also considered the possibility of spontaneous improvement as the weather changed to cooler temperatures (Wallengren and Sundler 2005). Regardless; capsaicin remains a safe alternative for treatment of brachioradial pruritus.

12.2.4 Lichen Simplex Chronicus and Prurigo Nodularis

Lichen simplex chronicus (LSC) and prurigo nodularis are dermatologic conditions that present in patients who chronically scratch or rub their skin due to intractable pruritus from a variety of primary sources. The causative source may be a dermatologic condition such as atopic dermatitis, scabies, or pemphigoid, or it may be related to pruritus associated with systemic illness, or malignancy. Lichen simplex chronicus and prurigo nodularis are not uncommon findings in patients with diabetes mellitus, obstructive biliary disease, chronic kidney disease, liver failure, endocrine dysfunction, or malignancies such as leukemia and lymphoma. Additionally, pruritus and secondary changes of lichen simplex chronicus and prurigo nodularis can be seen in patients with severe emotional stress or anxiety.

Lichen simplex chronicus presents as thickened, erythematous or hyperpigmented scaly plaques that may also show evidence of excoriation. Distribution is variable, and depends on the underlying source of pruritus. Regardless of the source, the lesions are usually located on easy-to-reach skin; that is, areas that the patient has access to rub or scratch repeatedly.

Prurigo nodularis is a similar condition in that it results from chronic mechanical irritation of the skin, however, it presents as discrete nodules of lichenification and excoriation rather than confluent plaques.

Treatment of both of these conditions is difficult. The pruritus is often intractable and the mechanical irritation caused by scratching or rubbing worsens the lichenification and inflammation, and subsequently, the pruritus. While treatment of the underlying condition can help significantly, often, that condition is not curable and therefore the pruritus persists. Therapeutic regimens aimed at easing the itch include topical medications such as emollients containing menthol and topical corticosteroids. These treatments are often insufficient on their own because as the stratum corneum thickens in these conditions, it inhibits penetration of the medication into the dermis. While intralesional steroids have been used with some success, the size of the plaque of LSC or the number of prurigo nodules may make this modality impractical. Systemic therapies that have been used with some success include antihistamines, ultraviolet light, corticosteroids, cyclosporine, thalidomide, and etretinate. Although these medications have been shown to be successful at ameliorating pruritus, each has side effects that limit the practicality of its use. Capsaicin is a reasonable alternative as it lacks systemic side effects and penetration through a thickened stratum corneum can be enhanced through occlusion.

To evaluate the efficacy of topical capsaicin in the treatment of prurigo nodularis, Stander et al. measured both the clinical and histologic features pre- and posttreatment in 33 patients. Each patient applied capsaicin to the lesional areas 4–6 times daily, starting with a concentration of 0.025 % and increasing as needed, to achieve complete cessation of pruritus. The highest concentration required was 0.3 % by a single patient. Treatment duration was also variable, lasting from 2 weeks to 33 months in one patient with poor compliance. However, all participants achieved complete remission within 12 days and 24 patients experienced flattening of lesions within 2 months. Although there was recurrence of pruritus once the capsaicin application was stopped in about half of the study patients, the majority experienced 2 weeks to 2 months of treatment-free remission. Patients also experienced relief when the medication was reinitiated following cessation and recurrence. The histologic changes accompanying the clinical changes showed thinning of the stratum corneum and epidermis, and decreased inflammation and scarring. Ultrastructurally, decreased reactivity to substance P was noted following treatment with capsaicin. The authors conclude that capsaicin is effective for symptomatic relief as well as clinical resolution of the nodules. They recommend regular application of topical capsaicin 4–6 times daily at a concentration that achieves complete cessation of pruritus with reapplication upon recurrence (Stander et al. 2001).

12.2.5 Pruritus Ani, Vulvae, and Scroti

Pruritus of the anogenital skin and mucosa may be idiopathic or secondary to an underlying disorder. It presents as intractable itching in the perianal or genital area, often with secondary lichenification. In order to diagnose primary or idiopathic pruritus ani, vulvae, or scroti, possible secondary causes should be ruled out. Potential causes of secondary anogenital pruritus include irritant or allergic contact dermatitis, primary cutaneous conditions (psoriasis, atopic dermatitis, seborrheic dermatitis, lichen planus, lichen sclerosus), malignancy (anogenital carcinoma, paget's disease), infection (pinworms, sexually transmitted diseases), hemorrhoids, rectal fistulas, or sinus tracts. In the absence of an underlying condition, idiopathic anogenital pruritus has been attributed to dietary causes such as excessive caffeine intake, personal hygiene, or psychogenic factors (Bolognia and Jorizzo 2012).

In cases of secondary anogenital pruritus, symptoms improve with treatment of the underlying condition. For idiopathic cases, treatment can be more challenging. In patients with a suspected psychogenic component, psychological evaluation, and counseling may be beneficial. Mild cases may respond to frequent sitz baths and mild-potency topical corticosteroids. However, severe cases with secondary lichenification may require more potent topical steroids, leading to increased risk of atrophy (Bolognia and Jorizzo 2012).

A randomized, placebo-controlled crossover study evaluating the efficacy of topical capsaicin use for patients with anogenital pruritus found that 31 of 49 participants experienced relief of symptoms during the treatment period. Participants applied 0.006 % capsaicin ointment or placebo ointment with menthol to the affected area 3 times daily for 4 weeks followed by a 1-week wash out and 4 week crossover period. Four patients withdrew from the study due to side effects. There was a statistically significant ($p < 0.001$) difference in response rate between the two groups. Responders required consistent treatment of at least one application of capsaicin daily to remain symptom-free (Lysy et al. 2003). For patients who are refractory to topical steroids, or have a risk of atrophy with continued treatment, topical capsaicin appears to be a safe and effective alternative.

12.2.6 Pruritus of Hemodialysis

Pruritus is the most common and most distressing dermatologic condition in patients undergoing chronic hemodialysis. Although prevalence has decreased recently because of improved dialysis techniques, it still occurs in 25–43 % of patients. The most common sites of involvement are the back, head, and abdomen, and frequently 1/3 of the total body surface area is involved (Weisshaar et al. 2003).

The pathogenesis of hemodialysis-associated itch is not well understood. Despite the well-established correlation of hyperuricemia and pruritus in patients with chronic renal failure, multiple studies have not shown an association between electrolyte levels and intensity of itch in patients undergoing hemodialysis. In a study involving 167 patients on hemodialysis, the only factor associated with increased pruritus was the presence of a preexisting neuropathy such as restless leg syndrome, paresthesias, decreased sensation, decreased deep tendon reflexes, or decreased muscle strength. The authors suggest that this association confirms the neurogenic origin of the pruritus of hemodialysis (Akhyani et al. 2005).

Multiple treatment modalities have found variable success in the treatment of hemodialysis-associated pruritus. Systemic therapy includes anti-histamines, cholestyramine, erythropoietin, ondansetron, and UVB phototherapy. Topical moisturizers and corticosteroids have also shown some efficacy in select patients. However, no specific therapy has shown consistent efficacy. In a 2003 study, no difference in pruritus was noticed between skin treated with capsaicin 0.05 % and untreated skin. However, topical capsaicin 0.05 % resulted in significantly decreased pruritus in hemodialysis patients compared with healthy controls (Weisshaar et al. 2003). In patients on chronic hemodialysis treatment, pretreatment with capsaicin may be helpful in decreasing dialysis-related pruritus.

12.2.7 Aquagenic Pruritus

Aquagenic pruritus is rare condition characterized by itching sensation of the skin following exposure to water of any temperature or salinity. No primary lesion or skin change is identified. Typically, itching, burning, or stinging sensation will begin within

30 min of exposure to water and last for up to 2 h. The lower extremities are affected first, with migration of symptoms to upper body but with sparing of the head, palms, and soles. While the etiology of idiopathic aquagenic pruritus is unclear, some studies have demonstrated elevated levels of neurotransmitters and peptides implicated in other pruritic conditions, including acetylcholine, histamine, serotonin, and prostaglandin E2 in the dermis and epidermis of affected skin. It is important to evaluate for and exclude underlying conditions that may lead to secondary aquagenic pruritus, such as hematologic malignancy (including Hodgkin disease), polycythemia vera, essential thrombocythemia, or myelodysplastic syndrome (Bolognia and Jorizzo 2012).

Overall, treatment options for idiopathic aquagenic pruritus have been dissatisfying. Systemic medications such as cyproheptadine, cimetidine, and cholestyramine have been used without much success. Ultraviolet light has been more effective with PUVA, demonstrating better results than with broadband UVB.

A study by Lotti et al. evaluated both the clinical and immunofluorescent changes in skin of patients with aquagenic pruritus before and after 4 weeks of treatment with capsaicin cream of three different concentrations (0.025, 0.5, 1.0 %). They found that prior to treatment, neuropeptidergic fibers in skin were filled with neuropeptides when evaluated with direct immunofluorescence and clinically patients experienced pruritus with exposure to water. Following capsaicin treatment, neuropeptidergic fibers were devoid of neuropeptide and water did not evoke pruritus. The authors conclude that aquagenic pruritus is mediated at least in part by neuropeptides, including substance P (Lotti et al. 1994). Thus, capsaicin is a reasonable treatment option for this rare condition. Currently, no standard for dosing or frequency of application exists and either parameter may be adjusted to achieve maximum efficacy while still being tolerable to the patient.

12.2.8 Apocrine Chromhidrosis

Apocrine chromhidrosis is a condition in which apocrine sweat is pigmented, usually yellow, green, or black. This results from the high lipofuscin concentration in apocrine sweat of some patients. One case report demonstrated effective treatment of facial apocrine chromhidrosis with topical capsaicin in a 30-year-old female. The patient applied capsaicin to half of her face 1–2 times daily, and vehicle to the other half. Resolution of her condition occurred only on the half treated with capsaicin and recurred within 2 days of cessation of the therapy (Marks 1989). While treatment options for apocrine chromhidrosis are limited, capsaicin is a valid option with few side effects.

12.2.9 Lipodermatosclerosis

Lipodermatosclerosis, a manifestation of chronic venous insufficiency, is a painful panniculitis that typically presents on the medial lower legs as a result of chronic venous insufficiency. In addition to pain, patients experience erythema progressing to hyperpigmentation, warmth, and induration of the site. It presents most commonly in women over the age of 40. Clinical manifestations are often bilateral. It is felt that in patients with venous insufficiency, venous hypertension leads to increased leakage of fibrinogen and other blood products from capillaries. Fibrinogen then polymerizes to form fibrin cuffs around vessels, further impairing oxygen exchange and leading to tissue hypoxia. This hypoxia results in the classic changes seen in the subcutaneous tissue in patients with lipodermatosclerosis: septal thickening and sclerosis with hyaline fibrosis and eventually lipomembranous change of fat lobules (Bolognia and Jorizzo 2012).

A number of therapeutic modalities have been attempted to treat this condition with variable success. Much depends on the stage of the disease. Compression and elevation are helpful in the early stages and are the mainstays of treatment. Anabolic steroids such as stanozolol have been used successfully for their fibrinolytic properties, however, significant side effects that limit its usefulness. Other treatments used in small studies and case reports with varying success include ultrasound, pentoxifylline, fasciotomy, and phlebectomy (Bolognia and Jorizzo 2012).

Typically, the pain associated with early lipodermatosclerosis is the most concerning symptom for patients. Yosipovitch et al. describe two patients with acute lipodermatosclerosis and one with acute lobular panniculitis and venous insufficiency who experienced relief of pain with topical capsaicin. They were each treated for 3 weeks with 0.075 % topical capsaicin 5 times per day, followed by continued treatment 3 times daily for an additional month in two of the cases. Each patient experienced resolution of pain and clinical panniculitis with no recurrence at follow-up of 2–6 months. While little is known about the fibrinolytic activity of capsaicin, Thai people who ingest chili pepper daily do show increased fibrinolytic activity (Visudhiphan et al. 1982). Additionally, capsaicin has been shown to increase bleeding time and inhibit platelet aggregation in mice. The authors postulate that substance P may have fibrinolytic properties, thus making topical capsaicin an useful treatment for early lipodermatosclerosis and other lobular panniculitides (Yosipovitch et al. 2005).

12.2.10 Alopecia Areata

This inflammatory alopecia is characterized by discrete round to oval areas of nonscarring hair loss, most commonly on the scalp. In many cases, the hair will regrow spontaneously, but often the condition recurs in a different area. There are chronic and more extreme forms of alopecia areata where a patient may lose all their scalp hair (alopecia totalis) or all of their body hair (alopecia universalis). The prognosis for complete regrowth in these cases is less promising. Alopecia areata may also affect the fingernails and toenails in a variety of ways, most common of which is pitting of the nail plate. Other nail changes include ridging, trachyonychia, onychomadesis, and red lunulae.

Alopecia areata is considered to be an autoimmune condition wherein T-cells target specific autoantigens on terminal anagen follicles. The histopathologic picture is that of a lymphocytic infiltrate tightly surrounding and sometimes infiltrating the follicular bulb, thus sparing the stem cells in the bulge region of the follicle and, therefore, the follicle's ability to regenerate intact. The main goal of treatment for alopecia areata is the reduction of the inflammatory response. For limited and localized disease, intralesional corticosteroids may speed regrowth of hair. Additional topical treatments include irritants such as azelaic acid and anthralin, or immunotherapy with agents such as squaric acid. For more widespread hair loss, systemic corticosteroids or immunosuppressants like cyclosporine have been used, but these options are limited due to side effects (Bolognia and Jorizzo 2012).

While the role of the immune system is well established in the etiology of alopecia areata, the clinic link between emotional stress and worsening of the condition has led some to search for a neurologic contribution. Previous studies have demonstrated decreased concentrations of substance P and calcitonin gene-related peptide in scalp biopsies of alopecia areata as well as changes in the structure and function of perifollicular nerves (Peters et al. 2001; Rossi et al. 1997). As capsaicin causes release and subsequent depletion of substance P, Ehsani et al. postulated its potential use in treating alopecia areata by transiently increasing the neuropeptide and the neurofollicular interface. They randomized 50 patients with less than 30 % scalp surface area involvement with alopecia areata to a control group or treatment group. The control group applied clobetasol ointment 0.05 % daily for 6 weeks while the treatment group applied capsaicin ointment daily for 2 weeks, then twice daily for 4 weeks. Although there was no statistically significant difference between the control and treatment group in terms of regrowth of terminal hairs, after 4 weeks, the treatment group demonstrated a significantly greater growth of vellus follicles. They concluded that capsaicin has a dual effect on the follicular unit: it inhibits hair shaft elongation and matrix proliferation but promotes vellus hair growth (Ehsani et al. 2009). While this does not appear to be an optimal treatment for alopecia areata, it does highlight a potential role for neuropeptides in the etiology of the condition and a potential target for treatment.

12.2.11 Psoriasis

Psoriasis is a common Th1/Th12-mediated inflammatory skin condition that presents in the classic form as variably sized erythematous and scaly plaques distributed on the extensor extremities, buttocks, and scalp. Presentation is variable, with involvement ranging from a few small plaques to complete erythroderma. Patients may have involvement with their hands, feet, scalp, or nails or isolation of disease to those areas. Twenty percent of patients have associated joint pain. While cutaneous pain and itch are not consistent symptoms, many patients experience such discomfort from their psoriatic plaques.

While recent psoriasis therapeutic research has focused on the inflammatory mechanisms involved in the pathogenesis of the disease, there is evidence to suggest that neurogenic pathways may also contribute to or exacerbate the condition. One double-blind study of topical capsaicin in the treatment of psoriasis-related pruritus demonstrated not only significant improvement of itch, but also reduction in combined psoriasis severity scores, as measured by degree of scaling, thickness, erythema, and pruritus, in patients using capsaicin 0.025 % cream for 4–6 weeks when compared to those using a vehicle control. The authors speculate that substance P plays a role not only in the driving the pruritus and pain associated with psoriasis, but also in influencing the inflammatory process by increasing perfusion and thus promoting accumulation of inflammatory markers at the site (Ellis et al. 1993).

An additional study supported the role of neurogenic factors in the pathogenesis of psoriasis. Krogstad, et al. found that lesional psoriatic skin treated with capsaicin showed immediate increase of histamine and overall perfusion. However, when measured at 24 h following application of capsaicin, there was a decrease below baseline of both perfusion and histamine levels (Krogstad et al. 1999). While capsaicin does not target specific inflammatory pathways—the feature that makes many of the new biologic medications and traditional immunosuppressant medications effective in the treatment of , the significant improvement in both pruritus and other psoriatic symptoms shown with topical capsaicin treatment make it a valuable adjuvant therapy in patients for whom systemic therapy is less desirable.

12.3 Treatment Limitations

12.3.1 Adverse Effects

The nature of capsaicin as a derivative of chili peppers and a substance P releaser makes it a powerful skin irritant. This has been known for generations among people who handle chili peppers and develop a contact dermatitis called "Hunan hand" as a result of chronic exposure. Its therapeutic effects are no different. All patients experience skin irritation in the form of burning with the application of even low concentrations of topical capsaicin. In the case of accidental inhalation, capsaicin can induce coughing and burning of the mucosa. This property is exploited in the formulation of personal protection sprays containing capsaicin (Bode and Dong 2011).

Reports of more severe side effects are rare. One report attributes a case of coronary vasospasm and acute myocardial infarction to the use of a topical capsaicin patch in the treatment of lower back pain (Akcay et al. 2009). Multiple studies done in mice also suggest that topical capsaicin may have carcinogenic potential, including skin cancer. The complete blockade of the transient receptor potential vanilloid subfamily member 1 (TRPV1) in the presence of a tumor promoter resulted in increased skin carcinogenesis in mice. The authors postulate that blockade of TRPV1 through chronic use of topical capsaicin, coupled with a tumor promoter such as ultraviolet light, could result in increased skin cancer (Bode and Dong 2011). Thus, caution should be taken into account when combining topical capsaicin with phototherapy.

12.3.2 Compliance

Perhaps the most significant limitation to using capsaicin to treat dermatologic conditions is compliance with the treatment. Because nearly every patient experiences immediate cutaneous discomfort, many patients are unable to continue treatment for a sufficient length of time to reach a point of therapeutic benefit. In fact, from reported clinical trials and experience, at least 30 % of patients or participants withdraw due to lack of tolerability (Papoiu and Yosipovitch 2010). As response rates for some dermatologic conditions are high, it may be necessary to counsel the patient about the expected transient cutaneous discomfort and the importance of compliance for a meaningful response.

12.4 Summary

Neurogenic pain and pruritus play a role in many dermatologic conditions, making topical capsaicin a viable treatment option that lacks the systemic side effects of the oral alternatives. Additionally, capsaicin is a reasonable alternative for the treatment of other diseases, including apocrine chromhidrosis, lipodermatosclerosis, and alopecia areata. Compliance can be difficult, especially with increased concentrations, as nearly as every patient experiences immediate cutaneous discomfort; however, this can be mitigated with appropriate dose escalation and education.

References

Akcay AB, Ozcan T, Seyis S, Acele A (2009) Coronary vasospasm and acute myocardial infarction induced by a topical capsaicin patch. Turk Kardiyol Dern Ars. 37(7):497–500

Akhyani M, Ganji MR, Samadi N, Khamesan B, Daneshpazhooh M (2005) Pruritus in hemodialysis patients. BMC Dermatol. 5:7

Backonja M, Wallace MS, Blonsky ER et al (2008) NGX-4010, a high-concentration capsaicin patch, for the treatment of postherpetic neuralgia: A randomised, double-blind study. Lancet Neurol 7(12):1106–1112

Bode AM, Dong Z (2011) The two faces of capsaicin. Cancer Res 71(8):2809–2814

Bolognia JL, Jorizzo JL (eds) (2012) Dermatology. 3rd edn. Elsevier, New York, pp 116–117, 1656–1658, 1100–1102

Ehsani AH, Toosi S, Seirafi H et al (2009) Capsaicin vs. clobetasol for the treatment of localized alopecia areata. J Eur Acad Dermatol Venereol 23(12):1451–1453
Ellis CN, Berberian B, Sulica VI et al (1993) A double-blind evaluation of topical capsaicin in pruritic psoriasis. J Am Acad Dermatol 29(3):438–442
Goodless DR, Eaglstein WH (1993) Brachioradial pruritus: Treatment with topical capsaicin. J Am Acad Dermatol 29(5 Pt 1):783–784
Knight TE, Hayashi T (1994) Solar (brachioradial) pruritus–response to capsaicin cream. Int J Dermatol 33(3):206–209
Krogstad AL, Lonnroth P, Larson G, Wallin BG (1999) Capsaicin treatment induces histamine release and perfusion changes in psoriatic skin. Br J Dermatol 141(1):87–93
Langley PC, Van Litsenburg C, Cappelleri JC, Carroll D (2013) The burden associated with neuropathic pain in western europe. J Med Econ. 16(1):85–95
Lotti T, Teofoli P, Tsampau D (1994) Treatment of aquagenic pruritus with topical capsaicin cream. J Am Acad Dermatol 30(2 Pt 1):232–235
Lysy J, Sistiery-Ittah M, Israelit Y et al (2003) Topical capsaicin–a novel and effective treatment for idiopathic intractable pruritus ani: A randomised, placebo controlled, crossover study. Gut 52(9):1323–1326
Marks JG Jr (1989) Treatment of apocrine chromhidrosis with topical capsaicin. J Am Acad Dermatol 21(2 Pt 2):418–420
McDermott AM, Toelle TR, Rowbotham DJ, Schaefer CP, Dukes EM (2006) The burden of neuropathic pain: Results from a cross-sectional survey. Eur J Pain 10(2):127–135
Metz M, Krause K, Maurer M, Magerl M (2011) Treatment of notalgia paraesthetica with an 8 % capsaicin patch. Br J Dermatol 165(6):1359–1361
Papoiu AD, Yosipovitch G (2010) Topical capsaicin. the fire of a 'hot' medicine is reignited. Expert Opin Pharmacother 11(8):1359–1371
Pellissier JM, Brisson M, Levin MJ (2007) Evaluation of the cost-effectiveness in the united states of a vaccine to prevent herpes zoster and postherpetic neuralgia in older adults. Vaccine. 25(49):8326–8337
Peters EM, Botchkarev VA, Botchkareva NV, Tobin DJ, Paus R (2001) Hair-cycle-associated remodeling of the peptidergic innervation of murine skin, and hair growth modulation by neuropeptides. J Invest Dermatol. 116(2):236–245
Rossi R, Del Bianco E, Isolani D, Baccari MC, Cappugi P (1997) Possible involvement of neuropeptidergic sensory nerves in alopecia areata. NeuroReport 8(5):1135–1138
Stander S, Luger T, Metze D (2001) Treatment of prurigo nodularis with topical capsaicin. J Am Acad Dermatol 44(3):471–478
Szallasi A, Blumberg PM (1999) Vanilloid (capsaicin) receptors and mechanisms. Pharmacol Rev 51(2):159–212
Tolle T, Dukes E, Sadosky A (2006) Patient burden of trigeminal neuralgia: Results from a cross-sectional survey of health state impairment and treatment patterns in six european countries. Pain Pract. 6(3):153–160
Visudhiphan S, Poolsuppasit S, Piboonnukarintr O, Tumliang S (1982) The relationship between high fibrinolytic activity and daily capsicum ingestion in thais. Am J Clin Nutr 35(6):1452–1458
Wallengren J, Klinker M (1995) Successful treatment of notalgia paresthetica with topical capsaicin: Vehicle-controlled, double-blind, crossover study. J Am Acad Dermatol 32(2 Pt 1):287–289
Wallengren J, Sundler F (2005) Brachioradial pruritus is associated with a reduction in cutaneous innervation that normalizes during the symptom-free remissions. J Am Acad Dermatol 52(1):142–145
Watson CP, Tyler KL, Bickers DR, Millikan LE, Smith S, Coleman E (1993) A randomized vehicle-controlled trial of topical capsaicin in the treatment of postherpetic neuralgia. Clin Ther 15(3):510–526
Weisshaar E, Dunker N, Gollnick H (2003) Topical capsaicin therapy in humans with hemodialysis-related pruritus. Neurosci Lett 345(3):192–194
Yosipovitch G, Mengesha Y, Facliaru D, David M (2005) Topical capsaicin for the treatment of acute lipodermatosclerosis and lobular panniculitis. J Dermatolog Treat. 16(3):178–180

Chapter 13
Use of Vanilloids in Urologic Disorders

Harris E. Foster Jr. and AeuMuro G. Lake

Abstract The bladder is an organ rich in vanilloid targets: dense unmyelinated c-fibers partially responsible for bladder sensation and response to noxious stimuli. Drugs such as capsaicin and resiniferatoxin (RTX) interact with the VR1 vanilloid receptor subtype to initially excite then subsequently desensitize the c-fibers. This chapter examines the literature describing the use of vanilloid receptor agonists in the treatment of the following urological disorders: neurogenic bladder (NGB), overactive bladder (OAB), and interstitial cystitis/painful bladder syndrome (IC/PBS). Review of the literature was performed using Pubmed and the following key words "capsaicin," "resiniferatoxin (RTX)," and "neurogenic bladder," "overactive bladder (OAB)," and "interstitial cystitis," "painful bladder syndrome." Articles focusing on randomized trials comparing intravesical administration of a vanilloid receptor agonist to placebo and those in English were reviewed. We conclude that capsaicin and RTX do appear to provide some acceptable treatment results in patients with neurogenic bladder, though larger studies are needed to confirm this. Although efficacy has been shown in some studies, currently the use of vanilloids cannot be recommended for routine use in patients with OAB as the need for catheterization may cause the risk to outweigh the benefit of treatment. Similarly, for the treatment of BPS, vanilloid receptor agonists lack strong evidence for efficacy or tolerability; larger studies are needed to define their role. Understanding how vanilloids are able to impact these disorders, however, may help further elucidate their underlying pathophysiological processes.

H. E. Foster Jr. (✉)
Department of Urology, Yale University School of Medicine, New Haven, CT 06520-8028, USA
e-mail: harris.foster@yale.edu

A. G. Lake
Department of Obstetrics and Gynecology, Section of Urogynecology and Reconstructive Pelvic Surgery, Yale University School of Medicine, New Haven, CT 06520-8028, USA

O. M. E. Abdel-Salam (ed.), *Capsaicin as a Therapeutic Molecule*, Progress in Drug Research 68, DOI: 10.1007/978-3-0348-0828-6_13, © Springer Basel 2014

13.1 Introduction

Vanilloids can be useful in a variety of clinical disorders, some involving those of urological origin. Most of the focus has revolved around treating disorders in which the bladder is the offending organ either directly or indirectly. The bladder is an organ rich in vanilloid targets, that being the dense unmyelinated c-fibers partially responsible for bladder sensation and response to noxious stimuli. Drugs such as capsaicin and RTX interact with the VR1 vanilloid receptor subtype to initially excite then subsequently desensitize the c-fibers. Although c-fibers are not the primary mediator of the bladder micturition reflex which ultimately eventuates in a bladder contraction, that primarily being the responsibility of their myelinated (faster) Aδ counterparts, in certain pathophysiological situations, where there is damage or dysfunction of the latter, they can significantly contribute to reflex bladder activity with negative consequences (Chancellor 2002). Furthermore, as pain associated with the bladder is mediated by these c-fibers, pharmacological methods to reduce their activity can be beneficial in the treatment of disease entities in which pain from the bladder is a primary symptom. The purpose of this chapter is not to discuss the detailed mechanisms by which vanilloids affect the neurological system in general as this is covered elsewhere in this text. The goal, however, is to describe how these agents perform in the treatment of certain urological disorders. In particular, the diseases/disorders to be discussed will include neurogenic bladder, overactive bladder (OAB), and interstitial cystitis/painful bladder syndrome (IC/PBS).

13.2 Neurogenic Bladder

Neurogenic bladder (NGB) can result from any neurological insult that interferes with the normal functioning of the lower urinary tract which requires intact pathways involving the central and peripheral neurological systems. Causes are many but most commonly include spinal cord injury (SCI), multiple sclerosis (MS), spina bifida, degenerative spinal disease, cerebrovascular accident and as a result of surgical extirpative procedures that affect peripheral bladder innervation such as radical hysterectomy and abdominal-perineal resection. Almost all patients with SCI and anywhere from 50 to 90 % of those with MS will develop some type of NGB dysfunction throughout the course of their disease (Burns et al. 2001; Fingerman and Finkelstein 2000). Depending on the specific location of the neurological insult, the effects on lower urinary tract function are varied. Typical manifestations of dysfunction are neurogenic detrusor overactivity (NDO), detrusor hyperreflexia with external sphincter dyssynergia, detrusor hypocontractility, detrusor areflexia, and loss of normal detrusor compliance. Urinary incontinence and/or urinary retention are the most likely clinical manifestations of NGB which primarily although not exclusively affect quality of life. The most disturbing and potentially life threatening complication to be prevented, however, is upper tract deterioration as manifested

Table 13.1 Treatment options for NGB

Route	Treatment	Proposed mechanism of action
Observation	Spontaneous voiding	–
Oral	Antimuscarinics	Suppresses detrusor muscle contractions
	Tricyclic antidepressant	Central and peripheral anticholinergic
Catheterization	Intermittent	Drainage of bladder/urinary tract
	Condom (male)	
	Suprapubic tube	
	Indwelling urethral	
Urinary diversion	Ileovesicostomy (continent or incontinent)	
	Ileal conduit	
Intravesical	Intradetrusor on a botulinum toxin A injection	Paralyzes detrusor muscle
	Antimuscarinics	Suppresses detrusor muscle contractions

by hydronephrosis which can ultimately result in chronic renal insufficiency. This is generally due to a loss in the low pressure storage capabilities of the bladder, overwhelming the propulsive effects of the ureter to transport urine from the kidneys. The primary goal when managing NGB is to establish a low pressure reservoir in the bladder with secondary goals including continence of urine if possible and reduction of other complications such as recurrent urinary tract infections and urolithiasis.

Management of NGB is varied and depends on multiple factors mainly related to the type of NGB dysfunction present and the capabilities and desires of the particular patient (Table 13.1). Most importantly, urodynamics, where the relationship between bladder filling and storage pressure along with an assessment of its ability to contract is required for adequate assessment. As mentioned previously, findings can range from an underactive or overactive detrusor along with different degrees of bladder compliance. Physical and social capabilities of the patient and their providers are almost as important as this will determine whether or not intermittent urethral catheterization is an option since this is generally the preferred method of management when bladder emptying is incomplete. Other options for managing the NGB include condom catheterization (in the male), spontaneous voiding (diapered if incontinent), suprapubic tube drainage, indwelling urethral catheter, continent or incontinent ileovesicostomy, and supravesical diversion with ileal conduit or continent catheterizable reservoir.

Pharmacologic intervention is often necessary to ameliorate involuntary bladder contractions secondary to NDO when intermittent catheterization is the preferred method of management in those with NGB. This is typically accomplished with the use of antimuscarinic agents of which a myriad are available commercially (i.e., oxybutynin, tolterodine, solifenacin, etc.). Antimuscarinic drugs are thought to suppress bladder contractions by the blockade of muscarinic receptors on the detrusor muscle, however, effects on the urothelium and central nervous system may also play a role. Use of these agents in combination or in conjunction with other drugs with anticholinergic effects such as the tricyclic antidepressant class may be of benefit when monotherapy is insufficient at achieving the clinical goal. In the case when oral therapies are unable to suppress the bladder effectively, options include various intravesical treatments, augmentation ileocystoplasty, or a change to another form of bladder management. Direct instillation or injection of different substances into the bladder have the advantage of obviating the need for oral administration and avoiding many of the associated side effects of antimuscarinic agents such as dry mouth, constipation, and less commonly, mental status changes. Currently, the only Food and Drug Administration (FDA)-approved drug for intravesical administration for NGB is botulinum toxin A which has performed well in multiple clinical trials with an acceptable side effect profile (Linsenmeyer 2013). The mechanism of action behind its efficacy is a selective blockade of acetylcholine-mediated detrusor muscle contractions (Schurch et al. 2000). Intravesical instillations of oxybutynin and lidocaine have also been described but are not used commonly for the management of NGB. It is in this clinical situation and administration route that vanilloids have shown some clinical efficacy in patients with NGB.

There have been numerous studies investigating the therapeutic benefit of intravesical vanilloids (capsaicin and RTX) in patients with NGB secondary to SCI and MS that are refractory to oral antimuscarinic therapy. A thorough review of the published randomized trials was performed by MacDonald et al. in 2007 (MacDonald et al. 2008). They compiled data from nine clinical trials (288 patients) comparing capsaicin and RTX to each other, placebo, or, in 1 trial, to botulinum toxin A (BTX-A). The majority of patients had either SCI or MS and nearly three quarters (71 %) were male. The main outcome measure was improvement in urinary incontinence as measured by the number of daily episodes. Doses of capsaicin ranged from 1 mM, 30 mg, and 2 mM and that of RTX was 0.005–1.0 μM, and 100 nM. Duration of treatment was 4 weeks to 18 months with the majority being at least 90 days duration. Many of the trials were placebo controlled and double blinded. Capsaicin reduced the number of daily urinary incontinence episodes by 3.8 episodes when compared to placebo. There was also a significant reduction in the numbers of pads used per day from 10 to 4. In the two trials comparing capsaicin to RTX, one showed no difference between treatment arms with both agents decreasing the urinary incontinence episodes at 30 days. As expected, the RTX groups had more durable responses at 90 days with the median number of daily incontinence episodes being 1 and 4 in the RTX and capsaicin groups, respectively. The side effect profile of capsaicin demonstrated greater incidences of pelvic pain/burning and flushing with the former occurring in 50–60 % of those treated with this agent. Although it was thought that the ethanol solvent may be responsible for this result, the effect was unchanged when glucidic acid was used as the solvent. Other side effects were similar to that of the placebo group. When capsaicin and RTX were compared to each other, capsaicin had a significantly higher incidence of pelvic pain (50 vs. 12 %).

Lazzeri et al. reported on their 10-year experience using intravesical vanilloids in 54 patients with neurogenic incontinence (Lazzeri et al. 2004). Doses of capsaicin and RTX were 10 mM and 10 nM–10 μM, respectively. A number of treatment outcomes were investigated including improvement in clinical status (dry on intermittent catheterization and bladder capacity 50 % higher at 3 months), number who continued therapy, number of instillations received, interval length between instillations, and alternative therapies when vanilloids failed. Over half (53.7 %) of those who received capsaicin had an improvement in their clinical symptoms and urodynamic parameters at 3 months. A higher response rate (73.33 %) was noted in those who received RTX at the 10 μM dose.

In summary, capsaicin and RTX do appear to provide acceptable treatment results in patient with neurogenic bladder, primarily due to SCI and MS. Randomized studies, however, are few and involve relatively small numbers of patients. The side effect profile generally favors RTX and durability of response is longer as would be expected. Although promising, at this point, use of these agents cannot be recommended as a standard treatment for NGB based on available data.

13.3 Overactive Bladder

OAB comprises a constellation of symptoms including urinary frequency, urgency with or without urinary incontinence in the absence of definable pathology such as urinary tract infection, bladder outlet obstruction, bladder cancer, or disorder of the neurologic system (i.e., SCI, MS, cerebrovascular accident, spina bifida, Parkinson's disease, etc.) which can result in a similar clinical presentation. The prevalence of OAB in the United States ranges from 7–27 % in men and 9–43 % in women (Gormley et al. 2012). It also disproportionately affects the elderly population and can heighten the risks of falls potentially resulting in hip fractures and skull injuries with their concomitant comorbidities (deep vein thrombosis, pulmonary embolus, intracranial hemorrhage etc.). Despite not having direct impact on duration of life, OAB can have tremendous negative effects on the quality of life. Many find that their ability to perform and/or enjoy daily activities and ability to obtain satisfactory sleep is encumbered by the frequent and urgent need to void. Furthermore, management of the often associated urinary (urgency type) incontinence can often be a costly venture requiring the use of various types of protective devices such as sanitary pads and diapers. In severe cases, chronic urethral catheterization may be chosen as the most pragmatic method of management, exposing the patient to some of the long-term consequences previously mentioned when used in the neurogenic population.

Evaluation of the patient with OAB revolves around diagnostic tests able to detect causative and potentially treatable etiologies. Simple urinalysis can detect evidence of urinary tract infection, glucosuria which may be causing an osmotic diuresis, and hematuria (microscopic or gross), a potential indicator of urinary tract pathology such as neoplasia or urolithiasis. Urine cytology while not highly sensitive does have good specificity (low false positives) and can be utilized when social data (tobacco use or exposure to chemicals) suggest predisposition to

Table 13.2 Treatment options for OAB

Route	Treatment	Proposed mechanism of action
Behavioral	Avoidance of bladder irritants, bladder retraining	Decreases irritation
Oral	Antimuscarinics	Suppresses detrusor muscle contractions
	Beta-3 Agonist	Relaxes detrusor smooth muscle
Transdermal	Antimuscarinics	Suppresses detrusor muscle contractions
Intravesical	Intradetrusor on a botulinum toxin A injection	Paralyzes detrusor muscle
Neuromodulation	Sacral	Unknown, electrically stimulates somatic afferent nerves in spinal nerve root
	Percutaneous tibial nerve	Unknown, electrically stimulates somatic afferent nerves in spinal nerve root

urothelial malignancy. Measurement of post-void residual urine can assist in the detection of bladder outlet obstruction and neurogenic vesicourethral dysfunction when elevated. Direct inspection of the bladder and urethra with cystourethroscopy may be indicated when there are reasons to suspect bladder neoplasm (primarily hematuria or suspicious urine cytology). Urodynamics, although not required for diagnosis, can be helpful in determining if bladder outlet obstruction or neurogenic bladder is the underlying pathophysiological process. Typical findings in patients with OAB are the presence of involuntary detrusor contractions of varying magnitudes during the filling phase, sometimes accompanied by the loss of urine. The absence of this pattern, however, is not sufficient to eliminate the diagnosis of OAB as the study can be normal in up to 50 % of affected patients.

Management and treatment of OAB is dictated primarily by the severity of the symptoms and the level of impact it has on the patient's quality of life (Table 13.2). Oftentimes behavioral modification by the moderation in fluid intake, reduction in the use of caffeinated products and others with diuretic properties (i.e. alcohol), and elimination of food stuffs with high spice content can be sufficient at satisfactorily ameliorating the symptoms of OAB. In most instances, however, this is not adequate and pharmacological or surgical options must be considered. The goal of these therapies is either reduction in the frequency or amplitude of the associated involuntary detrusor contraction or their elimination altogether. As with NGB, pharmacotherapy for OAB generally involves the use of agents with antimuscarinic properties that interfere with detrusor contractions. Many are commercially available with no significant differences in their efficacy. Oral preparations are most commonly used; however, agents that can be topically administered (transdermal patch, gel) exist. Recently, another agent with beta-3 agonist properties (mirabegron) has become commercially available that has similar efficacy to the antimuscarinics but without the typical side effects of dry mouth and constipation (Herschorn et al. 2013). Studies to investigate the potential benefit of combination therapy with the antimuscarinics and beta-3 agonists are currently in development and may provide an additional option for treatment. When pharmacotherapy fails to achieve significant clinical benefit, surgical options include intravesical injections of botulinum toxin or sacral neuromodulation utilizing the Interstim device made by Medtronic. Both have demonstrated acceptable results in patients in whom medical therapy is inadequate or side effects are intolerable. The advantages of botulinum toxin are its simplicity of administration and low side effect profile. Repeat injections (every 6–9 months), however, are necessary to maintain efficacy and there is the potential for transient urinary retention requiring catheterization (indwelling or intermittent) until resolution. Sacral neuromodulation typically requires two phases, one of which is a testing period with a stimulating lead in place to establish efficacy followed by surgical implantation of the generator when successful. Complications can include infection, pain, and lead displacement.

As mentioned above, OAB can have multiple etiologies; however, if its underlying pathophysiology is related to sensitization or recruitment of c-fibers resulting in involuntary bladder contractions, then functional desensitization of these fibers with a vanilloid would be expected to provide some benefit. Many studies have suggested efficacy of vanilloids in the treatment of OAB. Soontrapa et al. reported on 25 patients with either OAB or what they described as either a hypersensitive bladder or primary detrusor instability, who were treated with 1 mM of capsaicin diluted in 100 ml of 30 % ethanol solution (Soontrapa et al. 2003). In those with OAB it was found that daytime urinary frequency (16.5–8.6), incontinence episodes per day (9.7–2.4), bladder capacity (160.1–236.9 ml), and detrusor contraction pressure (71.1–57.3 cm H20) improved following treatment with capsaicin. Mahawong et al. reported efficacy when using capsaicin to treat Benign prostatic hypertrophy (BPH) with OAB symptoms (Mahawong et al. 2007). Urinary frequency, nocturia, and mean first desire to void improved at 1, 3, and 6 months and mean maximal cystometric capacity improved at 1 month. There were no significant differences in peak flow rate, detrusor pressure, and post-void residual volume compared to pretreatment values. However, in a randomized placebo controlled study of 58 female patients with OAB, Rios et al. found no difference in efficacy between a single 50 mM intravesical dose of RTX and placebo in any clinical or urodynamic parameters including urgency incontinence (Rios et al. 2007). Safety was not found to be concerning as RTX instillation was well tolerated with few and self-limited side effects.

Vanilloids have been found to be useful in patients with OAB for reasoning similar to that of NGB. When compared to standard therapies, disadvantages to their use primarily include the need for intravesical instillation via catheter and multiple treatments to maintain efficacy. The former is particularly problematic as the overwhelming majority of patients with OAB do not require intermittent catheterization and may be reluctant to submit to the procedure regularly. Although efficacy has been shown in some studies, currently the use of vanilloids cannot be recommended for routine use in patients with OAB. In fact, treatment with these agents is not included in the American Urological Association guidelines for the management of OAB (Gormley et al. 2012).

13.4 Interstitial Cystitis/Bladder Pain Syndrome

Bladder pain syndrome (BPS) (sometimes referred to synonymously as interstitial cystitis) is a condition that falls under a larger category of genitourinary pain syndromes, hypersensitivity, or sensory disorders of the urinary tract. It is described as "the complaint of suprapubic pain related to bladder filling, accompanied by other symptoms such as increased daytime and nighttime frequency, in the absence of proven urinary infection or other obvious pathology" (Abrams et al. 2002). Similar to other conditions in this class, BPS is a diagnosis of exclusion and lacks a clear pathophysiologic basis for the symptoms reported and therefore scientifically proven medical or surgical treatments for the diagnosis.

Understandably in BPS, as the hypotheses for etiologic nature are varied, so too are the diagnostic criteria. Over the last 3 decades, several urologic associations, conferences, and institutes have posited a range of criteria to be met and excluded for diagnosis of BPS (Gillenwater and Wein 1988; Hanno and Dmochowski 2009; Simon et al. 1997; van de Merwe et al. 2008). The most recent of these is from 2008, proposed by the European Society for the Study of Interstitial Cystitis (ESSIC) (Hanno and Dmochowski 2009). This criteria suggests that a diagnosis of BPS would be made "on the basis of chronic pelvic pain, pressure or discomfort perceived to be related to the urinary bladder accompanied by at least one other urinary symptom (persistent urge to void or urinary frequency). Classification of BPS types might be performed according to findings on cystoscopy with hydrodistension and morphologic findings in bladder biopsies…" (van de Merwe et al. 2008).

In 2011, the American Urologic Association (AUA) published a clinical guideline statement on the diagnosis and treatment of BPS in keeping with the ESSIC consensus (Hanno et al. 2011). The treatment guidelines are stratified from first-line to sixth-line and include: patient education, stress management, and behavioral modification (first-line), oral, transdermal, and intravesical analgesic and restorative regimens (second-line), cystoscopy under general anesthesia, fulguration of Hunner's ulcers (third-line), neuromodulation (fourth-line), intradetrusor botulinum toxin, immunomodulation (fifth-line), and lastly urinary diversion with or without substitution cystoplasty (sixth-line) (Hanno et al. 2011). Pain management is a component of symptom control throughout this treatment algorithm. Analgesic agents commonly used for BPS range from amitriptyline, hydroxyzine, and lidocaine to narcotic drug prescription (Table 13.3).

One consequence of long-term narcotic use is opioid addiction. For this reason, medical personnel are advised to involve the participation of a pain management specialist in administering and regulating this aspect of treatment. Comprehensive treatment of often associated pain syndromes, irritable bowel syndrome, fibromyalgia, and chronic fatigue syndrome, is also recommended in a multidisciplinary fashion (Hanno and Dmochowski 2009).

The above listed treatment options reflect the current working pathophysiologic theories that exist for BPS. It is believed that the etiology of BPS is multifactorial. Specific factors thought to play a role in this syndrome can be stratified into three

Table 13.3 Treatment options for PBS

Route	Treatment	Proposed mechanism of action
Behavioral	Stress reduction/avoidance of bladder irritants	Decreases pain sensitivity
Oral	Amitriptyline	Central and peripheral anticholinergic
	Hydroxizine	Stabilizes mast cells
	Pentosanpolysulfate sodium	Stabilizes glycosaminoglycan (GAG) layer of urothelial cells
Intravesical	Lidocaine*	Analgesic
	Heparin*	Mimics GAG layer
	Sodium bicarbonate*	Alkalinization, promotes penetration of lidocaine
	Dimethyl sulfoxide (DMSO)	Anti-inflammatory
	Hydrodistension (Normal saline)	Unknown, possibly increases bladder capacity

*These agents are typically mixed and administered together

categories: offensive foreign antigens, intrinsic structural abnormalities of the bladder, and neurogenically and biochemically mediated host immune response (Bologna and Whitmore 2007).

As stated previously in this chapter, vanilloid receptors in the bladder modulate activity of sensory neurons. RTX and capsaicin act at this receptor and may potentially offer a viable treatment modality for BPS. The following is a summary of the existing literature that includes studies focused on comparisons of intravesically administered vanilloid receptor agonists and a placebo or other active control.

Currently, there are three randomized placebo-controlled studies that have investigated the efficacy and/or safety and tolerability of intravesical RTX for the treatment of BPS. Lazzeri et al. reported their findings on 18 subjects (15 women), who received a single dose of 30 cc saline containing 10 nM of intravesically administered RTX in 1 % ethanol or placebo saline solution (Lazzeri et al. 2000). The primary outcome was voiding pattern and pain score at 30 days evaluated by patient diary of urinary frequency and nocturia and previously utilized pain scale (occurrence (0–5) and intensity of pain (0–4)). They reported a statistically significant decrease in frequency and nocturia at 30 days. This decrease remained statistically significant at 3 months for frequency but not nocturia. Pain scores decreased at 30 days to a level of statistical significance, but this did not persist to 3 months.

The second study by Chen et al., reported on the safety and tolerability of intravesical RTX for the treatment of BPS (Chen et al. 2005). In it, 22 subjects (17 women), received 0.05 or 0.10 μM of RTX or placebo (10 % ethanol in saline). An optional retreatment of the bladder included 50 cc of 2 % lidocaine in the bladder via a Foley catheter for 10 min, followed by a 50 cc rinse of the bladder with saline. The primary outcome was pain and voiding pattern assessed by visual analog scale and voiding diary, respectively at 1, 4, 8, and 12 weeks. Additional measures included cystoscopy and serum concentrations of RTX preinstillation as well as immediately and 4 weeks after therapy. No serious adverse event was reported. They found no statistically significant change in pain scores or voiding diary among the three groups.

The final, and largest study by Payne et al. comprised a cohort of 163 patients (86 % women) with IC who were randomized to a single dose of intravesical placebo (10 % ethanolic solution), or 0.01, 0.05, or 0.10 μM of RTX (Payne et al. 2005). Pretreatment included 50 mL of 2 % lidocaine intravesically for 10 min; this was increased during the study to 100 mL of 4 % lidocaine for 30 min to increase tolerability of the therapy. The primary efficacy endpoint was assessed using the Global Response Assessment (GRA) at 4 weeks. Twelve subjects discontinued the study, four from the placebo group. No change in GRA score was noted among the groups. A dose-dependent increase in treatment pain and urgency, however, was observed and one adverse event of lower abdominal pain (judged to be related to the study drug) requiring hospitalization was reported.

As elucidated in this study, instillation pain appears to be the main limitation in the use of RTX for the treatment of BPS. Additionally, sustained efficacy of RTX treatment has yet to be depicted in the current literature.

In summary, intravesically administered vanilloid receptor agonists lack strong evidence for efficacy or tolerability in the treatment of BPS. Further studies describing treatment schedules, long-term outcomes, and comparison to existing bladder instillation regimens are necessary to establish the role of this therapy in BPS.

13.5 Conclusions

Urologic disorders in which bladder function is negatively impacted such as neurogenic bladder, OAB, and IC/PBS are prevalent, challenging to treat, and can result in significant reduction in quality of life. As a result of the unique properties of the bladder urothelium, intravesical application of vanilloids may provide a novel method for the treatment of these disorders. A cadre of clinical studies exist, which have been described in this chapter, suggest some efficacy utilizing these agents in affected patients. At this point, current data do not support the routine use of vanilloids in these clinical situations. A better understanding of their limited efficacy, however, may help further elucidate underlying pathophysiology and help expand our armamentarium of treatments.

References

Abrams P, Cardozo L, Fall M, Griffiths D, Rosier P, Ulmsten U et al (2002) The standardisation of terminology of lower urinary tract function: Report from the standardisation sub-committee of the international continence society. Am J Obstet Gynecol 187:116–126

Bologna RA, Whitmore KE (2007) Painful bladder syndromes. In: Walters MD, Karram MM (eds) Urogynecology and reconstructive pelvic surgery. Mosby Elsevier, Philadelphia, pp 377–379

Burns AS, Rivas DA, Ditunno JR (2001) The management of neurogenic bladder and sexual dysfunction after spinal cord injury. Spine 16:S129–S136

Chancellor MB (2002) New frontiers in the treatment of overactive bladder and incontinence. Rev Urology 4:S50–S56

Chen TY, Corcos J, Camel M, Ponsot Y, le Tu M (2005) Prospective, randomized, double-blind study of safety and tolerability of intravesical resiniferatoxin (RTX) in interstitial cystitis (IC). Int Urogynecol J Pelvic Floor Dysfunct 16:293–297

Fingerman J, Finkelstein D (2000) The overactive bladder in multiple sclerosis. J Am Osteopath Assoc 100:59–63

Gillenwater JY, Wein AJ (1988) Summary of the national institute of arthritis, diabetes, digestive and kidney diseases workshop on interstitial cystitis, national institutes of health, bethesda, maryland, August 28–29, 1987. J Urol 140:203–206

Gormley EA, Lightner DJ, Burgio KL, Chai TC, Clemens JQ, Culkin DJ et al (2012) American urological association (AUA) guideline: diagnosis and treatment of overactive bladder (non-neurogenic) in adults: AUA/SUFU guideline. Am Urol Assoc Educ Res pp 1–36 (Copyright 2012)

Hanno P, Dmochowski R (2009) Status of international consensus on interstitial cystitis/bladder pain syndrome/painful bladder syndrome: 2008 snapshot. Neurourol Urodyn 28:274–286

Hanno PM, Burks DA, Clemens JQ, Dmochowski RR, Erickson D, Fitzgerald MP et al (2011) AUA guideline for the diagnosis and treatment of interstitial cystitis/bladder pain syndrome. J Urol 185:2162–2170

Herschorn S, Barkin J, Castro-Diaz D et al (2013) A phase III, randomized, double-blind, parallel-group, placebo-controlled, multicentre study to assess the efficacy and safety of the B3 adrenoceptor agonist, mirabegron, in patients with symptoms of overactive bladder. Urology 82:313–320

Lazzeri M, Beneforti P, Spinelli M, Zanollo A, Barbagli G, Turini D (2000) Intravesical resiniferatoxin for the treatment of hypersensitive disorder: a randomized placebo controlled study. J Urol 164:676–679

Lazzeri M, Spinelli M, Zanollo A, Turini D (2004) Intravesical vanilloids and neurogenic incontinence: ten years experience. Urol Int 72:145–149

Linsenmeyer TA (2013) Use of botulinum toxin in individuals with neurogenic detrusor overactivity: state of the art review. J Spinal Cord Med 36:402–419

MacDonald R, Mong M, Fin HA, Wilt TJ (2008) Neurotoxin treatments for urinary incontinence in subjects with spinal cord injury or multiple sclerosis: a systematic review of effectiveness and adverse effects. J Spinal Cord Med 31:157–165

Mahawong P, Chaiyaprasithi B, Soontrapa S, Tappayuthapijarn P (2007) A role of intravesical capsaicin instillation in benign prostatic hyperplasia with overactive bladder symptoms: the first reported study in the literature. J Med AssocThai 90:2301 2309

Payne CK, Mosbaugh PG, Forrest JB, Evans RJ, Whitmore KE, Antoci JP et al (2005) Intravesicalresiniferatoxin for the treatment of interstitial cystitis: a randomized, double-blind, placebo controlled trial. J Urol 173:1590–1594

Rios LA, Panhoca R, Mattos D Jr, Srugi M, Bruschini H (2007) Intravesicalresiniferatoxin for the treatment of women with idiopathic detrusor overactivity and urgency incontinence: a single dose, 4 weeks, double-blind randomized, placebo controlled trial. Neurourol Urodyn 26:773–778

Schurch B, Stohrer M, Kramer G, Schmid DM, Gaul G, Hauri D (2000) Botulinum-A toxin for treating detrusor hyperreflexia in spinal cord injured patients: a new alternative to anticholinergic drugs? preliminary results. J Urol. 164:692–697

Simon LJ, Landis JR, Erickson DR, Nyberg LM (1997) The interstitial cystitis data base study: concepts and preliminary baseline descriptive statistics. Urology 49:64–75

Soontrapa S, Ruksakul W, Nonthasood B, Tappayuthpijarn P (2003) The efficacy of Thai capsaicin in management of overactive bladder and hypersensitive bladder. J Med Assoc Thai 86:861–867

van de Merwe JP, Nordling J, Bouchelouche P, Bouchelouche K, Cervigni M, Daha LK et al (2008) Diagnostic criteria, classification, and nomenclature for painful bladder syndrome/interstitial cystitis: An ESSIC proposal. Eur Urol 53:60–67

Index

O. M. E. Abdel-Salam (ed.), *Capsaicin as a Therapeutic Molecule*, Progress in Drug Research 68, DOI: 10.1007/978-3-0348-0828-6, © Springer Basel 2014

MIX
Papier aus verantwortungsvollen Quellen
Paper from responsible sources
FSC® C105338

If you have any concerns about our products,
you can contact us on
ProductSafety@springernature.com

In case Publisher is established outside the EU,
the EU authorized representative is:
Springer Nature Customer Service Center GmbH
Europaplatz 3, 69115 Heidelberg, Germany

Printed by Libri Plureos GmbH
in Hamburg, Germany